Inflammation
and Antiinflammatories

Inflammation and Antiinflammatories

Edoardo Arrigoni-Martelli, M.D., Ph.D.
Department of Pharmacology
Leo Pharmaceutical Products Ltd.
Ballerup, Denmark

S P Books Division of
SPECTRUM PUBLICATIONS, INC.
New York

Distributed by Halsted Press
A Division of John Wiley & Sons

New York Toronto London Sydney

SPECTRUM PUBLICATIONS, INC.
175-20 Wexford Terrace, Jamaica, N.Y. 11432

Library of Congress Cataloging in Publication Data

Arrigoni-Martelli, Edoardo, 1930-
    Inflammation and antiinflammatories.

    Includes bibliographical references and index.
    1. Anti-inflammatory agents. 2. Inflammation.
I. Title. [DNLM: 1. Anti-inflammatory agents–
Pharmacodynamics. 2. Inflammation–Drug therapy.
QZ150 A776i]
RM405.A77   616'.047   77-24745
ISBN 0-89335-028-1

Distributed solely by the Halsted Press Division of John Wiley & Sons, Inc.,
New York
ISBN 0-470-99175-5

Contents

CONTENTS

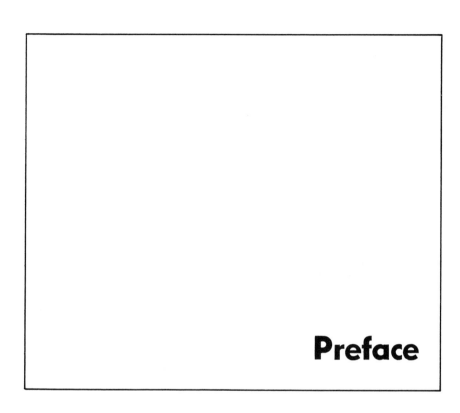

Preface

The aim of this volume is to summarize and review the continuously expanding knowledge concerning the physiopathology of inflammation and the many endeavors to developing suitable experimental models for evaluating new agents. Biological profiles are also provided of compounds either currently used in therapy or still at the investigational stage.

Hopefully, this monograph will prove useful to those interested in the problems of inflammation and its control, as they range from the laboratory to the clinical level.

I wish to thank Drs. E. Frederiksen and W. Godtfredsen, without whose encouragement this book would not have been written.

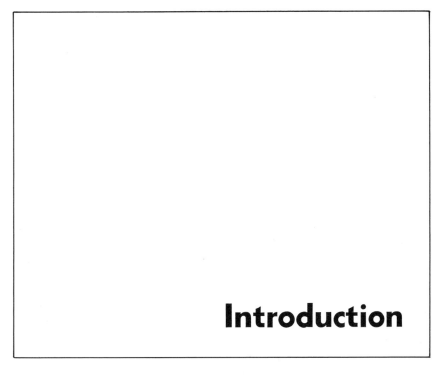

Introduction

Approximately 2000 years ago Celsus suggested the first fenomenologic description and definition of inflammation. Since that time the inflammatory reaction has been investigated from many points of view: by anatomists, biochemists, physiologists, pathologists, immunologists, pharmacologists and clinicians, and the formerly fenomenologic descriptions have been replaced by much more rigorous and quantitative approaches. Inflammation has become a discipline and it is likely to be the backbone of the pathology.

Inflammation may be considered as an essentially protective response to any noxious stimulus ranging from a transient, self-limited and localized response when the injury is caused by a single finite event to a complex, sustained response involving the whole organism when the injurious agent cannot be removed or concealed, or it is self-perpetuating, or it is not recognized as truly "foreign" by the organism. A vast array of substances—the so-called mediators of inflammation—are formed or released either concurrently or in successive time sequences at the site of injury from various plasma or cells sources in response to an etiological factor. Their duration of action is usually brief since they are efficiently disposed or inactivated either by dilution within extravascular fluids or by catabolic enzyme systems. At least some of these factors trigger other mechanisms and/or recruit previously uncommitted cells in the inflammatory reaction, or they are continuously produced because of the persistence of the causative factor.

Effector molecules have been characterized, the mechanisms whereby these mediators bring about tissue injury and cellular responses, and the existence of intra- and extracellular control mechanisms of the release process have been described, the role of immunological reactions as a trigger for the release of mediators has been ascertained.

Almost all the antiinflammatory drugs presently available are probably polycompetent being able to modulate more than one molecular or cellular event thought to be concerned in the inflammatory response, the inhibition of prostaglandin synthetase and of the membrane labilization representing primary modes of action. Antiinflammatory drugs are symptomatic therapy and probably do not constitute an adequate treatment for rheumatoid arthritis, since they are unlikely to remove the underlying cause of the disease. A chronic inflammation in fact cannot be treated as a surge of continuing acute inflammation.

The very slow increase in the number of drugs accepted for the treatment of rheumatoid arthritis may underscore the limitations in the strategy of drug testing to find anything other than an indomethacin-like drug and emphasizes how much effort is still needed in synthetizing new structures and developing appropriate assays.

Perhaps, as alternative approach, should be considered to stimulate the inflammatory and immunological responses associated with the chronic inflammatory disease instead of suppressing them. It is of interest to note that some new non acidic compounds have shown pharmacological profile distinct from those of aryl acids, and that few of them possess also certain immunoregulatory properties.

Inflammation
and Antiinflammatories

Chapter 1

Release of Mediators from Inflammatory Cells

Cell and tissue changes caused by mediating substances that originate from various cells or plasma are the salient features of the inflammatory process. Stimuli which trigger the latter activate these mediators or lead to their release. A variety of cells contain several potent mediators and, in some instances, inhibitors of the inflammatory response. The cells most studied in this respect are neutrophils (polymorphonuclear neutrophil leukocytes = PMN), basophils, mast cells and platelets and, to a lesser extent, macrophages and lymphocytes.

Mast cells, basophils and platelets have morphologically similar dense granules containing potent vasoactive amines; neutrophils and macrophages have within their lysosomes many potential mediators, including proteolytic enzymes; lymphocytes generate, when immunologically stimulated, the so-called lymphokines.

The release process can be subdivided in two main categories: (1) the cytotoxic release which occurs when the cell is destroyed by different causes and (2) the noncytotoxic release which shows

1

remarkable similarities with the secretory process in general.

Other features common to several cell types are represented by intra- and extracellular controls of the release process, which either inhibit or enhance the process itself and, ultimately, the inflammatory reaction.

1. MEDIATORS OF INFLAMMATION

Mediators vary widely in their nature from cell type to cell type and are primarily contained within membrane-bound, intracytoplasmic granules (Table 1). They will be discussed in detail in the following chapters.

The *basophil* has proved a useful model for developing an understanding of the cellular release process and may provide an important source of mediators in some forms of inflammatory injury (81). The basophil contains electron-dense, membrane-bound granules, morphologically different from those of mast cells. The prime mediator released is histamine (5,36,93). Moreover, the basophil is one of the main sources of slow-reacting substances of anaphylaxis (32,54,102). Rabbit and, probably, human basophils also liberate a platelet-activating factor (9).

The dominant mediator of the rat *mast cell* is histamine stored in the characteristic dense granules of this cell, bound through firm ionic linkage to the carboxyl group on granule protein. In other animal species (mouse), the mediator of prime importance is serotonin (3,5,10). Heparin, whose possible role as mediator is unknown, is also present in mast-cell granules and it has been suggested that an heparin-protein-histamine complex could exist (60). The presence of a chymotrypsin-like enzyme has been reported in rat, cat, dog, and human mast cells (15,65). Slow-reacting substance of anaphylaxis (SRS-A) also derives from the mast cells of several animal species, including man (53,54,63,79,93,102), as does the so-called eosinophil chemotactic factor of anaphylaxis (ECFA) (59). Phospholipase A is present on the mast-cell surface (106): this enzyme may be of some importance in triggering prostaglandin formation.

Two types of granules are predominant in *platelets* (116). The "dense bodies" have been shown to contain the vasoactive amine of the platelets—serotonin—in most species, and histamine and serotonin in the rabbit; they probably ionically linked to ATP (45,46, 62). Lysosomal enzymes are, in all likelihood, located in the so-called α-granules (68,117). Cationic substances able to induce an

TABLE 1. Mediators of inflammation and their distribution in cells and tissues

Basophils	Histamine, serotonin, SRS-A
Mast cells	Histamine, serotonin, SRS-A, Lysosomal enzymes
Platelets	Histamine, serotonin, (Lysosomal enzymes)
PMNs	Lysosomal enzymes, (SRS-A) Leukokinins
Macrophages	Lysosomal enzymes
Lymphocytes (activated)	Lymphokines
Reticuloendothelial cells	Complement
Plasma substrate	Kinins, plasmin, Hageman Factor
Ubiquitous intracellular precursors	Prostaglandins

increase in vascular permeability have been detected (74) and the capacity of platelets to synthetize prostaglandins has been described (107).

Neutrophil and *macrophage* mediators are represented by lysosomal hydrolases and some other non-enzymatic inflammatory materials, such as the cationic proteins. In addition, neutrophils participate in the release of SRS-A, at least in some circumstances (80), and give rise to kinin-like substances—leukokinins—when incubated with human plasma (34). This property is also shared by macrophages (33).

2. STIMULI OF MEDIATOR RELEASE

Stimuli for noncytotoxic mediator release vary greatly among the different types of cells. However, they have the common characteristic of acting at the external surface of the cell, which suggests the presence of receptors there. Several groups of stimuli have been described. The more important of these is probably represented by immunoglobulins which are able to produce the non-cytotoxic release from all cell classes, although the type of immunoglobulins may be different for each category of cells. Low molecular weight peptides or proteins are also stimuli for many cell types, while other cells respond to certain proteolytic enzymes (e.g., platelets to thrombin, mast cells to chymotrypsin). A further source of stimuli for mediator release is represented by the cell-to-cell interaction.

The stimulus most explored to date, which is able to induce *basophil* release has been the homocytotropic antibody (IgE) ; it is bound to the cell surface receptors by virtue of its Fc region and reacts with antigen or with anti-IgE antibody (54,58,61,76,102). The release of histamine and of SRS-A is a consequence of these reactions.

An identical stimulus triggers the release response from *mast cells* in purified preparations (54,58,61,76,102). This has been shown to also occur in intact lung or lung fragments rich in mast cells of different animal species, including man (53,63,78).

An example of the cell-to-cell cooperative effect in the release of inflammatory mediators is provided by a small cationic protein actively released by rabbit neutrophils (39,40), which induces non-cytotoxic secretion of vasoactive amines from mast cells (5). Small cationic fragments cleaved from the complement components (C3a and C5a) have the same effect (14,21,55).

A large number of low molecular weight, highly selective activators of mast cells have been described. Among them is compound 48/80—the prototype of these substances—(24) whose action is likely to be species dependent (71), and polymyxin B (85). A long list of these activators is provided in the "Handbook of Pharmacology" (Volume 18, 1966).

A wide variety of different stimuli may cause the *platelet* release reaction. These include both soluble and particulate materials, low molecular weight inducers and proteolytic enzymes (8,74).

Platelets adhere closely to collagen fibers, swell and undergo the release reaction: this phenomenon may be of great importance in inflammatory processes (90). A release reaction can also be induced by thrombin and trypsin but not by chymotrypsin (74) and, in high concentration, by ADP which is primarily an inducer of platelet aggregation (74).

Immunological reactions are of great importance as triggers for platelet release response (8). However, a distinction must be made between platelets from man, baboon, pig and sheep—which do not exhibit immune adherence and react directly with immunoglobulin—and those from rabbit, mouse, guinea pig, dog and cat—which have receptors for C3b and manifest immune adherence and, then, release reaction (8,44,87). The immunological responses have probably most relevance in cytotoxic release (8,83). Also endotoxin-induced release is the consequence of a platelet lysis in rabbit (8, 83). Endotoxin is, however, unable to induce release from human platelets (75). Both immune complexes (73) and endotoxin (12) act as releasers in vivo, as does the interaction of IgE-antigen-basophils (35). This interaction results in the release of a low molecular weight activator which, in turn, induces a release reaction in platelets (9).

Lysosomal enzyme secretion occurs primarily as result of the interaction between *neutrophil* and *macrophage* plasma membranes and immunological reactants. Neutrophils have separate receptors for C3 and the Fc region of immunoglobulins G and A (8). Human monocytes have receptors for the Fc portion of both IgG1 and IgG3 (37). The ability of these cells to uptake the immune complex is now well documented (6,23,26,38,40,41,42,88,89,101). They then release selectively a portion of their lysosomal content without a concomitant release of cytoplasmic constituents (13,38,40,47,48,49,50, 52,81,115,119). This release appears to be due to the extrusion of lysosomal material from as yet incompletely closed phagosomes open at their external border to tissue spaces but already joined at their internal border by lysosomes actively discharging their hydrolases into the vacuole (38,40,41,47,81,122). This process has been termed "regurgitation during feeding." Indeed, it is the uptake of antigen-antibody complex from the bulk phase of the circulation, tissue fluids or joint fluids that may account for removing inflammatory materials from leukocytes in the many forms of tissue injury associated with circulating, large molecular weight aggregates (114). When cells regurgitate their hydrolases after uptake of immune precipitates, they form the sort of inclusion found in the RA cells obtained from synovial fluid of patients with rheumatoid arthritis. The sequence of events described above applies not only to the uptake of immune complexes but also to the ingestion of other inert particles, such as zymosan of calcium pyrophosphate dihydrate (115).

However, endocytosis of particulate reactants is not a prerequisite for enzyme secretion, since the latter may also occur in the absence of phagocytosable particles, such as nonphagocytosable immune complex surfaces (38,40,48,50,81). When polymorphonuclear leukocytes make contact with various solid surfaces coated with immune complexes, they discharge their hydrolases onto these surfaces (40,41,42) by a mechanism which has been termed "reversed endocytosis" (114). In this process, phagocytosis "per se" does not take place. In experimental conditions, it is possible to inhibit phagocytosis of particles by neutrophils with cytochalasin B and, thus, transform "regurgitation during feeding" into "reverse endocytosis" (17,70,123). Cells exposed to cytochalasin B do not take up the particles which aggregate on the cell surface and directly cause the cells to extrude lysosomal hydrolases (123).

Lymphokines produced by activated lymphocytes (109) and endotoxin (108) stimulate macrophages to manufacture collagenase. Under such circumstances, synthesis of new enzyme seems to occur and not merely a discharge of preformed enzyme.

In other experimental conditions, certain substances—monosodium urate and silica are the best examples—gain access to the inside of the lysosomal system where they cause the lysosome membrane to rupture from within (1,115). Both these crystals appear to be membranolytic because of their capacity to form hydrogen bonds with the phosphate ester group, such as that present on the internal lysosomal membrane (1,115). The release of lysosomal enzymes occurs concomitantly with that of cytoplasmic enzymes and other intracellular constituents as the cell dies.

It is appropriate to mention that soon after the elucidation of the role of lysosomes in the intracellular digestion of autologous and heterologous materials (18,19), it was reported that vitamin A (19,22,25,67), vitamin E (20) as well as testosterone, progesterone and pregnanolone (110) labilize the lysosomes. Physical injury, such as freezing and thawing, ultraviolet and γ-irradiation (20, 103,111), and polyene antibiotics (4,96), has the same effect. Substantial evidence has also been presented for the role of lysosomal labilization in mediating tissue injury (2,113,120).

3. MECHANISMS OF MEDIATOR RELEASE

The exact mechanisms of what happens between stimulus and secretion are not yet known. Nevertheless some of the factors involved in this process have been identified (Fig. 1).

Activation of the precursor of serine esterase is a possible way in which cell reactions, including release, may be triggered (56). Release from most cells is blocked by a variety of phosphonate in-

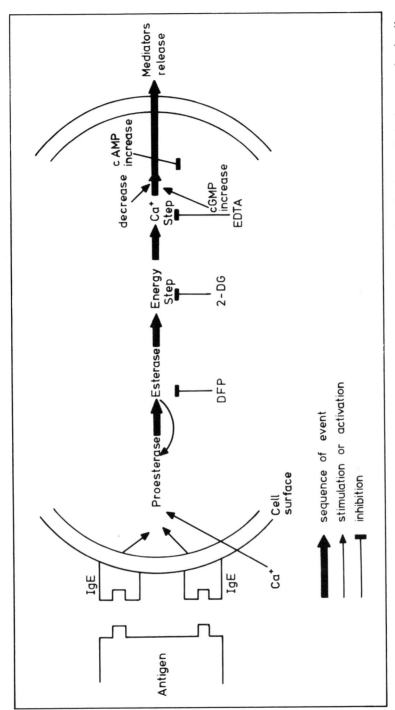

FIG. 1. Biochemical events in immunologically mediated mediator release

hibitors (8). The latter exhibit specific activity-structure profiles in inhibiting different known types of serine esterase; it has been suggested that in many cases different stimuli activate different esterases on one type of cell (8). The presence of serine esterase has been directly demonstrated in neutrophils (7) and, in the same cell type, the role of its activation for some cell functions has also been shown (86).

Ca^{++} in the external medium is generally required for mediator release, as it is for many secretory phenomena (94). The penetration of Ca^{++} into cells has, in fact, been shown to trigger the secretory reaction from mast cells (27) and rabbit neutrophils (118). Calcium influx into human neutrophils occurs during cell contact with immune reactants (98), but these cells may be also able to mobilize intracellular sources (8).

Cyclic nucleotides appear to play an important role in the release of mediators. This subject is discussed in detail in Chapter 9 and, therefore, we shall only deal with it briefly here. Generally, the increase of intracellular cyclic 3',5' adenosine monophosphate (cyclic AMP = cAMP) inhibits the release. Conversely, mechanisms which specifically decrease the latter enhance the release. This has been shown to occur in platelets (95), mast cells (78,99), basophils (11,66) and neutrophils (124). The opposite applies to cyclic guanosine monophosphate (cGMP)—its increase appears to enhance the release process in mast cells (57) and neutrophils (124). The relationship between levels of both cyclic nucleotides seems to have considerable bearing on mediator release (57,124), probably through an interaction with Ca^{++} (92) and microtubules (29).

Microtubules appear to play a role in secretion, as seen morphologically and through the inhibitory action of the specific microtubule-disrupting agent, colchicine (77,114). There is evidence suggesting that they act in directing the motion of either the whole cell or of its granules (28,105,114). Disruption of microtubules prevents mediator release (84) and their aggregation enhances it (30) in mast cells. The same phenomena occur in basophils. Colchicine and related drugs have been reported to partially inhibit degranulation of neutrophils (69), and to reduce the release of lysosomal enzymes during phagocytosis (124). In contrast, deuterium oxide, which promotes microtubule assembly, enhances enzyme release (124). Moreover cGMP, which also induces mediator release, appears to exert this effect by stimulating assembly of microtubules (31,124).

Actinomyosinoid material is present in most cells and in some of them—including those containing mediators—it was distinguished morphologically as microfilaments. It has been suggested that such contractile elements are involved in secretion and that their action, in part, requires the presence of Ca^{++} and cAMP (29). Neutrophils contain actinomyosinoid protein (97). Cytochalasin B enhances exocytosis of granules from neutrophils (8, 123), but whether this is entirely the result of microfilament disruption is not known since cytochalasin B also inhibits glucose uptake into neutrophils and may have other effects (121). Cytochalasin B prevents phagocytosis and enhances granule enzyme release also from macrophages (16).

It is not yet clearly known in what order the above factors and requirements are involved in the release process. It has been suggested that esterase activation is an early step in platelets, preceding the Ca^{++} requirement and the step modulated by cAMP (43). In mast cells, there are two Ca^{++} requiring steps (56); the early one would involve a proesterase which necessitates Ca^{++} for its function or activation; the second follows esterase activation and, perhaps, cAMP modulation (56). In basophils, cAMP modulation of release occurs before Ca^{++} requirement which itself precedes or accompanies steps requiring energy metabolism and microtubule function (64). In neutrophils, as in platelets, esterase activation is an early step. The possible controlling action of cAMP may be tied to microtubule function (124). It has been shown that low concentrations of cAMP enhance translocation of lysosome to phagosome, which is inhibited by high concentrations (112); it has also been suggested that an intracellular gradient of cAMP could exist, highest in the locally perturbed regions of the cell (114). cGMP, as mentioned, seems to play an influential although as yet undefined role. It may act in opposition to cAMP, thus, providing an important controlling influence on the release processes.

REFERENCES

1. Allison, A. C., Harington, J. S., and Birbeck, M.: J. Exp. Med. *124*:141, 1968.
2. Ali, S. Y.: Biochem. J. *93*:611, 1964.
3. Anderson, P., and Uvnäs, B.: Acta Physiol. Scand. *94*:63, 1975.
4. Arrigoni-Martelli, E., and Restelli, A.: Eur. J. Pharmacol. *19*:191, 1972.
5. Åborg, C. M., Novotny, J., and Uvnäs, B.: Acta Physiol. Scand. *69*:276, 1967.
6. Baehner, R. L., Karnovsky, M. J., and Karnovsky, M. L.: J. Clin. Invest. *48*:187, 1969.

7. Becker, E. L.: J. Exp. Med. *135*:376, 1972.
8. Becker, E. L., and Henson, P. M.: Adv. Immunol. *17*:93, 1973.
9. Benveniste, J., Henson, P. M., and Cochrane, C. G.: J. Exp. Med. *136*: 1356, 1973.
10. Bergqvist, U., Samuelsson, G., and Uvnäs, B.: Acta Physiol. Scand. *83*: 362, 1971.
11. Bourne, H. R., Lehrer, R. I., Lichtenstein, L. M., Weissmann, G., and Zurier, R.: J. Clin. Invest. *52*:698, 1973.
12. Brown, D. L., and Lachmann, P. J.: Int. Arch. Allergy *45*:193, 1973.
13. Cardella, C. J., Davies, P., and Allison, A. C.: Nature *247*:46, 1974.
14. Cohrane, C. G., and Müller-Eberhard, H. J.: J. Exp. Med. *127*:371, 1968.
15. Darzynkiewicz, Z., and Barnard, E. A.: Nature *213*:1198, 1967.
16. Davies, P., Allison, A. C., and Haswell, A. D.: Biochem. J. *134*:33, 1973.
17. Davis, A. T., Estensen, R., and Quie, P. G.: Proc. Soc. Exp. Biol. Med. *137*:161, 1971.
18. De Duve, C.: Harvey Lect. *59*:49, 1965.
19. De Duve, C., and Wattiaux, R.: Annu. Rev. Physiol. *28*:435, 1968.
20. De Duve, C., Wattiaux, R., and Wibo, M.: Biochem. Pharmacol. *9*:97, 1962.
21. Dias da Silva, W., and Lepow, I. H.: J. Exp. Med. *125*:921, 1967.
22. Dingle, J. T.: Biochem. J. *79*:509, 1961.
23. Dixon, F. J.: Harvey Lect. *58*:21, 1963.
24. Fawcett, D. W.: J. Exp. Med. *100*:217, 1954.
25. Fell, H. B., and Dingle, J. T.: Biochem. J. *87*:403, 1963.
26. Fennell, R. H., and Santamaria, A.: Am. J. Pathol. *41*:521, 1962.
27. Foreman, J. C., Mongar, J. L., and Gomperts, B. D.: Nature *245*:249, 1973.
28. Freed, J. J., and Lebowitz, M. M.: J. Cell Biol. *45*:334, 1970.
29. Gillespie, E.: J. Cell Biol. *50*:544, 1971.
30. Gillespie, E., Levine, R. J., and Malawista, S. E.: J. Pharmacol. Exp. Ther. *164*:158, 1968.
31. Goldstein, I. M., Hoffstein, S., Gallin, J., and Weissmann, G.: Proc. Natl. Acad. Sci. USA *70*:2916, 1973.
32. Grant, J. A., and Lichtenstein, L. M.: J. Immunol. *112*:808, 1966.
33. Greenbaum, L. M., Freer, R., Chang, J., Semente, G., and Yamafuji, K.: Br. J. Pharmacol. *36*:623, 1969.
34. Greenabum, L. M., and Kim, K. S.: Br. J. Pharmacol. *29*:238, 1967.
35. Halonen, M., Pinckard, R. V., and Meng, A. L.: J. Immunol. *111*:331, 1973.
36. Hastie, R. W.: Clin. Exp. Immunol. *8*:45, 1970.
37. Hay, F. C., Torrigiami, G., and Roitt, L. M.: Eur. J. Immunol. *2*:257, 1972.
38. Hawkins, D.: J. Immunol. *108*:310, 1972.
39. Hawkins, D., and Peeters, S.: Lab. Invest. *24*:483, 1971.
40. Henson, P. M.: J. Immunol. *107*:1535, 1971.
41. Henson, P. M.: J. Immunol. *107*:1547, 1971.
42. Henson, P. M.: J. Exp. Med. *134* (3,Pt 2) : 1145, 1971.
43. Henson, P. M., Oades, Z. G., and Gould, R.: Fed. Proc. *32*:1010, 1973.
44. Henson, P. M., and Spiegelberg, H. L.: J. Clin. Invest. *52*:1282, 1973.
45. Humphrey, F. H., and Jacques, R.: J. Physiol. (Lond.) *124*:305, 1954.
46. Humphrey, F. H., and Jacques, R.: J. Physiol. (Lond.) *128*:9, 1955.
47. Ignarro, L. J.: Nature (New Biol.) *245*:151, 1973.

48. Ignarro, L. J.: Arthritis Rheum. *17*:25, 1974.
49. Ignarro, L. J.: Proc. Natl. Acad. Sci. USA *71*:2027, 1974.
50. Ignarro, L. J.: J. Immunol. *113*:298, 1974.
51. Ignarro, L. J., and George, W. J.: J. Exp. Med. *140*:225, 1974.
52. Ignarro, L. J., Lint, T. F., and George, W. J.: J. Exp. Med. *139*:1395, 1974.
53. Ishizaka, T., Ishizaka, K., and Tomioka, H.: J. Immunol. *108*:513, 1972.
54. Ishizaka, K., Tomioka, H., and Ishizaka, T.: J. Immunol. *105*:1459, 1970.
55. Jensen, J.: Science *155*:1122, 1967.
56. Kaliner, M. A., and Austen, K. F.: J. Exp. Med. *138*:1077, 1973.
57. Kaliner, M. A., Orange, R. P., and Austen, K. F.: J. Exp. Med. *136*:556, 1972.
58. Kay, A. B., and Austen, K. F.: J. Immunol. *107*:899, 1971.
59. Kay, A. B., Stechschulte, D. J., and Austen, K. F.: J. Exp. Med. *133*:602, 1971.
60. Kerp, L.: Int. Arch. Allergy Appl. Immunol. *22*:112, 1963.
61. Kulczycki, A., Isersky, C., and Metzger, H.: J. Exp. Med. *139*:600, 1974.
62. Lecomte, J.: Acta Allergol. (Kbh.) *7* (Suppl.): 81, 1960.
63. Lewis, R. A., Wasserman, S. I., Goetzl, E. J., and Austen, K. F.: Clin. Res. *22*:422 A, 1974.
64. Lichtenstein, L. M.: J. Immunol. *107*:1122, 1971.
65. Lichtenstein, L. M.: Ann N. Y. Acad. Sci. *180*:123, 1971.
66. Lichtenstein, L. M., and Margolis, S.: Science *161*:902, 1968.
67. Lucy, J. A., Dingle, J. T., and Fell, H. B.: Biochem. J. *79*:500, 1961.
68. Lutzner, M. A.: Fed. Proc. *23*:441, 1964.
69. Malawista, S. E.: Blood *87*:519, 1971.
70. Malawista, S. E., Gee, J. B. L., and Bensch, K. G.: Yale J. Biol. Med. *44*: 286, 1971.
71. Mongar, J. L.: In "Ciba Symposium on Histamine," G. E. W. Wolstenholme, and C. M. O'Connor, eds. Churchill, London, 1956, p. 74.
72. Morse, H. C. III, Bloch, K. J., and Austen, K. F.: J. Immunol. *101*:658, 1968.
73. Movat, H. Z., Urinhava, T., Taichman, N. S., Roswell, H. C., and Mustard, J. F.: Immunology *14*:637, 1968.
74. Mustard, J. F., and Packam, M. A.: Pharmacol. Rev. *22*:97, 1970.
75. Nagayama, M., Zucker, M. B., and Beller, F. K.: Thromb. Diath. Haemorrh. *26*:467, 1971.
76. Norman, P. S., Lichtenstein, L. M., and Ishizaka, K.: J. Allergy Clin. Immunol. *52*:210, 1973.
77. Olmstead, J. B., and Borisy, G. C.: Annu. Rev. Biochem. *42*:507, 1973.
78. Orange, R. P., Austen, W. G., and Austen, K. F.: J. Exp. Med. *134*:136s, 1971.
79. Orange, R. P., Stechschulte, D. J., and Austen, K. F.: J. Immunol. *105*: 1087, 1970.
80. Orange, R. P., Valentine, M. D., and Austen, K. F.: J. Exp. Med. *127*: 767, 1968.
81. Oronsky, A. L., Ignarro, L. J., and Perper, R. J.: J. Exp. Med. *138*:461, 1973.
82. Osler, A. G., Lichtenstein, L. M., and Levy, D. A.: Adv. Immunol. *8*:183, 1968.
83. Osler, A. G., and Siraganian, R. P.: Prog. Allergy *16*:450, 1972.

84. Padawer, J.: J. Cell Biol. *40*:747, 1969.
85. Parratt, J. R., and West, G. B.: J. Physiol. (Lond.) *137*:179, 1957.
86. Pearlman, D. S., Ward, P. A., and Becker, E. L.: J. Exp. Med. *130*:745, 1969.
87. Pfueller, S. L., and Lüscher, E. F.: Immunochemistry *9*:1151, 1972.
88. Phillips-Quagliata, J. M., Levine, B. B., Quagliata, F., and Uhr, J. W.: J. Exp. Med. *133*:589, 1971.
89. Pruzansky, J. J., and Patterson, R.: Proc. Soc. Exp. Biol. Med. *124*:56, 1967.
90. Puett, D., Wasserman, B. K., Ford, J. D., and Cunningham, L. W.: J. Clin. Invest. *52*:2195, 1973.
91. Ranadive, N. S., and Cochrane, C. G.: J. Immunol. *106*:506, 1971.
92. Rasmussen, H.: Science *170*:404, 1970.
93. Riley, J. F., and West, G. B.: J. Physiol. (Lond.) *120*:528, 1953.
94. Rubin, R. P.: Pharmacol. Rev. *22*:389, 1970.
95. Salzman, E. W.: N. Engl. J. Med. *286*:358, 1972.
96. Sessa, G., and Weissmann, G.: J. Biol. Chem. *243*:4364, 1968.
97. Shibata, N., Tatsumi, N., Tanaka, K., Okamura, Y., and Senda, N.: Biochim. Biophys. Acta *256*:565, 1972.
98. Smith, R. J., and Ignarro, L. J.: Pharmacologist *16*:308, 1974.
99. Stechschulte, D. J., and Austen, K. F.: Int. Arch. Allergy Appl. Immunol. *45*:110, 1973.
100. Stechschulte, D. J., Austen, K. F., and Bloch, K. J.: J. Exp. Med. *125*:127, 1967.
101. Steinman, R. M., and Cohn, Z. A.: J. Cell Biol. *55*:616, 1972.
102. Sullivan, A. L., Grimley, P. M., and Metzger, H.: J. Exp. Med. *134*:1403, 1971.
103. Tappel, A. L., Sawant, P. L., and Shibko, S.: In "Ciba Foundation Symposium on Lysosomes." Churchill, London, 1963, p. 78.
104. Thomas, L., McCluskey, R. T., Potter, J. L., and Weissmann, G.: J. Exp. Med. *111*:705, 1960.
105. Ukena, T. E., and Berlin, R. D.: J. Exp. Med. *136*:1, 1972.
106. Uvnäs, B.: In "Biochemistry of Acute Allergic Reaction." K. F. Austen, and E. L. Becker, eds. Blackwell, Oxford, 1968, p. 130.
107. Vane, J. R.: Nature (New Biol.) *321*:232, 1971.
108. Wahl, L. M., Wahl, S. M., Mergenhagen, S. E., and Martin, G. R.: Proc. Natl. Acad. Sci. USA *71*:3598, 1974.
109. Wahl, L. M., Wahl, S. M., Mergenhagen, S. E., and Martin, G. R.: Science *187*:261, 1975.
110. Weissmann, G.: Biochem. Pharmacol. *14*:525, 1965.
111. Weissmann, G., and Dingle, J. T.: Exp. Cell Res. *25*:207, 1961.
112. Weissmann, G., Dukor, P., and Sessa, G.: In "Immunopathology of Inflammation," B. Forscher, and J. C. Houck, eds. Excerpta Medica, Amsterdam, 1971, p. 107.
113. Weissmann, G., and Spilberg, I.: Arthritis Rheum. *11*:162, 1968.
114. Weissmann, G., Zurier, R. B., and Hoffstein, S.: Am. J. Pathol. *68*:539, 1972.
115. Weissman, G., Zurier, R. B., Spieler, P. J., and Goldstein, I. M.: J. Exp. Med. *134*:1495, 1971.
116. White, J. G.: In "The Circulating Platelet." S. A. Johnson, ed. Academic

Press, New York, 1971, p. 46.
117. White, J. G., Krivit, W., and Vernier, R.: Fed. Proc. *23*:238, 1964.
118. Woodin, A. M., and Wieneke, A. A.: Biochem. J. *87*:487, 1963.
119. Wright, D. G., and Malawista, S. E.: J. Cell Biol. *53*:788, 1972.
120. Ziff, M., Gribetz, H. J., and Lo Spalluto, J.: J. Clin. Invest. *39*:405, 1960.
121. Zigmond, S., and Hirsch, J. G.: Exp. Cell Res. *73*:383, 1972.
122. Zucker-Franklin, D., and Hirsch, J. C.: J. Exp. Med. *120*:569, 1964.
123. Zurier, R. B., Hoffstein, S., and Weissmann, G.: Proc. Natl. Acad. Sci. USA *70*:844, 1973.
124. Zurier, R. B., Weissmann, G., Hoffstein, S., Kammerman, S., and Tai, H. H.: J. Clin. Invest. *53*:297, 1974.

Chapter 2

Histamine

Histamine is an endogenous substance found in most tissues and in many physiological fluids. Its wide distribution would appear to make it ideally suited as a mediator of acute inflammation and of acute anaphylactic reaction.

The release of histamine in anaphylaxis was conclusively demonstrated in 1932 (6,30). The extensive studies of Lewis (58) indicated that a substance with the properties of histamine is released by injurious nonimmunologic stimuli. Subsequently, the localization of histamine in mast cells was discovered (70). It is widely accepted today that histamine plays only a transitory role in the development of the inflammatory reaction, being one of the first mediators released by the injurious stimuli. Its participation in immunologically mediated inflammatory processes is a subject of intensive investigation. Recent investigations on histamine receptors also suggests an autoregulatory role for this amine, in concert with other substances involved in inflammatory and immune responses. Should any of the new antihistamine compounds specific for H_2 receptors (14) prove to exert an useful action within the overall context of the inflammatory state, the role of histamine will probably have to be reevaluated. Further research on the preferred conformation of histamine (54,55) is necessary to improve our understanding of its role and functions.

More extensive information is available in a number of monographs and reviews dealing with histamine and inflammation (36, 45,50,74,77,82).

1. CHEMISTRY, BIOSYNTHESIS AND DEGRADATION

Histamine, or 4-(2-aminoethyl)imidazole, $C_5H_9N_3$, has a molecular weight of 111 and functions as a bivalent radical in salt formation. It is a basic, highly hygroscopic substance, stable in acid solution even on prolonged boiling, but rapidly destroyed by heating in aqueous solutions. It has no absorption maximum in the 210-700 nm region, nor does it exhibit fluorescence in the ultraviolet region. In aqueous solution, it has pk_a values of 5.94 and 9.80. It undergoes reactions characteristic of primary amines and of imidazole compounds, including acylation and diazotization (Fig. 2).

Histamine is presumably synthetized in the cytoplasm of mast cells and basophils from l-histidine by a specific cytoplasmic histidine decarboxylase which can be inhibited by l-methylhistidine and 4-bromo-3-hydroxybenzyloxyamine. The pathway of histamine from its site of synthesis to that of its storage is unknown. Once inside the granule, it appears to be retained there for a long time through firm ionic linkage to carboxyl groups on granule protein (85). This conclusion is also supported by research with [22]NaCl (83), suggesting that histamine can be released from the granule matrix by sodium or other basic radicals, such as for instance biogenic amines (11), through ion-exchange. Histamine release is energy dependent since it can be blocked by anoxia and by a number of metabolic inhibitors (68,71). It can be induced both in vivo and in vitro by a variety of stimuli or agents (36) which trigger a process involving fusion of perigranular membranes with plasma membrane. The biological effects of histamine occur only after it has been released and they are fairly transient since it is rapidly converted to inactive derivatives. The metabolism of histamine has been the subject of extensive reviews (36,45). Two major steps are involved in the catabolism of this amine—acetylation and oxidative deamination. The former brings about the formation of acetylhistamine and occurs by bacterial action in the intestine. The latter is

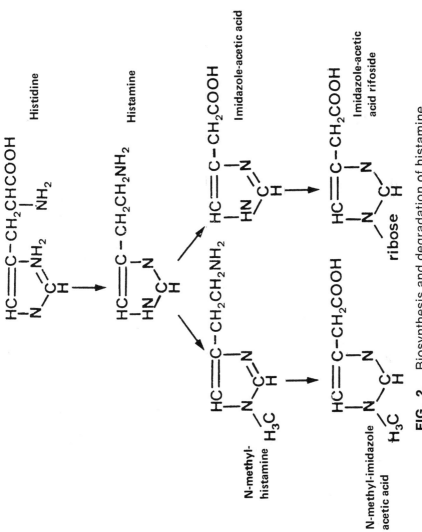

FIG. 2. Biosynthesis and degradation of histamine.

17

catalyzed by the enzyme, histaminase, leading to the formation of imidazole-acetaldehyde which is then further oxidized as imidazole acetic acid riboside. Histaminase is found in higher concentration in kidney, intestine and liver than in other tissues. Moreover, it may be significant that lymph nodes contain high levels of this enzyme which seems to have the same intracellular distribution as histamine. Both metabolic pathways, whose relative importance varies from species to species, abolish the pharmacological action of histamine. Study of the catabolism of histamine-^{14}C in man showed imidazole acetic acid to be the prevalent metabolic product in urine. Labeled imidazole acetic acid and methylimidazole acetic acid were also recovered but histamine-^{14}C was not found (9).

2. ROLE OF HISTAMINE IN INFLAMMATORY AND IMMUNOLOGICAL REACTIONS

The most striking effects of intravenous or subcutaneous injection of histamine, hypotension and edema, respectively, are the consequence of a generalized or localized vasodilatation. Electronmicroscopy studies contributed to localizing the site of action of histamine in postcapillary venules whose diameter ranges from 20 to 30 μm (64). The endothelial cells are made to contract by histamine, thus producing gaps between adjacent cells. These discontinuities allow the leakage of plasma which then filters through the semipermeable periendothelial basement membrane and into surrounding tissue space (34,63). The effects of histamine are believed to be mediated through its interaction with specific receptors located on the plasma membrane of cells in target tissues. Two different types of receptors have been hypothesized (3) : H_1 receptors mediating vasodilatation and smooth muscle contraction, and sensitive to the usual antihistamines (e.g., mepyramine), and H_2 receptors mediating histamine-induced secretion of gastric acid, increase in heart rate, uterine contractions and possibly, immunological release of histamine (60) ; H_2 receptors are insensitive to the above-mentioned antihistamines but respond to recently described thiourea derivatives (14). Human leukocytes have receptors for histamine (66), which have recently been identified as belonging to the H_2 type (60).

Histamine is one chemical mediator whose role in the inflammatory process, particularly its early phases, has clearly been established on the basis of its known effects on microvasculature and the many studies on different types of experimentally-induced inflammation (26,28,33,79,84).

Histamine is released at the site of local injury produced by various substances, such as dextran (35,49,53,67), ovalbumin (1, 37,67), turpentine (78,79,83), and carrageenin (28,84), or procedures, such as thermal injury (44,73) and aseptic trauma (13). This release is associated with a degranulation of the mast cells in the injured tissues and the development of local inflammatory reactions. Histamine is also released in a specific manner from rat mast cells in vitro (7,27). Theophylline, prostaglandin E₁, isoproterenol and norepinephrine inhibit this release (7). Adrenergic agents and theophylline also afford protection in vivo against the reaction to dextran (8).

If tissue stores of histamine are depleted by one means or another prior to the local injection of irritants or other procedures, the vascular response which usually occurs in the initial stages of an inflammatory reaction is reduced (12,28,35,67,80) and the latter's onset delayed (29).

It appears, therefore, that the role of histamine in the inflammatory response is transient, and other mediators and mechanisms are required to explain the continued vascular and cellular changes characterizing the progression and regression of this response.

Certain other inflammatory conditions exist where histamine release occurs as a consequence of immunological reactions, or in which mast cells and basophils appear to play a significant role. One such example is the allergic or immediate hypersensitivity reaction. When certain individuals encounter antigens in their surroundings—clinically the most important being those causing pollinosis—they respond by producing antibodies of several immunoglobulin classes, particularly the IgE type capable of binding firmly and for prolonged periods to the surface of mast cells and basophils (15,46). The interaction of the antigen with its specific antibody results in the release of histamine and of other mediators as well. For a more complete discussion on the immunological release of chemical mediators see Chapter 1. Biochemical and morphological data suggest that histamine release is a secretory event and is not the result of a cytolytic lesion (61,62). It occurs without the simultaneous loss of other intracellular components (48) and is accompanied by active cellular motility and ruffling (38). Much of the pathophysiology of the hypersensitivity reaction, mediated by IgE antibodies, can be explained by the pharmacological effect of histamine. Further evidence is provided by the finding of a close correlation between antigen-induced histamine release from leukocytes in vitro and the intensity of patients symptoms in the hay-fever season (61). In addition, human lung tissue (20) and nasal polyps (52) from allergic individuals release histamine in vitro upon contact with specific antigen. Similar release has been demonstrated from passively sensitized human and monkey lung (4,5,47).

The release reaction can be modulated with hormones and drugs which are capable of changing the intracellular cyclic nucleotide levels, such as theophylline, β-adrenergic catecholamines and prostaglandin E (16,17,19). It is of great interest that exogenous histamine, at concentrations equivalent to those in leukocytes, can increase intracellular levels of cAMP and inhibit antigen-induced release of endogenous histamine (59). Standard H_1-type antihistamines do not interfere with these phenomena which are, however, blocked by burimamide and other H_2-receptor antagonists (60). It appears, therefore, that immunologically released histamine interacting with H_2-receptors leads to activation of adenylate cyclase. The resulting increase in cAMP levels is associated with a diminished endogenous histamine release. Conversely, the selective rise in cGMP enhances the immunological release of histamine (51). Further evidence for a feedback mechanism modulating cell function is the finding that methiamide, an H_2-receptor antagonist, is able to stimulate IgE-mediated histamine release from lung fragments (21). These observations are consistent with the hypothesis that histamine, in concert with other substances, acts in vivo to regulate the intensity and character of inflammatory and immune responses (18). They also suggest that antigen-induced release of histamine may be thought of as an effector mechanism by which an immunologic response is directly linked to inflammation.

Another inflammatory condition in which histamine appears to be involved as a chemical mediator is the so-called immune complex disease. This form of immune injury is initiated when antigen reacts with precipitating antibody in tissue fluids, forming microprecipitates in and around small blood vessels, or when antigen, present in excess, reacts in the blood stream with potentially precipitating antibody, producing soluble circulating complexes, which are deposited in the walls of blood vessels, including the glomerular capillaries of the kidney. These complexes initiate an intricate series of reactions leading to tissue injury (22,23,72). It has been suggested by observation of experimental immune complex disease in rabbits that the passive deposition of immune complexes depends on a state of enhanced vascular permeability resulting from a release of histamine by platelets (24). Several immunological mechanisms can lead to such a release (41,42), one of them requiring an interaction of IgE-sensitized basophils with platelets (40,43). Preliminary evidence for the existence of a similar mechanism in man has been obtained (10). The administration of cyproheptadine, an antagonist of both histamine and serotonin, reduced the severity of chronic glomerulonephritis induced by immune complex in rabbit (57) and rat (56).

Recent studies have drawn attention to the possible role of basophils and mast cells and, therefore, of histamine in several immunological reactions previously considered as involving primarily lymphocytes and monocytes (31,32). Microscopic examination of biopsy specimens from patients undergoing acute cellular rejection of human allografts showed that basophils accounted for 40% of infiltrating granulocytes (25). The existence of an interaction between basophils or mast cells and thymus derived lymphocytes has, therefore, been hypothesized. Some evidence also exists (39,69) suggesting that histamine released from mast cells and basophils may modulate the functions of thymus-derived lymphocytes.

3. METHODS OF ASSAY

Histamine can be determined either by bioassay or by chemical means (36). In either case, it must be separated from other pharmacologically or chemically reactive substances, deproteinizing tissue samples or extracting them with an organic solvent.

Bioassays are based on the effect of histamine on blood pressure and smooth muscle. The Schultz-Dale method is still widely used. When exposed to histamine, the guinea-pig ileum contracts and then relaxes rapidly. The intensity of contraction is quantitatively related to the histamine concentration. The sensitivity ranges from 1 to 10 ng.

The most used chemical assay is that of Shore et al. (75), as modified by May et al. (65). It is based on the fluorescence of the O-phtal-dialdehyde derivative of histamine. The intensity of fluorescence is proportional to the histamine concentration over a wide range of values (5-500 ng/ml). This method can also be used for the histochemical detection of histamine. A technique with greater sensitivity and specificity than the assays previously mentioned is the enzymatic isotope assay (76,81). It allows measurement of 0.1 ng of histamine in 0.02 ml of tissue extract. This method depends on the transfer of the ^{14}C-methyl of ^{14}C-S-adenosylmethionine to histamine to form ^{14}C-methylhistamine. The reaction is catalyzed by histamine-N-methyltransferase. Tracer amounts of ^{3}H-histamine are added and the final product is ^{14}C-^{3}H-histamine. After separation of histamine, the radioactivity is counted, the ratio ^{14}C : ^{3}H being linearly related to histamine content.

REFERENCES

1. Arrigoni-Martelli, E., and Kramer, M.: Boll. Soc. Ital. Biol. Sper. *34*:1130, 1958.
2. Asboe-Hansen, G., and Wegelius, O.: Nature *178*:262, 1956.
3. Ash, A. S. F., and Schild, H. O.: Br. J. Pharmacol. *27*:427, 1966.
4. Assem, E. S. K., and Schild, H. W.: Nature *224*:1028, 1969.
5. Austen, K. F.: J. Allergy Clin. Immunol. *51*:106, 1973.
6. Bartosch, R., Feldberg, W., and Nagel, E.: Pfluegers Arch. Ges. Physiol. *230*:129, 1932.
7. Baxter, J. M.: Proc. Soc. Exp. Biol. Med. *141*:576, 1972.
8. Baxter, J. M., Beaven, M. A., and Horakova, Z.: Biochem. Pharmacol. *23*: 1211, 1974.
9. Beall, G. N., and Van Arsdel, P. P., Jr.: J. Clin. Invest. *39*:676, 1960.
10. Benveniste, J.: Fed. Proc. *33*:797 (Abst.), 1974.
11. Bergvist, U., Samuelsson, G., and Uvnäs B.: Acta Physiol. Scand. *83*:362, 1971.
12. Bhatt, K. G. S., and Sanyal, R. K.: J. Pharm. Pharmacol. *15*:78, 1963.
13. Bhatt, K. G. S., and Sanyal, R. K.: J. Pharm. Pharmacol. *16*:385, 1964.
14. Black, J. M., Duncan, W. A. M., Durant, C. J., Grimellin, C. R., and Parson, E. M.: Nature *236*:385, 1972.
15. Bloch, K. J.: In "Mechanism in Allergy," L. Goodfriend, A. H. Schon, and R. P. Orango, eds. Dekker, New York, 1973, p. 11.
16. Bourne, M. R., Lehrer, R. I., Cline, M. J., and Melmon, K. L.: J. Clin. Invest. *50*:920, 1971.
17. Bourne, H. R., Lichtenstein, L. M., and Melmon, K. L.: J. Immunol. *108*: 695, 1972.
18. Bourne, H. R., Lichtenstein, L. M., Melmon, K. L., Henney, C. S., Weinstein, Y., and Shearer, G. M.: Science *184*:19, 1974.
19. Bourne, H. R., Melmon, K. L., and Lichtenstein, L. M.: Science *173*:743, 1971.
20. Brocklehurst, W. E.: J. Physiol. (Lond.) *151*:416, 1960.
21. Chakrin, L. W., Krell, R. D., Mengel, J., Young, D., Zaher, C., and Wardell, J. R., Jr.: Agents Actions *4*:297, 1974.
22. Cochrane, C. G.: Prog. Allergy *11*:1, 1967.
23. Cochrane, C. G.: J. Allergy *42*:113, 1968.
24. Cochrane, C. G., Koffler, D.: Adv. Immunol. *16*:185, 1973.
25. Colvin, R. B., Dvorak, H. F.: Lancet *1*:212, 1974.
26. Crunkhorn, P., Meacock, S. C. R.: Br. J. Pharmacol. *42*:392, 1971.
27. Dias da Silva, W., and Lemos Fernandes, A. D.: Experientia *21*:96, 1965.

28. Di Rosa, M., Giroud, J. P., and Willoughby, D. A.: J. Pathol. *104*:15, 1971.
29. Di Rosa, M., Papadimitriou, J. M., and Willoughby, D. A.: J. Pathol. *105*: 239, 1971.
30. Dragstedt, C. A., and Gebauer-Fuelnegg, E.: Am. J. Physiol. *102*:512, 1932.
31. Dvorak, H. F.: J. Immunol. *106*:279, 1971.
32. Dvorak, H. F., Mihm, M. C., Jr.: J. Exp. Med. *135*:235, 1972.
33. Giroud, J. P., and Willoughby, D. A.: J. Pathol. *101*:241, 1970.
34. Gotran, R. S., and Maino, G.: Ann. N. Y. Acad. Sci. *116*:750, 1964.
35. Halpern, B. N., Liacopoulos, P., and Liacopoulos-Briot, M.: Arch. Int. Pharmacodyn. Ther. *119*:56, 1959.
36. Eichler, O., and Farah, A. (eds.): "Handbuch der experimentellen Pharmakologie," XVIII. Springer-Verlag, Berlin, 1966.
37. Harris, J. M., and West, G. B.: Nature *191*:399, 1961.
38. Hastie, R.: Clin. Exp. Immunol. *8*:45, 1971.
39. Henney, S. C., Bourne, H. R., and Lichtenstein, L. M.: J. Immunol. *108*: 1526, 1972.
40. Henson, P. M.: J. Immunol. *105*:490, 1970.
41. Henson, P. M., and Cochrane, C. G.: J. Exp. Med. *129*:153, 1969.
42. Henson, P. M., and Cochrane, C. G.: J. Immunol. *105*:476, 1970.
43. Henson, P. M., and Cochrane, C. G.: J. Exp. Med. *133*:554, 1971.
44. Horakova, Z., and Beaven, M. A.: Eur. J. Pharmacol. *27*:305, 1974.
45. CIBA Foundation Symposium: "Histamine," G. E. W. Wolstenholme and C. M. O'Connor, eds. Little Brown, Boston, 1955.
46. Ishizaka, K.: Ann. Rev. Med. *21*:187, 1970.
47. Ishizaka, T., Ishizaka, R., Orange, R. P., and Austen, K. F.: J. Immunol. *106*:1267, 1971.
48. Johnson, A. R., and Moran, N. C.: Fed. Proc. *28*:1716, 1969.
49. Jori, A., Bentivoglio, A. P., and Garattini, S.: J. Pharm. Pharmacol. *13*: 617, 1961.
50. Judah, J. D., and Ahmed, K.: Biol. Rev. *39*:160, 1964.
51. Kaliner, M., Orange, R. P., and Austen, K. F.: J. Exp. Med. *136*:556, 1972.
52. Kaliner, M., Wasserman, S. I., and Austen, K. F.: N. Engl. J. Med. *289*: 277, 1973.
53. Kató, L., and Göszy, B.: Am. J. Physiol. *199*:657, 1960.
54. Kier, L. B.: J. Med. Chem. *11*:441, 1968.
55. Kier, L. B.: "Molecular Orbital Theory in Drug Research." Academic Press, New York, 1972.
56. Kline-Botton, W., Spargo, B., and Lewis, E. J.: J. Lab. Clin. Med. *83*:695, 1974.
57. Knicker, W. T.: In "Inflammation: Mechanisms and Control," I. H. Lepow and P. A. Ward, eds. Academic Press, New York, 1972, p. 335.
58. Lewis, T.: "Blood Vessels of the Human Skin and Their Response." Shaw, London, 1927.
59. Lichtenstein, L. M.: In "Clinical Immunobiology," F. H. Bach and R. A. Good, eds. Academic Press, New York, 1972, Vol. 1, p. 243.
60. Lichtenstein, L. M., and Gillespie, E.: Nature *244*:287, 1973.
61. Lichtenstein, C. M., and Osler, A. G.: J. Exp. Med. *120*:507, 1964.
62. Lichtenstein, L. M., and Osler, A. G.: J. Immunol. *96*:159, 1966.
63. Majno, G.: In "Handbook of Physiology," Vol. 3, Sect. 2, J. Field, ed.

Williams and Wilkins, Baltimore, 1965, p. 2293.

64. Majno, G., and Palade, G. E.: J. Biophys. Biochem. Cytol. *11*:607, 1961.
65. May, D. C., Lyman, M., Alberto, R., and Chang, J.: J. Allergy *46*:12, 1970.
66. Melmon, K. L., Bourne, M. R., Weinstein, J., and Sela, M.: Science *177*: 707, 1972.
67. Parratt, J. R., and West, G. B.: J. Physiol. *139*:27, 1957.
68. Peterson, C.: Acta Physiol. Scand. *92* Suppl n. 413, 1974.
69. Plaut, M., Lichtenstein, L. M., Gillespie, E., and Henney, S. C.: J. Immunol. *111*:389, 1973.
70. Riley, J. F.: Science, *118*:332, 1953.
71. Rothschild, A. M., Vugman, I., and Rocha e Silva, M.: Biochem. Pharmacol. *7*:248, 1961.
72. Ruddy, S., Gigli, I., and Austen, K. F.: N. Engl. J. Med. *287*:489, 1972.
73. Schayer, R. W., and Ganley, O. M.: Am. J. Physiol. *197*:721, 1959.
74. Shanes, A. M.: Pharmacol. Rev. *10*:156, 1958.
75. Shore, P. A., Burkhalter, A., and Cohn, V. M., Jr.: J. Pharmacol. Exp. Ther. *127*:182, 1959.
76. Snyder, S. H., Baldessarini, R. J., and Axelrod, J.: J. Pharmacol. Exp. Ther. *153*:544, 1966.
77. Spector, W. G.: Pharmacol. Rev. *10*:475, 1958.
78. Spector, W. G., and Willoughby, D. A.: J. Pathol. *74*:57, 1957.
79. Spector, W. G., and Willoughby, D. A.: J. Pathol. *77*:1, 1959.
80. Spector, W. G., and Willoughby, D. A.: J. Pathol. *78*:121, 1959.
81. Taylor, K. M., and Snyder, S. M.: J. Neurochem. *19*:1343, 1972.
82. Zweifach, B. W., Grant, L., and McCluskey, R. T. (eds.): "The Inflammatory Process." Academic Press, New York, 1973.
83. Uvnäs, B.: In "Inflammation Biochemistry and Drug Interaction," A. Bertelli and J. C. Houck, eds. Excerpta Medica, Amsterdam, 1969, p. 221.
84. Willis, A. L.: J. Pharm. Pharmacol. *21*:126, 1969.
85. Åborg, C. H., Novotny, J., and Uvnäs, B.: Acta Physiol. Scand. *69*:276, 1967.

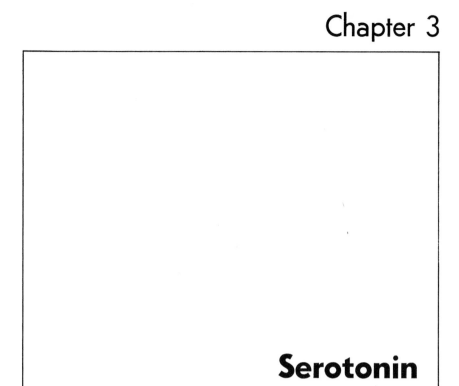

Chapter 3

Serotonin

Serotonin is an endogenous biogenic amine which, like histamine, has potent effects on small blood vessels and smooth muscles in certain mammalian species. Its role in inflammation still needs further clarification. Its most important function probably pertains to the nervous system and gastrointestinal tract (13,22,25).

The chemical structure of serotonin is 5-hydroxytryptamine (5-HT), or 3-(2-aminoethyl)-5-indolol; it can be assayed fluorometrically or by bioassay with rat colon or estrous rat uterus. In case of the latter, serotonin is identified by showing that lysergic acid can inhibit muscle contractions induced by the test sample.

Serotonin originates from tryptophan which is hydroxylated to give 5-hydroxytryptophan. This compound, in turn, is decarboxylated to serotonin. After its release, 5-HT is oxidized by monoamine oxidase to 5-hydroxyindole acetic acid which is then excreted in urine (Fig. 3).

In mammalian tissues, serotonin is localized in enterochromaf-

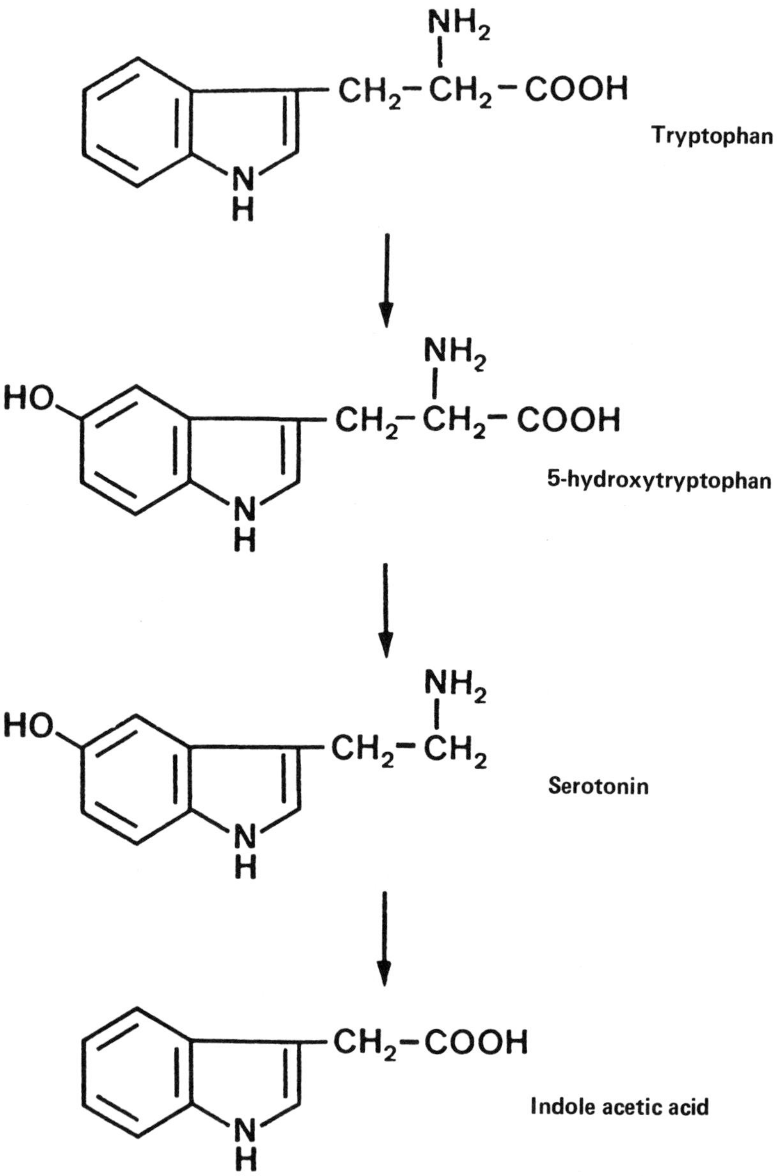

FIG. 3.   Biosynthesis and degradation of serotonin

fin cells of the mucosal layer of the gastrointestinal tract. The gut contains about 1 μg of serotonin/g tissue; carcinoid tumors of the enterochromaffin cells may have 1000 times this amount. Part of the brain, the hypothalamus for example, also contains about 1 μg/g tissue of serotonin. Rat, rabbit and mouse lung, but not that of man or guinea pig, represents another site of serotonin storage. In most mammals, platelets are the reservoir of serotonin in the blood. Rat, mouse and rabbit mast cells, but not those of many other species, are rich in serotonin (5,10,18,31). Rat peritoneal mast cells contain from 0.2 to 6 μg of serotonin/10^6 cells. This amine is stored in the same cytoplasmic granules that contain histamine (1,22). Serotonin is also found in basophils (2). Rabbit platelets release serotonin together with histamine when exposed to immune complexes in the presence of complement (8,12,28). This process, which is calcium dependent, occurs both in vitro and in vivo (8,14,29). Also the IgE antibody-mediated, complement-independent mechanisms may release serotonin from rabbit platelets (3). Rat peritoneal mast cells release serotonin when challenged with several agents, including IgE and IgG antibodies, anaphylatoxins, compound 48/80 and polymyxin B (16). There is also both direct and indirect evidence supporting the hypothesis that serotonin may participate in anaphylactic reactions in rat and mouse (6,7,21,24). In other species, the role of 5-HT in these reactions is probably of very scarce importance. It may participate, however, along with histamine, in the mediation of immune complex disease in rabbits and humans (3,11).

The possible role of serotonin in acute inflammation has been the subject of numerous investigations. As mentioned before, in many animal species, mast cells and platelets contain relatively large amount of serotonin which is released along with histamine by agents, such as dextran (9,19), turpentine (23) and egg albumen (17), which cause local inflammatory reactions. Serotonin increases vascular permeability when injected subcutaneously in low amounts: 0.1 — 1 μg in rats (20,26) and mice (27,30). Furthermore, some studies seem to indicate that the depletion of serotonin stores reduces the intensity of local inflammatory reactions produced by different agents (4,15).

It can be concluded that the role of serotonin in acute inflammation, if any, is very modest and limited to the early phases, mainly characterized by histamine release.

REFERENCES

1. Austen, K. F.: In "Immunological Diseases," 2nd ed., M. Samter ed. Little Brown, Boston, 1971, p. 332.
2. Åborg, C. M., Novotny, J., and Uvnäs, B.: Acta Physiol. Scand. *69*:276, 1967.
3. Cochrane, C. G., and Koffler, D.: Adv. Immunol. *16*:185, 1973.
4. Craps, L., and Inderbitzin, T.: Int. Arch. Allergy *18*:268, 1961.
5. Day, S. M., and Green, J. P.: Fed. Proc. *18*:1505, 1959.
6. Donaldson, R. M., Jr., Malkiel, S., and Gray, S. J.: Proc. Soc. Exp. Biol. Med. *103*:261, 1960.
7. Gershon, M. D., and Ross, L. L.: J. Exp. Med. *115*:367, 1962.
8. Gocke, D. J., and Osler, A. G.: J. Immunol. *95*:1526, 1965.
9. Halpern, B. N., Liacopoulos, P., and Liacopoulos-Briot, M.: Arch. Int. Pharmacodyn. Ther. *119*:56, 1959.
10. Keller, R.: Helv. Physiol. Pharmacol. Acta *15*:371, 1957.
11. Knicker, W. T.: In "Inflammation: Mechanism and Control," J. H. Lepow and P. A. Ward, eds. Academic Press, New York, 1972, p. 335.
12. Lecomte, J.: Acta Allergol. (Kbh.) *7*: (Suppl.) 81, 1960.
13. Lecomte, J.: Acta Allergol. (Kbh.) *15*:61, 1960.
14. Lecomte, J., and Lapiére, C. M.: C. R. Soc. Biol. (Paris) *154*:2386, 1960.
15. Mathies, H.: Med. Exp. *4*:12, 1961.
16. Morrison, D. C., Roser, J. F., Henson, P. M., and Cochrane, C. G.: J. Immunol. *112*:573, 1974.
17. Morsdorf, K.: Med. Exp. *4*:293, 1961.
18. Parratt, J. R., and West, G. B.: J. Physiol. (Lond.) *137*:179, 1957.
19. Parratt, J. R., and West, G. B.: J. Physiol. (Lond.) *139*:27, 1957.
20. Rowley, D. A., and Benditt, E. P.: J. Exp. Med. *103*:399, 1956.
21. Sanyal, R. K., and West, G. B.: J. Physiol. (Lond.) *144*:525, 1958.
22. Spector, W. G.: Pharmacol. Rev. *10*:475, 1958.
23. Supek, Z., Jonic, M., and Kreckes, S.: Arzneim. Forsch. *11*:132, 1961.
24. Tokuda, S., and Weiser, R. S.: J. Immunol. *86*:292, 1961.
25. Udenfriend, S., and Waalkes, T. P.: In "Mechanisms of Hypersensitivity," J. H. Schaffer, G. A. Lo Grippo and M. W. Chase, eds. Little Brown, Boston, 1959, p. 219.
26. Ungar, G., Kobrin, S., and Sezesny, B. R.: Arch. Int. Pharmacodyn. Ther. *123*:71, 1959.
27. Vogin, E. E., Rossi, G. V., Chase, G. D., and Osol, A.: Experientia *18*:191, 1962.
28. Waalkes, T. P., and Coburn, H.: J. Allergy *30*:394, 1959.
29. Waalkes, T. P., Coburn, H., and Terry, L. L.: J. Allergy *30*:408, 1959.
30. Weis, J.: Med. Exp. *8*:1, 1963.
31. West, G. B.: J. Pharm. Pharmacol. *11*:513, 1959.

Chapter 4

Bradykinin

Bradykinin, as one member of the family of plasmakinins, can be defined as an endogenous substance of polypeptide nature, producing a slow contraction of the guinea-pig ileum, relaxation of the rat duodenum, fall in blood pressure due to vasodilatation, and increase in capillary and venule permeability. These effects are resistant to atropine, to some of the most specific antihistamines and to antiserotonin agents. It would be impossible to review the large number of papers devoted to the study of the action of bradykinin on the mammalian organism, including that of man. Table 2 summarizes the main effects observed. This matter has been the subject of several reviews and symposia (20,33,35,84,90,96). We will confine our discussion to the role of bradykinin in inflammation.

TABLE 2. Actions of bradykinin

Effect		Dose	References[(')]
Contraction:	rat uterus	0.03 ng/ml	64
	rabbit duodenum	1.0 ng/ml	64
	guinea pig ileum	1.0 ng/ml	27
	guinea pig isolated vesicles	0.5 ng/ml	64
Relaxation:	rat duodenum	1.0 ng/ml	27
Constriction:	bronchioles, cat	0.8 μg/kg	64
	guinea pig	12 μg/kg	64
Hypotension:	cat	0.4 μg/kg	27, 64
	rat	1.5 μg/kg	18
	guinea pig	0.2 μg/kg	105
	rabbit	0.2 μg/kg	105
Increased vascular permeability:			
	guinea pig	5 ng	27,64
	rabbit	1 ng	18,40
	rat	15 ng	4
Pain induction:	cat	2 μg	47
	dog	2 μg	47
	man (blister base)	1 μg	27

[(')] In addition to the papers quoted, see also 20, 33, 35, 84, 90, 96.

1. CHEMISTRY, BIOSYNTHESIS AND DEGRADATION

Bradykinin is a linear nonapeptide first discovered by Rocha e Silva et al. (85). Its structure and those of the related deca- and endecapeptide (named kallidin or l-lysyl-bradykinin and 1-methionyl-lysyl-bradykinin, respectively) are reported in Table 3. Bradykinin has been obtained in pure form from plasma globulin by action of trypsin, serum kallikrein and snake venoms (28,29,49,50); it was synthetized later on (8,9). The synthetic nonapeptide was compared with the natural product and found to share all its biological properties (9,64,94,105). l-Lysyl-bradykinin is released by pancreatic or urinary kallikreins (49,75). An enzyme which is able to transform l-lysyl-bradykinin into bradykinin has been isolated from brain tissues (14). So far, no enzymatic system has been described able to release only the endecapeptide from plasma kininogen.

TABLE 3. Structure of bradykinin and related kinins

H	—	Arg	—	Pro	—	Pro	—	Gly	—	Phe	—	Ser	—	Pro	—	Phe	—	Arg	—	OH
		1		2		3		4		5		6		7		8		9		

Bradykinin (kallidin I)

H	—	Lys	—	Arg	—	Pro	—	Pro	—	Gly	—	Phe	—	Ser	—	Pro	—	Phe	—	Arg	—	OH
		1		2		3		4		5		6		7		8		9		10		

I-Lysylbradykinin (kallidin II)

H	—	Met	—	Lys	—	Arg	—	Pro	—	Pro	—	Gly	—	Phe	—	Ser	—	Pro	—	Phe	—	Arg	—	OH
		1		2		3		4		5		6		7		8		9		10		11		

I-Methionyllysylbradykinin

Met	=	Methionine
Lys	=	Lysine
Arg	=	Arginine
Pro	=	Proline
Gly	=	Glycine
Phe	=	Phenylalanine
Ser	=	Serine

The pathway leading to the formation of bradykinin is initiated by the activation of Hageman factor (clotting factor XII) and causes the conversion of a series of proenzymes to their active form, with the resultant generation of several biological activities in addition to those of bradykinin (Fig. 4).

Early observations of the activation of Hageman factor by non-biological surfaces (2,3) have been extended to such negatively charged surface as articular cartilage (71), collagen (114), renal vascular basement membrane (16), sodium urate crystal of gout and pyrophosphate crystal of pseudogout (61). The enzymes kallikrein, plasmin and trypsin also activate Hageman factor (16). In vitro activation with soluble immune complexes has been reported (60) but more recent investigations failed to confirm previous results (17).

Once activated, Hageman factor converts three plasma proenzymes into their active forms: clotting factor XI, initiating the intrinsic coagulation mechanism (78); plasminogen proactivator, leading to plasmin formation (58); and prekallikrein which liberates kinin (57). As mentioned before, these three enzymes further activate Hageman factor (16), thus providing positive feedback loops in the system, with kallikrein being more active than the other two (80).

In addition, plasmin is able to break down the activated Hage-

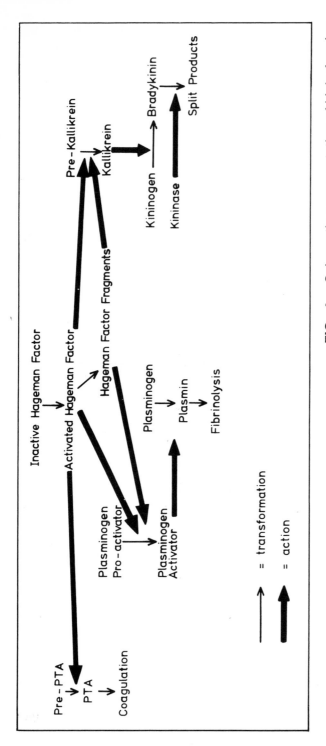

FIG. 4. Schematic representation of kinin-forming pathway and of its relationship to coagulation and fibrinolysis

man factor into the so-called Hageman factor prealbumin fragments (57,58,92). These act on the same enzyme precursors as the parent factor. However, clotting factor XI is more rapidly activated by the intact Hageman factor, whereas the fragments are more effective in respect to prekallikrein (57). The prealbumin factor activities have been found in rabbit (119), guinea pig (107) and man (72).

It is now recognized that forms of activated Hageman factor are functionally synonymous with the so-called "PF/dil" (52,56, 79), i.e., the factor present in human and guinea-pig plasma after dilution with saline and contact with glass, and which increases vascular permeability when injected intradermally (68,104).

Kallikrein has been found in saliva, urine, plasma and certain tissues (39), including lymphnodes (111), synovia (1) and leukocytes (69). It has been highly purified and characterized with several physicochemical methods (59,118). This enzyme cleaves a plasma substrate, kininogen, to release the nonapeptide, bradykinin (111). Earlier findings suggested the existence of two different kininogens (5,74,110). Subsequently, a model of a single kininogen (60,100,118) has been proposed with the kinin moiety located internally (63), susceptible to both urinary and plasma kallikrein.

Bradykinin is rapidly inactivated simply by pass through the lungs (37,89), as well as in plasma and other biological fluids. Two enzymes which metabolize bradykinin have been characterized and purified from human plasma or serum: kininase I, an arginine carboxypeptidase (34), and kininase II which cleaves the carboxyterminal phenylalanyl arginine dipeptide from bradykinin (110). Kininase I is the same protein as the anaphylatoxin inactivator (10), whereas kininase II appears to be identical to the carboxydipeptidase angiotensin I converting enzyme (31).

2. ROLE OF BRADYKININ IN INFLAMMATION

One of the most striking properties of bradykinin is its capacity to increase vascular permeability in most animals tested and also in man. In contrast, serotonin acts only in mice and rats, and is completely inert in rabbits and guinea pigs. Histamine is the only other endogenous substance that may be induced to participate in inflammatory reactions in all the species studied, although its effect on the vascular permeability of rabbits and rats is much weaker than that of bradykinin (18,27,40,113,115). The latter in-

TABLE 4. Relative potency in increasing vascular permeability in
some animal species of bradykinin, histamine, serotonin
and their releasers

Mediators	Guinea Pig	Rat	Rabbit
Bradykinin	2-10.000.000	10-100.000	700.000
Histamine	32.000	1.500	37.000
Serotonin	60	16.200	
48/80	3.500	7.000	30
Polymyxin B	1.000	15.000	0
Kallikreins	2.500	900	600

Data reported in 18, 27, 40, 105, 113.

creases capillary permeability after both intradermal and subcutaneous administration (55,115), causing gap formation in the
capillary endothelium (55) or raising the pressure in the proximal
venules (88), which produces edema or exudate accumulation, for
example, in the pleural cavity (98). The relative potencies of bradykinin, histamine, serotonin and of some of their releasers are listed
in Table 4.

The finding that antihistamines diminish the bradykinin-induced increase of vascular permeability in the skin of several species (6) raised the possibility of bradykinin releasing histamine
from cellular stores. This possibility has been examined using rat
peritoneal mast cells (53), and the above observation was recently
confirmed and expanded (54).

Bradykinin also seems to act as mediator of certain forms of
pain both in man (2,21,67,94) and animals (30,48,65). It is of
interest that, when bradykinin is injected into the splenic artery, a
kind of visceral pain is evoked, characterized by a so-called pseudo-
affective reflex-vocalization, transient hypertension and hyperpnea,
and discharge of potentials in splenic nerves (47,66). This discharge, associated with the sensation of pain, is blocked by acetylsalicylate but not by morphine, whereas the pseudo-affective response is inhibited by both narcotic and non-narcotic analgesics
(65).

Considerable research has been devoted to the involvement of
kinins in the swelling produced in the rat's paw by several substances or procedures. An acute inflammatory reaction occurs in the
rat's paw exposed for 30 min to a temperature of 45-46°—so-called
thermic edema (83,103). The exudate, collected by means of coaxial

perfusion (83), contains bradykinin-like material while histamine appears in the perfusate only when the paw is exposed to higher temperatures (5,42,82,83,103). A large number of sulfated polysaccharides can produce edema when injected subcutaneously and almost invariably a kinin-like substance has been found in the exudate (86,87). This substance has been also found in exudate produced by serotonin (12), kaolin (11), brewer yeast (42), and carrageenin (109).

Direct experimental evidence, however, suggests that bradykinin could be responsible only for the intermediate phase of carrageenin edema, the earlier and more advanced phases being mediated by histamine and prostaglandins, respectively (5,13,23,25,24) (Fig. 5).

Bradykinin involvement has also been claimed in human and experimental animal gout (36,93,97). Kinin levels are increased in the synovial fluid of gouty joints (71) ; here a possible mechanism could be activation of Hageman factor by urate microcrystals in synovial fluid (62). Moreover, in a relatively high percentage of joint exudates obtained from rheumatic patients, high bradykinin levels (26,71) have been shown but they seem to correlate more with articular pain than with other arthritic symptoms (26).

In spite of the many advances made in characterizing the components and interactions of the kinin system, its exact role in an in vivo inflammatory response has yet to be determined. Studies of models of inflammation are difficult to interpret because of the complexity of the kinin-forming system and its interactions with other plasma systems. Artifactual activation of the kinin system and the short half-life of bradykinin ($t_{1/2} = 20$ sec) complicate matters further. Available evidence would suggest a secondary role for the kinin-forming pathway (5,13,23,25,24), possibly dependent on the activation of enzymes capable of converting Hageman factor to an active form (2,3,16,60,61,71,114). Subsequent conversion of the Hageman factor substrates to their active enzymatic forms could then result in several biological activities capable of contributing to an inflammatory response either directly or by interaction with other systems (6,7,53,54,73).

3. COMPONENTS OF THE KININ SYSTEM IN WHITE BLOOD CELLS

Kinins may possibly be given another lease on life as prominent mediators of inflammation by the discovery of a certain type of

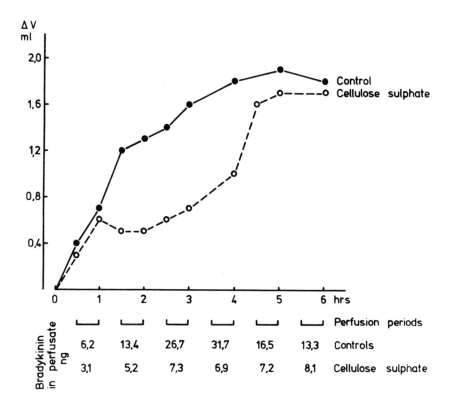

FIG. 5. Carrageenin edema development and bradykinin content in paw perfusate in untreated rats (controls) and in rats pretreated with cellulose sulfate (total dose 3 mg/kg, i.v., 3 hr before carrageenin). The perfusates were collected by means of paw coaxial perfusion during the indicated periods (10 ml of saline) and the total bradykinin content determined by bioassay on rat uterus

kinins formed by leukocytes, the so-called leukokinins. When whole-cell lysates—lysosomal and extralysosomal cell fractions from rabbit peritoneal polymorphonuclear leukocytes—were incubated at acid pH with partially purified human kininogen, a material contracting guinea-pig ileum was produced (43,46). This was confirmed using human lymphocytes (32), and rabbit alveolar and peritoneal macrophages (45). The active factor is destroyed by carboxypeptidase B and chymotrypsin (43,46). It is likely that different kinins are formed, depending on the source of enzymes, the substrates used and the conditions of incubation (32,45,46,70). The two peptides so far characterized do not contain the bradykinin sequence (15) and their relative potency in several bioassay systems differs from that of bradykinin (38) although they are able to increase vascular permeability (44). The experimental conditions for the formation of leukokinins, the concomitant presence of kininases in the same cell types and the poor characterization of substrates have so far made it difficult to understand their possible in vivo role in the inflammatory process. However, their participation in the latter cannot be excluded and, at least, they may well enhance the contribution of leukocytes to inflammation.

4. METHODS OF ASSAY

Several functional assays for the various components of the kinin system have been described. Hageman factor has been measured by its ability to activate prekallikrein or hydrolyze N-a-acetylglycine lysine methyl ether (58,108); kallikrein—by reasing bradykinin from kininogen or cleaving certain synthetic esters, such as the methyl-ester of benzoyl-l-arginine = BAME (20,111,117); kininogen—by serving as a substrate for kinin-generating enzymes (22, 76); bradykinin—by a variety of bioassays based on its pharmacological properties, in particular those of contracting the guineapig ileum or estrous rat uterus, or lowering blood pressure in isolated limb preparations (106).

Because of the ease with which the various components can be activated, the presence of inhibitors of the enzyme component and of kininases, the functional assays suffer certain limitations. However, non-specific antibodies have been developed which make it possible to measure several components of the kinin system. Preparations of antibodies against human Hageman factor (17,77), kininogen (99-101), and bradykinin (102) have been described. Antibody against kininogen has been utilized for radioimmunodiffusion assay (116) and that against bradykinin for radioimmunoassay (42,81,116).

REFERENCES

1. Antonio, A.: Br. J. Pharmacol. *32*:78, 1968.
2. Armstrong, D., Jepson, J. B., Keele, C. A., and Stewart, J. W.: J. Physiol. *135*:350, 1957.

3. Armstrong, D., Keele, C. A., Jepson, J. B., and Stewart, J. W.: Nature *174*:721, 1954.

4. Arrigoni-Martelli, E.: J. Pharm. Pharmacol. *19*:617, 1967.

5. Arrigoni-Martelli, E., Corsico, N., and Fogagnolo, E.: In "Inflammation Biochemistry and Drug Interaction," A. Bertelli and J. C. Houck, eds. Excerpta Medica, Amsterdam, 1969, p. 185.

6. Becker, E. L., Mota, I., and Wong, D.: Br. J. Pharmacol. *34*:330, 1968.

7. Blombäck, B., Blombäck, M., Edman, P., and Hessel, B.: Biochim. Biophys. Acta *115*:371, 1966.

8. Biossonas, R. A., Gutmann, S., and Jaquenod, P. A.: Helv. Chim. Acta *43*:1349, 1960.

9. Biossonas, R. A., Gutmann, S., Jaquenod, P. A., and Pless, J.: Ann. N. Y. Acad. Sci. *104*:5, 1963.

10. Bokisch, V. A., and Müller-Eberhard, H. J.: J. Clin. Invest. *49*:2427, 1970.

11. Bonta, I. L., and De Vos, C. J.: Experientia *21*:34, 1965.

12. Bonta, I. L., and De Vos, C. J.: Eur. J. Pharmacol. *1*:222, 1967.

13. Briseid, K., Arntzen, F., and Dyrud, O. K.: Acta Pharmacol. Toxicol. (Kbh.) *29*:265, 1971.

14. Camargo, A. C. M., Ramalho-Pinto, F. J., and Greene, L. J.: J. Neurochem. *19*:37, 1972.

15. Chang, J., Freer, R., Stella, R., and Greenbaum, L. M.: Biochem. Pharmacol. *21*:3095, 1972.

16. Cochrane, C. G., Revak, S. D., Aiken, B. S., and Wuepper, K. P.: In "Inflammation: Mechanism and Control," I. H. Lepow and P. A. Ward, eds. Academic Press, New York, 1972, p. 119.

17. Cochrane, C. G., and Wuepper, K. P.: J. Exp. Med. *134*:986, 1971.

18. Collier, H. O. J.: Actual. Pharmacol. (Paris) *14*:51, 1961.

19. Colman, R. W., Mattler, L., and Sherry, S.: J. Clin. Invest. *48*:11, 1969.

20. "Proceedings of the Conference on Structure and Functions of Biologically Active Peptides, Bradykinin, Kallidin and Congeners." Ann. N. Y. Acad. Sci. *104*:1, 1963.

21. Cormia, F. E., and Daugherty, J. W.: J. Invest. Dermatol. *35*:21, 1960.

22. Diniz, C. R., and Carvahlo, I. F.: Ann. N. Y. Acad. Sci. *104*:77, 1963.

23. Di Rosa, M., Giroud, J. P., and Willoughby, D. A.: J. Pathol. *104*:15, 1971.

24. Di Rosa, M., and Sorrentino, L.: Eur. J. Pharmacol. *4*:340, 1968.

25. Di Rosa, M., and Sorrentino, L.: Br. J. Pharmacol. *38*:214, 1970.

26. Eisen, V.: In "Scientific Basis of Medicine, Annual Review" Athlone Press, London, 1969, p. 146.

27. Elliot, D. F., Horton, E. W., and Lewis, G. P.: J. Physiol. (Lond.) *153*: 473, 1960.

28. Elliot, D. F., Horton, E. W., and Lewis, G. P.: Biochem, J. *78*:60, 1961.

29. Elliot, D. F., Lewis, G. P., and Horton, E. W.: Biochem. J. *74*:15p, 1960.

30. Emele, J. F., and Shanaman, J.: Proc. Soc. Exp. Biol. Med. *114*:680, 1963.

31. Engel, S. L., Schaeffer, T. R., Gold, B. L., and Rubin, B.: Proc. Soc. Exp. Biol. Med. *140*:240, 1972.

32. Engelmann, E. G., and Greenbaum, L. M.: Biochem. Pharmacol. *20*:922, 1971.

33. Erdös, E. G., Back, N., and Sicuteri, F. (Eds.) : "Hypotensive Peptides." Springer-Verlag, Berlin, 1966.

34. Erdös, E. G., and Sloane, E. M.: Biochem. Pharmacol. *11*:585, 1962.

35. Erdös, E. G., and Yang, H. Y. T.: In "Handbook of Experimental Pharmacology," Vol. 25, E. G. Erdös, ed. Springer-Verlag, Berlin, 1970, p. 289.
36. Faires, J. S., and McCarty, D. J.: Lancet 2: 682, 1962.
37. Ferreira, S. H., and Vane, J. R.: Br. J. Pharmacol. *29*:367, 1967.
38. Freer, R., Chang, J., and Greenbaum, L. M.: Biochem. Pharmacol. *21*: 3107, 1972.
39. Frey, E. K., Kraut, H., and Werle, E.: "Das Kallikrein—Kinin system und seine Inhibitoren." Enke-Verlag, Stuttgart, 1968.
40. Frimmer, M.: Arch. Exp. Pathol. Pharmakol. *242*:390, 1961.
41. Gilfoil, T. M., and Klavins, I.: Am. J. Physiol. *208*:867, 1965.
42. Goodfriend, L., and Ball, D. B.: J. Lab. Clin. Med. *73*:501, 1969.
43. Greenbaum, L. M.: Am. J. Path. *68*:613, 1972.
44. Greenbaum, L. M., Freer, R., Chang, J., Semente, G., and Yamafuji, K.: Br. J. Pharmacol. *36*:623, 1969.
45. Greenbaum, L. M., and Kim, K. S.: Br. J. Pharmacol. Chemother. *29*: 238, 1967.
46. Greenbaum, L. M., and Yamafuji, K.: In "Hypotensive Peptides," E. G. Erdös, N. Back, and F. Sicuteri, eds. Springer-Verlag, Berlin, 1966, p. 252.
47. Guzman, F., Braun, C., and Lim, R. K. S.: Arch. Int. Pharmacodyn. Ther. *136*:353, 1962.
48. Guzman, F., Braun, C., Lim, R. K. S., Potter, G. D., and Rodgers, D. W.: Arch. Int. Pharmacodyn. Ther. *149*:571, 1964.
49. Habermann, E., and Blennemann, G.: Arch. Exp. Pathol. Pharmakol. *249*:357, 1964.
50. Hamberg, U., Bumpus, F. F., and Page, I. H.: Biochim. Biophys. Acta *52*:533, 1961.
51. Jacobsen, S., and Kriz, M.: Br. J. Pharmacol. *29*:25, 1967.
52. Johnson, A. R., Cochrane, C. G., and Revak, S. D.: J. Immunol. *113*:103, 1974.
53. Johnson, A. R., and Erdös, E. G.: Proc. Soc. Exp. Biol. Med. *142*:1252, 1973.
54. Johnson, A. R., Hugli, T. E., and Müller-Eberhard, H. J.: Immunology *28*:1057, 1975.
55. Kaller, H., Hoffmeister, F., and Kroneberg, G.: Arch. Int. Pharmacodyn. Ther. *161*:389, 1966.
56. Kaplan, A. P., and Austen, K. F.: J. Immunol. *105*:802, 1970.
57. Kaplan, A. P., and Austen, K. F.: J. Exp. Med. *133*:696, 1971.
58. Kaplan, A. P., and Austen, K. F.: J. Exp. Med. *136*:1378, 1972.
59. Kaplan, A. P., Kay, A. B., and Austen, K. F.: J. Exp. Med. *135*:81, 1972.
60. Kaplan, A. P., Spragg, J., and Austen, K. F.: In "Second International Symposium on the Biochemistry of the Acute Allergic Reactions," K. F. Austen and E. L. Becker, eds. Blackwell, Oxford, 1971, p. 279.
61. Kellermeyer, R. W., and Breckenridge, R. T.: J. Lab. Clin. Med. *65*:307, 1965.
62. Kellermeyer, R. W., and Breckenridge, R. T.: J. Lab. Clin. Med. *67*:455, 1966.
63. Komiya, M., Kata, H., and Suzuki, T.: Biochem. Biophys. Res. Commun. *49*:1438, 1972.
64. Konzett, H., and Stürmer, E.: Nature *188*:998, 1960.
65. Lim, R. K. S., Guzman, F., Rodgers, D. W., Gotto, K., Braun, C., Dicker-

son, G. D., and Engle, R. J.: Arch. Int. Pharmacodyn. Ther. *152*:25, 1964.
66. Lim, R. K. S., Liu, C. N., Guzman, F., and Braun, C.: J. Comp. Neurol. *118*:269, 1962.
67. Lim, R. K. S., Miller, D. G., Guzman, F., Rodgers, D. W., Rodgers, R. W., Wang, S. K., Chao, P. Y., and Shih, T. Y.: Clin. Pharmacol. Ther. *8*:521, 1967.
68. Mac Kay, M. W., Miles, A. A., Schachter, M., and Wilhelm, D. L.: Nature *172*:714, 1953.
69. Melmon, K. L., and Cline, M. J.: Nature *213*:90, 1967.
70. Melmon, K. L., and Cline, M. J.: Biochem. Pharmacol. *17* (Suppl.): 271, 1968.
71. Melmon, K. L., Webster, M. E., Goldfinger, S. E., and Seegmiller, J. E.: Arthritis Rheum. *10*:13, 1967.
72. Moskowitz, R. W., Schwartz, H. J., Michel, B., and Ratnoff, A. R.: J. Lab. Clin. Med. *76*:790, 1970.
73. Northover, B. J., and Subramanian, G.: Br. J. Pharmacol. *17*:107, 1961.
74. Osbahr, A. J., Gladner, J. A., and Laki, K.: Biochem. Biophys. Acta *86*: 535, 1964.
75. Pierce, J. V.: Fed. Proc. *27*:52, 1968.
76. Pierce, J. V., and Webster, M. E.: Biochem. Biophys. Res. Commun. *5*: 353, 1961.
77. Pierce, J. V., and Webster, M. E.: In "Hypotensive Peptides," E. G. Erdös, N. Back, and F. Sicuteri, eds. Springer-Verlag, Berlin, 1966, p. 130.
78. Ratnoff, O. D.: J. Lab. Clin. Med. *80*:704, 1972.
79. Ratnoff, O. D., Davie, E. W., and Mallett, D. L.: J. Clin. Invest. *40*:803, 1961.
80. Ratnoff, O. D., and Miles, A. A.: Br. J. Exp. Path. *45*:328, 1964.
81. Revak, S. D., Cochrane, C. G., and Johnstone, A. R.: Fed. Proc. *32*:845 (Abstr.) 1973.
82. Rinderknecht, H., Haverback, B. J., and Aladiem, F.: Nature *213*:1130, 1967.
83. Rocha e Silva, M.: Ann. N. Y. Acad. Sci. *116*:899, 1964.
84. Rocha e Silva, M.: "Kinin Hormones," Charles C. Thomas, Springfield, Ill., 1970.
85. Rocha e Silva, M., and Antonio, H.: Med. Exp. *3*:371, 1960.
86. Rocha e Silva, M., Beraldo, W. T., and Rosenfeld, G.: Am. J. Physiol. *156*:261, 1949.
87. Rocha e Silva, M., Cavalcanti, R. R., and Reis, M. L.: Biochem. Pharmacol. *18*:1285, 1969.
88. Rocha e Silva, M., Garcia Leme, J., and De Sonza, J. M.: In "Inflammation Biochemistry and Drug Interaction," A. Bertelli and J. C. Houck, eds. Excerpta Medica, Amsterdam, 1969, p. 170.
89. Rowley, D. A.: Br. J. Exp. Pathol. *45*:56, 1964.
90. Ryan, J. W., Roblero, G., and Stewart, J. M.: Biochem. J. *110*:795, 1968.
91. Schachter, M. (Ed.): "Polypeptides which Affect Smooth Muscle and Blood Vessel," Pergamon Press, Oxford, 1960.
92. Schachter, M.: In "Proceedings of the 1st International Pharmacology Meeting," Vol. 9. Pergamon Press, Oxford, 1963, p. 87.
93. Schreiber, A. D., Kaplan, A. P., and Austen, K. F.: J. Clin. Invest. *52*: 1402, 1973.

94. Seegmiller, J. E., Howell, R. R., and Malawitta, S. E.: J. Am. Med. Assoc. *180*:469, 1962.
95. Shorley, P. G., and Collier, H. O. J.: Nature *188*:999, 1960.
96. Sicuteri, F., Fanciullacci, M., Franchi, G., and Del Brianco, P. L.: Life Sci. *4*:309, 1965.
97. Sicuteri, F., Rocha e Silva, M., and Back N. (Eds.): "Bradykinin and Related Kinins: Cardiovascular, Biochemical and Neural Actions." Plenum Press, New York—London, 1970.
98. Sokoloff, L.: Metabolism *6*:230, 1957.
99. Spector, W. G.: In "Injury, Inflammation and Immunity," L. Thomas, J. W. Uhr, and L. M. Grant, eds. Williams and Wilkins, Baltimore, 1964, p. 178.
100. Spragg, J., and Austen, K. F.: J. Immunol. *107*:1512, 1971.
101. Spragg, J., and Austen, K. F.: Biochem. Pharmacol. *23*:781, 1974.
102. Spragg, J., Haber, E., and Austen, K. F.: J. Immunol. *104*:1348, 1970.
103. Spragg, J., Talamo, R. C., and Austen, K. F.: In "Handbook of Experimental Pharmacology," Vol. 25 E. G. Erdös, ed. Springer-Verlag, Berlin, 1970, p. 372.
104. Starr, M. S., and West, G. B.: Br. J. Pharmacol. *31*:178, 1967.
105. Stewart, P. B., and Bliss, J. R.: Br. J. Exp. Path. *38*:462, 1957.
106. Stürmer, E., and Cerletti, A.: Am. Heart J. *62*:149, 1961.
107. Trautschold, L.: In "Handbook of Experimental Pharmacology," Vol. 25, E. G. Erdös, ed. Springer-Verlag, Berlin, 1970, p. 52.
108. Treloar, M. P., and Movat, H. Z.: Fed. Proc. *29*:576 (Abstr.) 1970.
109. Ulevitch, R. J., and Letchford, D. J.: Fed Proc. *32*:845 (Abstr.) 1973.
110. Van Arman, C. G., Begany, A. J., Miller, L. M., and Pless, H. H.: J. Pharmacol. Exp. Ther. *150*:328, 1965.
111. Vogt, W., Garbe, G., and Schmidt, G.: Arch. Exp. Pathol. Pharmakol. *256*:127, 1967.
112. Webster, M. E., and Pierce, J. V.: Ann. N. Y. Acad. Sci. *104*:91, 1963.
113. Werle, E., and Vogel, R.: Arch Int. Pharmacodyn. Ther. *131*:257, 1961.
114. Wilhelm, D. L.: Pharmacol. Rev. *14*:251, 1962.
115. Wilner, G. D., Nossel, H. L., and Le Roy, E. C.: J. Clin. Invest. *47*:2608, 1968.
116. Witte, S., Schricker, T., and Schmid, E.: Arzneim. Forsch. *11*:619, 1961.
117. Wintroub, B. U., Spragg, J., Stechschulte, R. J., and Austen, K. F.: "Control Mechanisms in Reagin Mediated Hypersensitivity," L. Goodfriend, A. Sehon, and R. P. Orange, eds. Marcel Dekker, New York, 1973, p. 495.
118. Wuepper, K. D., and Cochrane, C. G.: In "2nd International Symposium on the Biochemistry of the Acute Allergic Reaction," K. F. Austen and E. L. Becker, eds. Blackwell, Oxford, 1971, p. 299.
119. Wuepper, K. D., and Cochrane, C. G.: J. Exp. Med. *135*:1, 1972.
120. Wuepper, K. D., Tucker, E., and Cochrane, C. G.: J. Immunol. *105*:1307, 1970.

Chapter 5

Prostaglandins

Since it was first observed that human semen induces rhythmic contractions of human myometrium (36,62,103), and the active principle responsible for this effect was shown to consist of hydroxy fatty acids (7,8,36,103), we have learned a great deal about prostaglandins. However, despite intensive studies, their physiological role is not yet clear. They appear to be almost ubiquitous and are found in many tissues, each of which has the capacity for synthetizing prostaglandins from essential fatty acids. It, therefore, seems unlikely that these agents are part of a classical endocrine-target organ system. They may, however, serve as local regulators of cell functions. In fact, prostaglandins possess a broad spectrum of pharmacological activities (104) which in some cases appear to involve changes in cAMP concentrations (48). Even mild stimulation of cells and tissues results in increased biosynthesis of prostaglandins (82). This has impeded investigation on the role of prostaglandins in physiologically normal organisms since even a minor

8,11,14 Eicosatrienoic Acid

(dihomo -γ- linolenic acid)

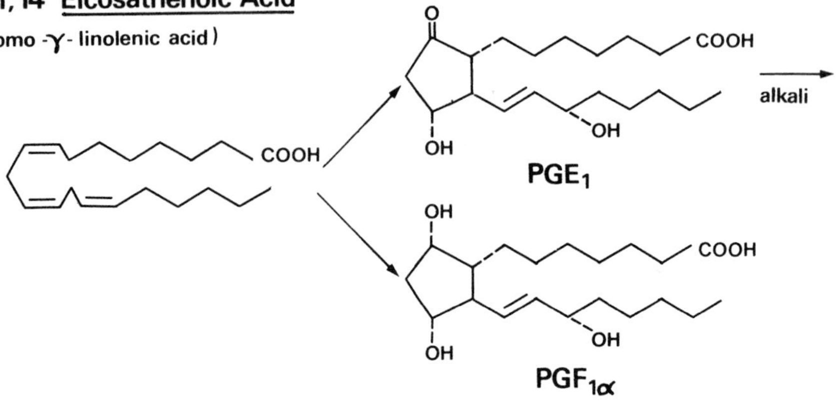

PGE$_1$

PGF$_{1\alpha}$

alkali

5,8,11,14 Eicosatetraenoic Acid

(Arachidonic Acid)

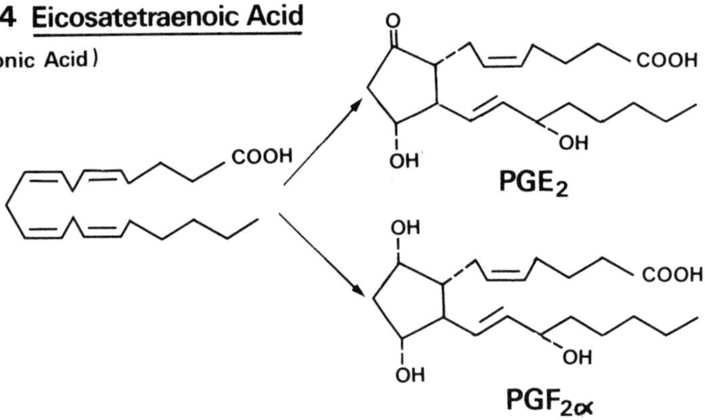

PGE$_2$

PGF$_{2\alpha}$

5,8,11,14,17 Eicosapentaenoic Acid

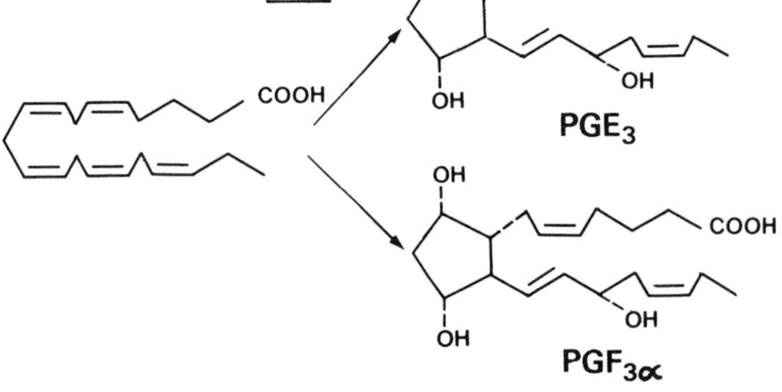

PGE$_3$

PGF$_{3\alpha}$

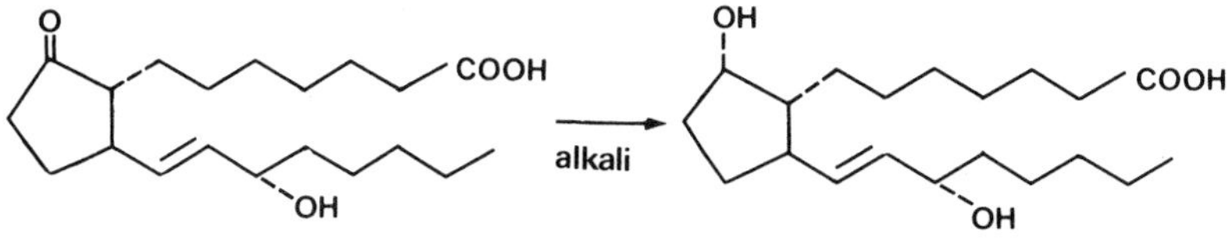

FIG. 6. Prostaglandins and their precursors

manipulation is sufficient to induce their synthesis—which would not occur under resting conditions. It has been suggested that one stimulus of prostaglandin synthesis is inflammation, in the course of which phospholipids of the cell membrane are cleaved to yield the precursor, arachidonic acid (1) (Fig. 6).

1. PROSTAGLANDINS AS "MEDIATORS" OF INFLAMMATION

Intradermal injections of PGE_1 and PGE_2 into normal human (19,56,59,92,95) and animal skin (18,19,50,57) increase vascular permeability. The potency of prostaglandins of the E class is several times higher than that of histamine and bradykinin. A wheal and flare response in human skin is also induced by $PGF_{1\alpha}$ and $PGF_{2\alpha}$ (19,95). PGE_1 injections elicit inflammatory edema in rat paw in a dose-dependent manner (32), and repeated injections of PGE_2 cause persistent swelling of the paw (109). Disabling arthritis has been observed in dogs injected into knee joints with PGE_1 and PGE_2 (86). Additive effects, rather than synergism, were also demonstrated between E-type prostaglandins and histamine, bradykinin or carrageenin in the paw edema induced in rats (32, 71). These results have been confirmed in guinea pigs; it was also observed that PGA_1 and $PGF_{2\alpha}$ are devoid of such an additive effect (106) (Table 5).

$PGE_{1\alpha}$ and $PGE_{2\alpha}$ injected either intradermally or applied to blister base (51) have been reported not to elicit pain in humans. According to more recent investigations (28), PGE_1 is supposed to produce long-lasting pain when injected intradermally whereas his-

TABLE 5. Effect of prostaglandins on vascular permeability in rats

Compounds	Relative Potency
PGE_1	100
PGE_2	100
PGA_1	20
PGF_{1a}	10
PGF_{2a}	10
Bradykinin	40
Histamine	30

tamine, bradykinin and acetylcholine evoke only transitory pain. Moreover, PGE_1 (but not PGE_2) induces writhing when injected intraperitoneally in mice (16). Prostaglandins are thermogenic in man (29), cats, rabbits and rats (27,70).

In respect to their role in inflammation, prostaglandins (mainly PGE_2) were first identified in carrageenin edema fluid and in carrageenin air bleb fluid (107,108). The presence of prostaglandins was then confirmed in various inflammatory exudates (17,22,23,24, 31,35,72,101,110) where they occur in the more advanced phases of the inflammatory reaction (17,22,23,24,35), following the appearance of histamine and bradykinin. Similar observations have been made in lymph collected from scalded dog paws (5), suggesting a role for PGE_2 in the pathophysiology of the human burn syndrome. Prostaglandins have also been found in relatively high concentrations in joint fluid from rabbits with ovalbumin-induced arthritis (9,10) and in inflamed eyes of rabbits with immunogenic uveitis (25) (Fig. 7).

Prostaglandins are released from guinea-pig isolated lung by a variety of stimuli. In addition to anaphylaxis, (65,67,77,78), these include injection into the pulmonary artery of bradykinin, SRS-A, arachidonic acid, and histamine (75,77,78,79,100). The mechanism of prostaglandin release from guinea-pig lung during anaphylaxis is not clear; presumably stimulation of adenyl cyclase is the underlying process. It has been suggested that prostaglandins may play a role in bronchial asthma (52,66,79) ; $PFG_{2\alpha}$ is a bronchoconstrictor while PGE compounds are bronchodilators (94). PGE_1 and PGE_2 increase the forced expiratory volume only in asthmatic patients (21). Prostaglandins of both E and F type are released from human lungs passively sensitized with reaginic antibody when exposed to appropriate antigen (80).

PGE_1, PGE_2, $PGF_1\alpha$, and $PGF_2\alpha$ have been identified in the inflamed skin of patients with allergic contact dermatitis (38) and in areas of delayed cutaneous inflammation caused by ultraviolet irradiation (37).

Explants of synovium obtained at surgery from patients with rheumatoid arthritis and maintained in culture produce larger amounts of prostaglandins than synovium from patients with osteoarthritis (85). In agreement with these observations, prostaglandins, mainly of the E type, have been found in higher concentrations in the joint fluid from patients with rheumatoid arthritis than in that from patients with degenerative joint disease (45,84).

PGE_1 has been shown to be chemotactic for rabbit polymorphonuclear leukocytes (58,68). This was confirmed and it has been demonstrated that the chemotactic activity of PGE_1 is at least 100 times higher than that of $PGF_2\alpha$ and PGE_2 (44). Other investigators, however, claimed that PGE_2 is also endowed with potent chemotactic activity (69). These results suggest that the released prostaglandins might help perpetuate the inflammatory reaction by calling forth additional leukocytes.

There is evidence that prostaglandins, at variance with other mediators, are not stored within any subcellular compartment but are formed on physiological demand (4,49), probably to act closely to the site of synthesis (3). They are then inactivated by the ubiquitous prostaglandin dehydrogenases (3). Most processes which disturb membrane function or alter its structure activate the hydrolysis of arachidonic acid from phospholipids (34), the rate-limiting step in prostaglandin biosynthesis (87). Phospholipase A, which is able to cleave arachidonic acid, seems, therefore, to play a central role in prostaglandin formation (6,61,102). In an inflamed area, polymorphonuclears lysosomes, mast cells and platelets are possible sources of phospholipase A (26,89). It has been observed that the release of lysosomal enzymes in an inflamed area parallels prostaglandin appearance in the exudate (1), that phagocytosing polymorphonuclear leukocytes produce up to ten times as much prostaglandins as do resting cells (44,46), and that inflammatory exudates rich in leukocytes are also rich in prostaglandins (1,101, 110). The role of polymorphonuclear leukocytes as a source of prostaglandins has been recently disputed (31) since they appear in at least one type of inflammatory exudate after both PGE_2 and $PGF_2\alpha$, and two symptoms of inflammation, nociception and temperature

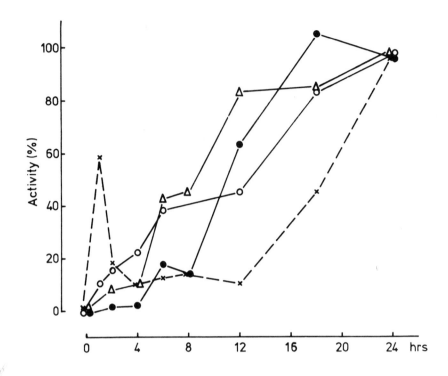

FIG. 7. β-glucuronidase O——O, acid phosphatase ●——●, prostaglandins △——△, histamine *——* in carrageenin exudate in rats

rise have been observed at the site of inflammation before the immigration of polymorphonuclear leukocytes and of monocytes (31). It has, therefore, been proposed that platelets may be a more likely source of prostaglandins in acute inflammation (31), since they appear early in the joint fluid (31), are known to release PGE_2 and $PFG_{2\alpha}$ (90), and were also present in all the experiments relating prostaglandin synthesis to polymorphonuclear leukocytes (1,46, 101).

2. PROSTAGLANDINS AS "MODULATORS" OF INFLAMMATION

Although there is strong experimental evidence that prostaglandins (mainly PGE_1 and PGE_2) are local mediators of inflammation, effects on mediator release, which suggest an antiphlogistic or a modulator action, have also been described.

PGE$_1$ and PGE$_2$ elicited acute antidematous effects (33) and also reduced the local levels of β-glucuronidase in carrageenin air blebs in rats (113), inhibited chemotaxis (83), produced immuno-suppressant-like reaction in a variety of systems (41,81), reduced the discharge of histamine and SRS-A from basophils and lung fragments (64,73), and prevented lymphocyte-mediated cytoxicity (41). In many cases, the mechanisms by which prostaglandins elicit these reactions are thought to involve the cyclic nucleotides. PGE$_1$, PGE$_2$ and PGE$_{2}\alpha$ have been reported to stimulate adenylate cyclase activity, to elevate cAMP levels in human leukocytes (11, 12,88) and to inhibit lysosomal enzyme discharge (105,114). There is evidence for a biphasic action of PGE$_1$ on enzyme release; thus low levels of PGE$_1$ which decrease cAMP enhance histamine release from challenged human lungs, while high levels of prostaglandin produce opposite effects (97). A similar biphasic action has been described for PGF$_2\alpha$ which accelerated enzyme discharge and increased cGMP levels at a high concentrations whereas when these were low, it inhibited enzyme release and raised cAMP levels (53). The above findings suggest a modulatory function for prostaglandins, possibly through an involvement of cyclic nucleotides in the inflammatory process (Fig. 8).

It is not clear whether this mechanism might explain the suppression of adjuvant-induced arthritis observed by many authors (2,33,112,113,115) with large doses—up to 1 mg/kg per day—of PGE$_1$ and PGE$_2$. Prostaglandins of the E type cause a reduction of circulating lymphocytes (113), prevent phytohemoagglutinin-induced transformation of lymphocytes (91), reduce the humoral antibody response (115), and inhibit lymphocyte-mediated destruction of allogeneic cells (41). It is, therefore, possible to speculate that these effects may be involved in the inhibition of tissue injury mediated by a delayed hypersensitivity reaction, such as adjuvant disease.

Whether they act as mediators or modulators, or both, the prostaglandins appear to play a complex central role in inflammation. These agents may provide a balance in the inflammatory reaction in that they appear capable of both mediating and suppressing the inflammatory response. The possibility of feedback regulation has been discussed. Alternatively or additionally, prostaglandins may also serve to restrain the inflammatory response through an equilibrium in local concentration of E and F compounds. Thus, for instance, PGE$_2$ enhances platelet aggregation

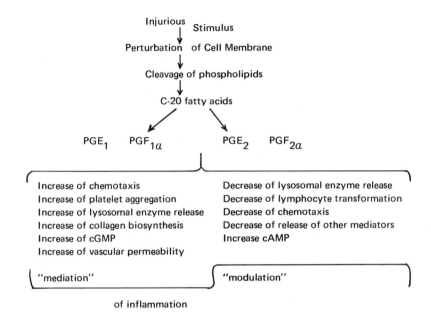

FIG. 8. Prostaglandins in the inflammatory response

while PGE_1 inhibits it (60), and it is known that, in the presence of complement, immune complexes induce release of vasoactive amines and lysosomal enzymes from platelets (42,43). Moreover, $PGF_{2\alpha}$ inhibits the increase in vascular permeability elicited in skin by PGE_1 and PGE_2 (20). The formation of both compounds follows a common pathway until the final stage of biosynthesis, and there is no evidence for interconversion between E and F prostaglandins. Local control of inflammation may, therefore, result also from a preferential biosynthesis of one or another of the prostaglandins (111).

3. METHODS OF ASSAY

In addition to bioassays (98), a variety of techniques have been employed for quantitative determinations of prostaglandins. These include: spectrophotometry (30,96), gas-liquid chromatography-mass spectrometry (39,40) and immunochemistry (14,63).

In recent years, radioimmunoassays have been developed and have gained wide acceptance. Most of them have been aimed at prostaglandins of the F type (15,47,54,74,76,99), but several assays have also been developed for prostaglandins of the E, A and B type (55, 93,116,117). To produce antisera, prostaglandins have been rendered antigenic by coupling the carboxyl group to a protein molecule or a polypeptide. A high degree of specificity is commonly exhibited towards structures in the cyclopentane ring and the C-12 side chain. In contrast, antibodies often cannot distinguish between compounds of the PG_1 and PG_2 type because of the vicinity of the 5,6 position to the site of coupling. It is also difficult to obtain antisera specifically directed against prostaglandin of the E, A, and B type, and a chromatographic separation has been included in the processing of the sample.

REFERENCES

1. Anderson, A. J., Brocklehurst, W. E., and Willis, A. L.: Pharmacol. Res. Commun. *3*:13, 1971.
2. Aspinall, R. L., and Cammarata, P. S.: Nature *224*:1320, 1969.
3. Anggard, E.: Ann. N. Y. Acad. Sci. *180*:200, 1971.
4. Anggard, E., Bohman, S. D., Griffin, J. E., Larsson, C., and Maunsbach, A. B.: Acta Physiol. Scand. *84*:231, 1972.
5. Anggard, E., and Jonsson, C. E.: In "Prostaglandins in Cellular Biology," P. W. Ramwell and B. B. Pharris, eds. Plenum Publishing Corp., New York, 1972, p. 269.
6. Bartles, J., Kunze, H., Vogt, W., and Wille, G.: Arch. Exp. Pathol. Pharmakol. *266*:199, 1970.
7. Bergström, S., and Sjövall, J.: Acta Chem. Scand. *11*:1086, 1957.
8. Bergström, S., and Sjövall, J.: Acta Chem. Scand. *14*:1701, 1960.
9. Blackham, A., Farmer, J. B., Radziwonik, H., and Westwick, J.: Br. J. Pharmacol. *48*:343P, 1973.
10. Blackham, A., Farmer, J. B., Radziwonik, H., and Westwick, J.: Br. J. Pharmacol. *51*:35, 1974.
11. Bourne, H. R., Lehrer, R. I., Cline, M. J., and Melmon, K. L.: J. Clin. Invest. *50*:920, 1971.
12. Bourne, H. R., and Melmon, K. L.: J. Pharmacol. Exp. Ther. *178*:1, 1971.
13. Brune, K., and Glatt, M.: Agents Actions *4*:95, 1974.
14. Burke, G.: Prostaglandins *2*:413, 1972.
15. Cladwell, B. V., Speroff, L., Brock, W. A., Auletta, F. J., Gordon, J. W., Andersen, G. G., and Hobbins, J. C.: J. Reprod. Med. *9*:361, 1972.
16. Collier, H. O. J., and Schneider, C.: Nature (New Biol.) *236*:141, 1972.
17. Crunkhorn, P., and Meacock, S. C. R.: Br. J. Pharmacol. *42*:392, 1971.
18. Crunkhorn, P., and Willis, A. L.: Br. J. Pharmacol. *36*:216P, 1969.
19. Crunkhorn, P., and Willis, A. L.: Br. J. Pharmacol. *41*:49, 1971.
20. Crunkhorn, P., and Willis, A. L.: Br. J. Pharmacol. *41*:507, 1971.

21. Cuthbert, M. F.: Br. Med. J. *4*:723, 1969.
22. Di Rosa, M., Giroud, J. P., and Willoughby, D. A.: J. Pathol. *104*:15, 1971.
23. Di Rosa, M., and Willoughby, D. A.: Arch. Exp. Pathol. Pharmakol. *269*: 482, 1971.
24. Di Rosa, M., and Sorrentino, L.: Br. J. Pharmacol. *38*:214, 1970.
25. Eakins, K. E., Whitelocke, R. A. F., Perkins, E. S., Bennett, A., and Ungar, W. G.: Nature (New Biol.) *239*:248, 1972.
26. Elsbach, P., and Kizack, A. M.: Am. J. Physiol. *205*:1154, 1963.
27. Feldberg, W., and Saxena, P. N.: J. Physiol. (Lond.) *217*:547, 1971.
28. Ferreira, S.: Nature (New Biol.) *240*:200, 1972.
29. Filshie, G.: Ann. N. Y. Acad. Sci. *180*:553, 1971.
30. Flower, R. J., Cheung, H. S., and Cushman, D. W.: Prostaglandins *4*: 325, 1973.
31. Glatt, M., Peskar, B., and Brune, K.: Experientia *30*:1257, 1974.
32. Glenn, E. M., Bowman, B. J., and Rohloff, N. A.: In "Prostaglandins in Cellular Biology," P. W. Ramwell and B. B. Phariss, eds. Plenum Publishing Corp. New York, 1972, p. 329.
33. Glenn, E. M., and Rohloff, N. A.: Proc. Soc. Exp. Biol. Med. *139*:290, 1972.
34. Gilmore, N., Vane, J. R., and Wyllie, J. H.: In "Prostaglandins, Peptides and Amines," P. Mantegazza and E. W. Horton, eds. Academic Press, New York—London, 1969, p. 21.
35. Giroud, J. P., and Willoughby, D. A.: J. Pathol. *101*:241, 1970.
36. Goldblatt, M. W.: J. Soc. Chem. Industr. *52*:1056, 1933.
37. Greaves, M. W., and Søndergard, J. S.: J. Invest Dermatol. *54*:365, 1970.
38. Greaves, M. W., and Søndergard, J. S.: Br. Med. J. *2*:258, 1971.
39. Hamberg, M.: Biochem. Biophys. Res. Commun. *49*:720, 1972.
40. Hamberg, M., and Samuelsson, B.: J. Biol. Chem. *247*:3195, 1972.
41. Henney, C. S., Bourne, H. R., and Lichtenstein, L. M.: J. Immunol. *108*: 1526, 1972.
42. Henson, P. M.: J. Immunol. *105*:476, 1970.
43. Henson, P. M.: J. Immunol. *105*:490, 1970.
44. Higgs, G. A., McCall, E., and Youlten, L. J. F.: Br. J. Pharmacol. *53*: 539, 1975.
45. Higgs, G. A., Vane, J. R., Hart, F. D., and Wojtulewski, J. A.: In "Prostaglandin Synthetase Inhibitors," H. J. Robinson and J. R. Vane, eds. Raven Press, New York, 1974, p. 165.
46. Higgs, G. A., and Youlten, L. J. F.: Br. J. Pharmacol. *44*:330P, 1972.
47. Hillier, K., and Dilley, S. R.: Prostaglandins *5*:137, 1974.
48. Hinman, J. W.: Ann. Rev. Biochem. *41*:161, 1972.
49. Hopkin, J. M., Horton, E. W., and Whittaker, V. P.: Nature *217*:71, 1968.
50. Horton, E. W.: Nature *200*:892, 1963.
51. Horton, E. W.: Experientia *21*: 113, 1965.
52. Horton, E. W.: Physiol. Rev. *49*:122, 1969.
53. Ignarro, L. J.: Agents Actions *4*:241, 1974.
54. Jubiz, W., Frailey, J., and Bartholomew, K.: Clin. Res. *20*:178, 1972.
55. Jubiz, W., Frailey, J., Child, C., and Bartholomew, K.: Prostaglandins *2*: 471, 1972.
56. Juhlin, L., and Michaelsson, G.: Acta Derm. Venereol. (Stockh.) *49*:251, 1969.
57. Kaley, G., and Weiner, R.: In "Prostaglandin Symposium of the Wor-

cester Foundation for Experimental Biology," P. W. Ramwell and J. E. Shaw, eds. Interscience, New York, 1968, p. 321.
58. Kaley, G., and Weiner, R.: Nature (New Biol.) *234*:114, 1971.
59. Kaley, G., and Weiner, R.: Ann. N. Y. Acad. Sci. *180*:338, 1971.
60. Kloeze, J.: In "Prostaglandins," S. Bergström and B. Samuelsson, eds. Almqvist and Wiksell, Stockholm, 1967, p. 241.
61. Kunze, H., and Vogt, W.: Ann. N. Y. Acad. Sci. *180*:123, 1971.
62. Kurzrock, R., and Lieb, C. C.: Proc. Soc. Exp. Biol. Med. *28*:268, 1930.
63. Levine, L.: Biochem. Biophys. Res. Commun. *47*:888, 1972.
64. Lichtenstein, L. M., and De Bernardo, R.: J. Immunol. *107*:1131, 1971.
65. Liebig, R., Bernauer, W., and Peskar, B. A.: Arch. Pharmacol. *284*:279, 1974.
66. Mathé, A. A., Hedqvist, P., Holmgren, A., and Svanborg, N.: Br. Med. J. *1*:193, 1973.
67. Mathé, A. A., and Levine, L.: Prostaglandins *4*:877, 1973.
68. McCall, E., and Youlten, L. J. F.: J. Physiol. (Lond.) *234*:98P, 1973.
69. McClatchey, W., and Snydermann, R.: Clin. Res. *22*:423A, 1974.
70. Milton, A. S., and Wendlandt, S.: J. Physiol. (Lond.) *207*:76P, 1970.
71. Moncada, S., Ferreira, S. H., and Vane, J. R.: Nature *246*:217, 1973.
72. Moncada, S., Ferreira, S. H., and Vane, J. R.: In "Prostaglandin Synthetase Inhibitors," H. J. Robinson and J. R. Vane, eds. Raven Press, New York, 1974, p. 189.
73. Orange, R. P., Austen, W. G., and Austen, K. F.: J. Exp. Med. *134*:136S, 1971.
74. Orzyk, C. P., and Behrman, H.: Prostaglandins *1*:3, 1972.
75. Palmer, M. A., Piper, P. J., and Vane, J. R.: Br. J. Pharmacol. *49*:226, 1973.
76. Patrono, C. J.: J. Nucl. Biol. Med. *17*:25, 1973.
77. Piper, P. J., and Vane, J. R.: In "Prostaglandins, Peptides and Amines," P. Mantegazza and E. W. Horton, eds. Academic Press, New York, 1969, p. 15.
78. Piper, P. J., and Vane, J. R.: Nature *223*:29, 1969.
79. Piper, P. J., and Vane, J. R.: Ann. N. Y. Acad. Sci. *180*:363, 1971.
80. Piper, P. J., and Walker, J. L.: Br. J. Pharmacol. *47*:291, 1973.
81. Quagliata, J. F., Lawrence, V. J. W., and Phillips-Quagliata, J. M.: Cell. Immunol. *6*:457, 1973.
82. Ramwell, P. W., and Shaw, J.: Recent Prog. Horm. Res. *26*:37, 1970.
83. Rivkin, I., and Becker, E. L.: Fed. Proc. *31*:657, 1972.
84. Robinson, D. R., and Levine, R.: J. Clin. Invest. *53*:65a, 1974.
85. Robinson, D. R., Smith, H., and Levine, L.: Arthritis Rheum. *16*:129, 1973.
86. Rosenthale, M. E., Dervinis, A., Kassarich, J., and Singer, S.: J. Pharm. Pharmacol. *24*:89, 1972.
87. Samuelsson, B.: In "Proceedings of the 4th International Congress of Pharmacology" *4*:12, 1970.
88. Scott, R. E.: Blood *35*:514, 1970.
89. Smith, A. D., and Winkler, H.: Biochem. J. *108*:867, 1968.
90. Smith, J. B., Ingermann, G., Kocsis, J. J., and Silver, M. J.: J. Clin. Invest. *52*:965, 1973.
91. Smith, J. W., Steiner, A. L., and Parker, C. W.: J. Clin. Invest. *50*:442, 1971.

92. Solomon, L. M., Juhlin, L., and Kirschenbaum, M. B.: J. Invest. Dermatol. *51*:280, 1968.
93. Stylos, W., and Rivetz, B.: Prostaglandins *2*:103, 1972.
94. Sweatman, W. J. F., and Collier, H. O. J.: Nature *217*:69, 1968.
95. Søndergard, J., and Greaves, M. W.: Br. J. Dermatol. *84*:424, 1971.
96. Takeguchi, G., and Sih, C. J.: Prostaglandins *2*:169, 1972.
97. Tauber, A. L., Kaliner, M., Stechschulte, D. J., and Austen, K. F.: J. Immunol. *111*:27, 1973.
98. Vane, J. R.: Nature (New Biol.) *231*:232, 1971.
99. Van Orden, D. E., and Farley, D. B.: Prostaglandins *4*:215, 1973.
100. Vargaftig, B. B., and Dao Hai, N.: Eur. J. Pharmacol. *18*:43, 1972.
101. Velo, G. P., Dunn, C. J., Giroud, J. P., Timsit, J., and Willoughby, D. A.: J. Pathol. *111*:149, 1973.
102. Vogt, W., Meyer, U., Kunze, H., Luft, E., and Babilli, S.: Arch. Exp. Pathol. Pharmakol. *262*:124, 1969.
103. Von Euler, U. S.: J. Physiol. (Lond.) *88*:213, 1936.
104. Weeks, J. R.: Ann. Rev. Pharmacol. *12*:317, 1972.
105. Weissmann, G., Zurier, R. B., Spieler, P. J., and Goldstein, I. M.: J. Exp. Med. *134*:149S, 1971.
107. Willis, A. L.: In "Prostaglandins, Peptides and Amines," P. Mantegazza and E. W. Horton, eds. Academic Press, New York—London, 1969, p. 31.
108. Willis, A. L.: J. Pharm. Pharmacol. *21*:126, 1969.
109. Willis, A. L., and Cornelson, M.: Prostaglandins *3*:353, 1973.
110. Willoughby, D. A., Dunn, G. J., Yamamoto, S., Capasso, F., Deporter, D. A., and Giroud, J. P.: Agents Actions *5*:35, 1975.
111. Zurier, R. B.: Arch. Intern. Med. *133*:101, 1974.
112. Zurier, R. B., and Ballas, A. M.: Arthritis Rheum. *16*:251, 1973.
113. Zurier, R. B., Hoffstein, S., and Weissmann, G.: Arthritis Rheum. *16*: 606, 1973.
114. Zurier, R. B., Hoffstein, S., and Weissmann, G.: J. Exp. Med. *58*:27, 1973.
115. Zurier, R. B., and Quagliata, F.: Nature *234*:304, 1971.
116. Zusman, R., Caldwell, B., and Speroff, L.: Prostaglandins *2*:41, 1972.
117. Yu, S., and Burke, G.: Prostaglandins *2*:11, 1972.

Chapter 6

Complement
and Properdin

The term *complement* has been originally used to indicate a heat-labile substance present in serum and necessary for killing certain bacteria. Today, it designates a group of serum proteins which interact sequentially to effect a variety of inflammatory events, including bacterial lysis. The availability of highly advanced separative techniques has permitted the isolation and partial identification of most of the constituents of the complement (37). The availability of purified components has, in turn, made it possible to elucidate their interaction mechanisms and their multiple biological activities (49).

The term *properdin* was initially used to denote the activity of all the factors subsequently described as necessary in order for zymosan to destroy the third component of complement in whole serum. It is now employed to indicate a single protein which is central to this reaction (43).

Products formed during complement and properdin reactions

attract polymorphonuclear and mononuclear leukocytes, enhance phagocytosis, mediate increase of vascular permeability, damage cell membranes, and influence the release of lysosomal enzymes.

1. NOMENCLATURE AND GENERAL FEATURES

The symbol for the components of complement is a capital C, followed by a number identifying each discrete protein: C1, C2, C3, C4, etc. A bar over the number denotes the activated state of the component in the fluid phase: $\overline{C1}$, $\overline{C42}$, etc. The molecular subunits of C1 are indicated as C1q, C1r, C1s, whereas the cleavage fragments of the various components are suffixed with a,b,c,d,e,g. (2, 4,30).

Almost all the components of the complement system are glycoproteins (44) with a molecular weight between 100.000-200.000 and β-motility on electrophoresis. Their concentrations in serum range from a few micrograms to a milligram per milliliter. In addition to the similarities just mentioned, there appear to be definite homologies in the structure of certain of the components, accounting for the difficulty with which these proteins are separated from one another. Nevertheless, almost all the components have been isolated and characterized. The molecular subunits of C1, which is a multimolecular complex, have been obtained and identified (60,70). C3 was the first component to be purified (36) and its relatively easy availability accounts for the fact that it is frequently measured in clinical medicine. C6 and C7 are the last two components to have been successfully purified (1). Greater difficulties have been encountered in the separation of the other constituents although C2 and C4 have been purified to homogeneity, and antibodies against them have been prepared (45,46) (Table 6).

Properdin has also been purified: it appears to consist of four subunits of 45.000 molecular weight (34) as well as of two control proteins, the C1 inhibitor (44) and the C3b inactivator (26,50).

Complement activation results in a series of specific and limited proteolytic reactions which catalyze the cleavage of certain of the complement proteins, and cause the development of active enzymes from the latter's precursors and the formation of protein-protein complexes between two or more cleavage products (1). The first step is the binding and activation of C1 by the different subclasses of IgG and by IgM. The activated subcomponent $\overline{C1s}$ splits C4, its natural substrate, into two fragments, the larger of which becomes bound to the cell membrane to form C14 (6) or remains free but

TABLE 6. Properties of human complement system

Component	Molecular Weight	Electrophoretic Mobility	Serum Concentration μg/ml
C1g	400'000	$\gamma\,2$	180
C1r	180'000	β	
C1s	90'000	a	120
C2	117'000	$\beta\,1$	25
C3	180'000	$\beta\,2$	1600
C4	240000	$\beta\,1$	640
C5	185000	$\beta\,1$	80
C6	95000	$\beta\,2$	75
C7	120000	$\beta\,2$	60
C8	150000	$\gamma\,1$	80
C9	79000	a	230

inactive in the fluid phase (38). C1 also cleaves C2 and the major cleavage product forms complex $C\overline{42}$ with C4b (39) which, in turn, is capable of splitting C3. In the cleavage of the latter, the properdin system certainly plays an important role which includes an activation pathway and an amplification loop (18,34,56). The cleavage of C3 is a limited proteolytic reaction typical of the complement system. A small peptide C3a, is released and the major fragment C3b binds to the cell surface or remains in the fluid phase as inactive product C3i. C3b modifies the substrate specificity of $C\overline{42}$, rendering it capable of cleaving C5b from C5; C5b, in turn, interacts with C6 to form $C\overline{56}$ (17,59). Reaction of cell-bound $C\overline{56}$ with C7 leads to the formation of $C\overline{567}$ which is capable of binding directly to the surface of cells that have not reacted with antibody or the earlier complement components. Cells bearing $C\overline{567}$ interact with C8 and then with C9 (24), completing the formation of the membrane-damaging complex C5-C9.

2. COMPLEMENT AND INFLAMMATION

More than 70 years ago, the term *anaphylatoxin* was introduced to indicate a substance formed in homologous serum when exposed to immune complex and able to induce anaphylactic shock upon injection into guinea pig (14). Later on, it was demonstrated

TABLE 7. Properties of human anaphylatoxins

Properties	C3a	C5a
Electrophoretic mobility pH 8.5 (x 10^{-5}cm^{2}V^{-1}sec^{-1})	+2.1	$\div$1.7
Molecular weight	8900	16500
Biological activities:		
Minimal effective concentration in vitro: guinea pig ileum	1.3 x 10^{-8}M	7.5 x 10^{-10}M
Minimal effective dose in vivo: Wheal and erythema	2.1 x 10^{-12}mol	1 x 10^{-15}mol

that anaphylatoxins are formed from complement components (28, 41) and that their effects depend on their ability to release histamine (19,35). Today, it is accepted that the cleavage products, peptide C3a and C5a—the minor fragments of C3 and C5—are both anaphylatoxins (Table 7).

Any of a number of proteolytic enzymes, including C$\overline{42}$, trypsin and plasmin can split C3a from the parent molecule (4). C3a has a molecular weight of 8900, with a C-terminal arginine and an N-terminal serine (8). It is active in concentrations of 10^{-8}M on the guinea-pig ileum and 2×10^{-12}M when injected into human skin, where it causes local edema and mast cell degranulation (31).

C5a may be split from C5 by C$\overline{423}$ or by trypsin (9). Its molecular weight is approximately 16.000, and like C3a its activity depends on C-terminal arginine. Although it has properties similar to those of C3a, C5a has a different biological specificity: it is not possible to achieve cross-desensitization with the two anaphylatoxins on the guinea-pig ileum (9). Human anaphylatoxins do not desensitize the guinea-pig ileum toward guinea-pig anaphylatoxins (9), whereas they do share common properties with those of rat and pig (9,57).

Although both C3a and C5a are readily produced by digestion of purified C3 and C5, their formation and activity are difficult to demonstrate in whole human serum because of the presence of an anaphylotoxin inactivator. This appears to be the same protein as kininase I, an α-globulin with a molecular weight of 325.000, which cleaves the carboxy-terminal arginine from bradykinin, and from C3a and C5a (5).

The complement components exert several effects which are relevant in the inflammatory reaction, either directly or through an

TABLE 8. Biological effects of complement components

Effects	Components
Anaphylatoxin, chemotactic	C3a
Immune adherence, phagocytosis, reaction with lymphoid cells	C3b
Anaphylatoxin, chemotactic	C5a
Reaction with unsensitized cells, chemotactic	C5̄6̄7̄
Increase of vascular permeability	Cleavage product of C2
Membrane damage	C5-C9
Inhibition of Hageman factor fragments	C1INH
Anaphylatoxin inactivator, Kininase	Control protein (a-globulin)

interplay with other factors (Table 8). Three different *chemotactic factors* have been identified among the complement components. The first described was C$\overline{567}$ (40,64,65). Although nascent C$\overline{567}$ has the capacity to attach to cell membranes, rendering them susceptible to lysis by C8 and C9 (17), this characteristic rapidly disappears, leaving the chemotactic C567 complex (25). Both cleavage peptides, C3a and C5a, were found to have chemotactic properties, the latter being more active in most systems (4,52,61,67). Although the polymorphonuclear neutrophil leukocytes were the first cell type found to respond to chemotactic factors derived from complement, it was subsequently demonstrated that eosinophils (23) and mononuclears (55) respond in similar fashion. Activation of an identical intracellular serine esterase appears to be the initial step in the chemotactic response common to all these complement-derived chemotactic factors (62). A lysosomal enzyme obtained from rabbit polymorphonuclear leukocytes is capable of cleaving, at neutral pH, human C5 (but not C3) into chemotactically active fragments (66). A similar enzyme has been described in human polymorphonuclear leukocytes (58) which is able to split both C3 and C5 into large and small fragments. More recently, a proteinase, with an acid pH optimum, has been isolated from macrophages; it is capable of cleaving C5 into fragments chemotactic for polymorphs and mononuclears (54).

Immune complexes to which complement has become bound adhere to formed elements in the blood and in the reticuloendothelial system. This phenomenon, termed *immune adherence* occurs with erythrocytes, platelets, leukocytes and B lymphocytes in most species.

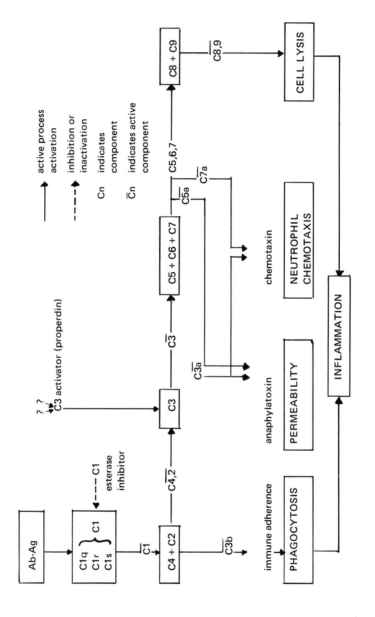

FIG. 9. Role of complement components in inflammation

60

The adherence of immune complexes to the cells is one of the more common stimuli triggering the release of intracellular mediators. This aspect has been discussed in Chapter 1.

The hallmark of complement action is cell *membrane damage*. The relevance of such a phenomenon for the development and maintenance of an inflammatory process is obvious. It has been shown that, in addition to cell membranes, complement is able to damage artificial bilayer structures, such as those of liposomes (20,27). This observation and certain direct additional findings (10,53) suggest an action of one or more terminal components of the complement system on the lipid constituents of the membranes (32).

Evidence for the release, during activation of the complement system, of a peptide with permeability-enhancing properties, the so-called *"C-kinin"* is largely indirect (3,29) and the hypothesis that C-kinin is a cleavage product of some components of the complement system still awaits definitive proof.

It should also be mentioned that the control proteins of the complement system, namely C1 inhibitor (C$\overline{1}$INH) and C3b inactivator (C3bINA) block, respectively, the biological effects of components of the kinin and complement systems. Thus C$\overline{1}$INH inhibits the action of Hageman factor fragments on their proenzyme substrates (51), the esterase activity of kallikrein (22), and its action on kininogen (15,33); on the other hand, CbINA blocks all the known biological effects of C3b.

A number of findings indirectly suggest the participation of complement in nonimmunologically mediated inflammatory reactions (11,16,68,69), including carrageenin edema (7,12,63). Of more direct interest is, however, the fact that complement levels in the synovial fluid of rheumatoid patients are lower than those in osteoarthritic and gouty patients (13,21,42). These observations are consistent with more recent data (47,48) suggesting an activation of the complement system by intraarticular immunological processes (Fig. 9).

REFERENCES

1. Arroyave, C. M., and Müller-Eberhard, H. J.: J. Immunol. *111*:302, 1973.
2. Austen, K. F., Becker, E. L., and Borsos, T.: Bull. WHO *39*:935, 1968.
3. Austen, K. F., and Sheffer, A. L.: N. Engl. J. Med. *272*:649, 1965.
4. Bokisch, V. A., Müller-Eberhard, H. J., and Cochrane, C. G.: J. Exp. Med. *129*:1109, 1969.
5. Bokisch, V. A., and Müller-Eberhard, H. J.: J. Clin. Invest. *49*:2427, 1970.
6. Borsos, T., Rapp, H. J., and Mayer, M. M.: J. Immunol. *87*:310, 1961.

7. Brocklehurst, W. E.: Proc. R. Soc. Med. *64*:4, 1971.
8. Budzko, D. B., Bokisch, V. A., and Müller-Eberhard, H. J.: Biochemistry *10*:1166, 1971.
9. Cochrane, C. G., and Müller-Eberhard, H. J.: J. Exp. Med. *127*:371, 1968.
10. De Lage, J. M., Lehner-Netsch, G., and Simard, J.: Immunology *29*:671, 1973.
11. Di Rosa, M., Giroud, J. P., and Willoughby, D. A.: J. Pathol. *104*:15, 1971.
12. Di Rosa, M., and Sorrentino, L.: Br. J. Pharmacol. *38*:214, 1971.
13. Fostiropoulos, G., Austen, K. F., and Block, K. J.: Arthritis Rheum. *8*:219, 1965.
14. Friederberger, E.: Z. Immunitätsforsch. *4*:636, 1910.
15. Gigli, I., Mason, J. W., Colman, R. W., and Austen, K. F.: J. Immunol. *104*:574, 1970.
16. Giroud, J. P., and Willoughby, D. A.: J. Pathol. *101*:241, 1970.
17. Goldman, J. N., Ruddy, S., and Austen, K. F.: J. Immunol. *109*:353, 1972.
18. Götze, O., and Müller-Eberhard, H. J.: J. Immunol. *111*:288, 1973.
19. Hahn, F., and Oberdorf, A.: Z. Immunitätsforsch. *107*:528, 1950.
20. Haxby, J. A., Götze, O., and Müller-Eberhard, H. J.: Proc. Natl. Acad. Sci. USA *64*:290, 1969.
21. Hedberg, H.: Acta Rheum. Scand. *9*:165, 1963.
22. Kagan, L. J.: Br. J. Exp. Pathol. *45*:604, 1964.
23. Kay, A. B.: Clin. Exp. Immunol. *7*:723, 1970.
24. Kolb, W. P., Haxby, J. A., Arroyave, C. M., and Müller-Eberhard, H. J.: J. Exp. Med. *135*:549, 1972.
25. Lachmann, P. J., Kay, A. B., and Thompson, R. A.: Immunology *19*:895, 1970.
26. Lachmann, P. J., and Müller-Eberhard, H. J.: J. Immunol. *100*:691, 1968.
27. Lachmann, P. J., Munn, E. A., and Weissmann, G.: Immunology *19*:37, 1970.
28. Lepow, I. H.: J. Allergy *28*:52, 1957.
29. Lepow, I. H.: In "Biochemistry of the Acute Allergic Reaction," K. F. Austen and E. L. Becker, eds. Blackwell, London, 1971, p. 205.
30. Lepow, I. H., Naff, G. B., Todd, E. W., Pensky, I., and Hinz, C. F.: J. Exp. Med. *117*:983, 1963.
31. Lepow, I. H., Wilms-Kretschemer, K., Patrick, R. A., and Rosen, F. S.: Am. J. Pathol. *61*:13, 1970.
32. Mayer, M. M.:Proc. Natl. Acad. Sci. USA *69*:2954, 1972.
33. McConnell, D. J.: J. Clin. Invest. *51*:1611, 1972.
34. Minta, J. O., and Lepow, I. H.: J. Immunol. *111*:286, 1973.
35. Mota, I.: Immunology *2*:403, 1959.
36. Müller-Eberhard, H. J.: Acta Soc. Med. Upsala. *66*:152, 1961.
37. Müller-Eberhard, H. J.: Adv. Immunol. *8*:1, 1968.
38. Müller-Eberhard, H. J., and Biro, C. E.: J. Exp. Med. *118*:447, 1963.
39. Müller-Eberhard, H. J., Polley, M. J., and Calcott, M. A.: J. Exp. Med. *125*:359, 1967.
40. Nilsson, U. R., and Müller-Eberhard, H. J.: J. Exp. Med. *122*:277, 1965.
41. Osler, A. G., Randall, H. G., Hill, B. M., and Ovary, Z.: J. Exp. Med. *110*:311, 1959.
42. Pekin, T. J., and Zvaifler, N. J.: J. Clin. Invest. *43*:1372, 1964.
43. Pensky, J., Hinz, E. F. Jr., Todd, E. W., Wedgwood, R. J., Boyer, J. R.,

and Lepow, I. H.: J. Immunol. *100*:142, 1968.
44. Pensky, J., and Schwick, H. G.: Science *163*:698, 1969.
45. Polley, M. J., and Müller-Eberhard, H. J.: J. Exp. Med. *128*:533, 1969.
46. Rosenfeld, S. I., Ruddy, S., and Austen, K. F.: J. Clin. Invest. *48*:2283, 1969.
47. Ruddy, S., and Austen, K. F.: Arthritis Rheum. *13*:713, 1970.
48. Ruddy, S., and Colten, H. R.: N. Engl. J. Med. *290*:1284, 1974.
49. Ruddy, S., Gigli, I., and Austen, K. F.: N. Engl. J. Med. *287*:489, 545, 592, 642, 1972.
50. Ruddy, S., Hunsicker, L. G., and Austen, K. F.: J. Immunol. *108*:657, 1972.
51. Schreiber, A. D., Kaplan, A. P., and Austen, K. F.: J. Clin. Invest. *52*:1394, 1973.
52. Shin, H. D., Snyderman, R., Friedman, E., Mellors, A., and Mayer, M. M.: Science *162*:361, 1968.
53. Smith, J. K., and Becker, E. L.: J. Immunol. *100*:459, 1968.
54. Snyderman, R., Shin, H. S., and Dannenberg, A. M., Jr.: J. Immunol. *109*: 896, 1972.
55. Snyderman, R., Shin, H. S., and Hausman, M. H.: Proc. Soc. Exp. Biol. Med. *138*:387, 1971.
56. Spitzer, R. E., and Stitzel, A. E.: J. Immunol. *111*:212, 1973.
57. Stegemann, H., Hillebrecht, R., and Rien, W.: Hoppe Seyler's. Z. Physiol. Chem. *340*:11, 1965.
58. Taubman, S. B., Goldschmidt, P. R., and Lepow, I. H.: Fed. Proc. *29*:434, 1970.
59. Thompson, R. A., and Lachmann, P. J.: J. Exp. Med. *131*:629, 1970.
60. Valet, G., and Cooper, N. R.: J. Immunol. *111*:292, 1973.
61. Ward, P. A.: J. Exp. Med. *126*:189, 1967.
62. Ward, P. A., and Becker, E. L.: J. Exp. Med. *127*:693, 1968.
63. Ward, P. A., and Cochrane, C. G.: J. Exp. Med. *121*:215, 1965.
64. Ward, P. A., Cochrane, C. G., and Müller-Eberhard, H. J.: J. Exp. Med. *122*:327, 1965.
65. Ward, P. A., Cochrane, C. G., and Müller-Eberhard, H. J.: Immunology *11*:141, 1966.
66. Ward, P. A., and Hill, H. L.: J. Immunol. *104*:535, 1970.
67. Ward, P. A., and Zvailer, N. J.: Clin. Res. *16*:325, 1968.
68. Willoughby, D. A., Coote, E., and Turk, J. L.: J. Pathol. *97*:295, 1969.
69. Willoughby, D. A., and Giroud, J. P.: J. Pathol. *98*:53, 1969.
70. Yonemasu, K., and Stroud, R. M.: J. Immunol. *106*:304, 1971.

Chapter 7

Slow-Reacting
Substances

The term *slow-reacting-substance* (SRS) was first applied to the active lipids produced from lung tissues and egg yolk by cobra venom (13). Anaphylactic shock of guinea-pig lung was then shown to release material with the same activity (24). In addition, the perfusion of cat paw with compound 48/80 resulted in the yield of a similar agent (9,40). These three substances have a common activity, i.e., they induce a prolonged contraction of the guinea pig ileum (55) and of a few other smooth-muscle preparations, with the exclusion of those sensitive to prostaglandins, serotonin and bradykinin (29).

The material generated by cobra venom—and designated SRS-C—was found to include oxidation products of unsaturated fatty acids, such as prostaglandin precursors, subsequently converted to prostaglandins by tissue synthetases (54).

The material produced from tissues by an anaphylactic reaction—termed slow-reacting substance of anaphylaxis, SRS-A—was first identified as being functionally distinct from histamine (6). Studies of its physicochemical properties clearly differentiate it from prostaglandins but also suggest at least a strict similarity with SRS (7,8,34). In addition, SRS-A was found to be resistant to proteolytic enzymes, such as trypsin, chymotrypsin, pepsin (7), peptidases, phospholipase A,B,C,D (1), pronase, neuramidase (34), and 15-hydroxyprostaglandin dehydrogenase (50).

Lipid-soluble, smooth-muscle-stimulating materials are also released from several tissues—the richest source being cat paw—perfused with compound 48/80 (1). The in vitro release of these materials, termed SRS, requires calcium ion for maximum yield (9,49), and is inhibited by anoxia, absence of glucose, and N-ethyl-maleimide (48). Investigations of its structure suggest that SRS is a carboxylic acid with hydroxyl groups and one or more double bonds (9,50).

1. PHARMACOLOGICAL ACTIVITY

The slow, prolonged contraction of the guinea-pig ileum in a standard bioassay resulted in the original discovery of SRS-A (24). Since that time, this bioassay was accepted as a suitable means for identifying and quantitating this substance (6,7,29,34). Other smooth-muscle preparations sensitive to SRS-A are: rabbit jejunum and duodenum, fowl rectal cecum and human bronchioles (7,12,29). The intensity of effect on guinea-pig bronchioles seems dependent on the SRS-A preparation (3,16).

The quantitation of SRS-A action on vascular permeability is not precise: it seems, however, that approximately 50 ng can induce an increase in vascular permeability in guinea pig and monkey while in rat it is substantially unaltered even by doses of 125 ng. (35). In the Konzett-Rössler preparation, anesthetized guinea pigs show a marked rise in lung resistance to inflation following intravenous administration of 40-160 ng of SRS-A (4). This observation has been recently confirmed with a different methodology (6). Only preliminary data exist on the effect of SRS-A on respiratory mechanics in man.

2. RELEASE MECHANISM AND ITS CONTROL

The general aspects of mediator release and its mechanism have been discussed in Chapter 1. Therefore, here only some aspects of this process will be examined which are of particular relevance to the subject under consideration. It has long been known that when a specific antigen is introduced into the skin of an appropriately sensitive individual, it will produce an immediate allergic reaction characterized by wheal and flare formation; this occurs in consequence of the interaction of antigen with immunoglobulin specifically bound to the cell-surface receptors of mast cells and basophils (18,25,51). The interaction initiates a series of biochemical responses within the cells, resulting in the secretion of several biologically active chemical mediators—including histamine, SRS-A and prostaglandins—responsible for the typical symptomatology. Functional (23), histological (18,51) and clinical (19,28) findings indicate that IgE is the immunoglobulin class essential for the acute allergic reaction. Immunoglobulins of IgG class also have a similar function in a number of experimental animals and, probably, in man (39,46). Evidence relating mast cells and basophils to the IgE-dependent immediate hypersensitivity reaction includes: the detection of IgE on the surface of these cells (18,51), the observation that most of the tissue and leukocyte histamine is stored within the granules of these cells (41), and the demonstration with phase-contrast microscopy of basophil degranulation in response to antigen challenge (15). Mast cells were implicated as a source of SRS-A because their removal from rat peritoneal cavity prevented release (36). Subsequently, SRS-A has been detected after antigen challenge in the supernatant of an IgE-sensitized basophil-rich fraction of human leukocytes (14) and in a cell suspension containing mast cells derived from monkey lung (16).

Guinea-pig lung tissue has been proved to be a reliable source of SRS-A (24). Biochemical investigations suggest that in this tissue the mast cell is the source of both histamine and SRS-A (5). Human lung tissue also has been identified as a source of SRS-A (6,38,45) as well as of other mediators (23,32). The finding that human lung cell suspensions rich in mast cells release both histamine and SRS-A, when challenged with mono-specific antisera against IgE (26), and similar observations with primate lung cells (17) clearly focus attention on the tissue mast cell. Certain investigations, however, suggest the possibility that polymorphonuclear leukocytes participate in the release of this substance (37).

The liberation of SRS-A after immunological activation of mast cells and basophils is recognized to be a secretory process (15,27). The biochemical prerequisites for the reaction include different phases: activation of the cells, SRS-A formation—it is not detectable in the tissue prior to the challenge in contrast to histamine which is stored in active form (6,10)—and release of the mediator. The biochemical requirements comprise an intact glycolytic pathway, the availability of calcium ions, and the activation of a serine esterase from its precursor state (31). The reaction sequence has been partially delineated as follows (20): union of antigen with two IgE antibodies upon the surface of the target cells; extracellular calcium-ion-dependent activation of a serine esterase from proesterase, inhibited by diisopropylfluorophosphate; autocatalytic feedback activation of the proesterase; energy-requiring stage, inhibited by 2-deoxyglucose; intracellular calcium-ion-dependent step, inhibited by ethylendiamine tetraacetate.

The release process of SRS-A, as well as that of other mediators, is modulated by intracellular cyclic nucleotides. This aspect will be discussed in detail in Chapter 9. It is, however, pertinent here to briefly mention some of the findings more directly relevant to the subject of this chapter. Forty years ago, it was observed that adrenaline suppressed the IgE-dependent wheal and flare reaction in human skin (53), and the immunologic release of histamine from guinea-pig lung (43). A number of recent investigations attribute this effect to the elevation of tissue cAMP: β-adrenergic agents (33), prostaglandins E_1 and F_{2a} (52), cholera toxin (57), methylxantines (32), and dibutyryl cyclic AMP (32) which are known to increase cAMP levels inhibit the immunologic release of chemical mediators. It should be noted, however, that the effects of cAMP are not limited to controlling the secretion of preformed mediators, like histamine, but extend to determining the quantity of SRS-A formed. Thus, it would appear that this nucleotide modulates specific immunologic activation of at least two sites; formation of SRS-A and release of SRS-A and histamine. Further data support the concept that a reciprocal relationship exists between the intracellular levels of cAMP and the ability of the cells to discharge mediators upon immunologic activation. They include the results of experiments where the reduction of cAMP levels, obtained by different means, was accompanied by greater mediator release (21,33,52).

Enhancement of guanylate cyclase activity, through cholinergic stimulation (47), produces a rise in cGMP levels and augments antigen-induced release of SRS-A and histamine (21,22); thus, an increase in cGMP has the opposite effect of one in cAMP.

Indirect evidence suggests that the endogenous production of one mediator could modulate the liberation of another. In fact, indomethacin, which blocks prostaglandin synthesis, completely inhibits the IgE-mediated release of prostaglandin from passively sensitized fragments of human lung: the release of SRS-A, however, is doubled (56). Interference with prostaglandin synthesis, therefore, seems to remove an inhibitory influence on SRS-A formation or release.

The pharmacological control of SRS-A release from human lung tissue has been extensively investigated. Diethylcarbamazine, initially observed to inhibit the discharge of SRS-A in rat peritoneal cavity (37), also prevents the liberation of histamine and SRS-A from human lung (30). Disodium chromoglycate blocks the IgE-mediated release of both histamine and SRS-A, by acting at a stage in the allergic pathway subsequent to antigen-antibody combination, but preceding mediator release (2,11,31). It has been suggested that disodium chromoglycate inhibits the discharge of cAMP phosphodiesterase from human lung more efficiently than does theophylline (42), therefore, increasing intracellular cAMP levels. The mechanism of its action requires further definition but certainly this compound appears to be unique in selectively suppressing the immunological pathways leading to the release of pharmacological mediators (11).

REFERENCES

1. Anggard, E., Bergqvist, U., Högberg, B., Johansson, K., Thon, I. L., and Uvnäs B.: Acta Physiol. Scand. *59*, 97, 1963.
2. Assem, E. S. K., and Mongar, J. L.: Int. Arch. Allergy Appl. Immunol. *38*:68, 1970.
3. Berry, P. A., and Collier, H. O. J.: Br. J. Pharmacol. *23*:201, 1964.
4. Berry, P. A., Collier, H. O. J., and Holgate, J. A.: J. Physiol. (Lond.) *165*: 41P, 1963.
5. Boreus, L. O., and Chakravarty, N.: Acta Physiol. Scand. *48*:315, 1960.
6. Brocklehurst, W. E.: J. Physiol. (Lond.) *151*:416, 1960.
7. Brocklehurst, W. E.: Prog. Allergy *6*:539, 1962.
8. Chakravarty, N.: Acta Physiol. Scand. *48*:167, 1960.
9. Chakravarty, N., Högberg, B., and Uvnäs, B.: Acta Physiol. Scand. *45*: 255, 1959.
10. Chakravarty, N., and Uvnäs, B.: Acta Physiol. Scand. *48*:302, 1959.
11. Cox, J. S. G.: Br. J. Dis. Chest *65*:189, 1971.
12. Drazen, J. M., and Austen, K. F.: J. Clin. Invest. *53*:1679, 1974.
13. Feldberg, W., and Kellaway, C. H.: J. Physiol. (Lond.) *94*:187, 1938.
14. Grant, J. A., and Lichtenstein, L. M.: J. Immunol. *112*:879, 1974.
15. Hastie, R. W.: Clin. Exp. Immunol. *8*:45, 1970.
16. Ishizaka, T., Ishizaka, K., Orange, R. P., and Austen, K. F.: J. Immunol. *104*:335, 1971.
17. Ishizaka, T., Ishizaka, K., and Tomioka, H.: J. Immunol. *108*:513, 1972.

18. Ishizaka, K., Tomioka, H., and Ishizaka, T.: J. Immunol. *105*:1459, 1970.
19. Johansson, S. G. O.: Lancet *2*:951, 1967.
20. Kaliner, M. A., and Austen, K. F.: J. Exp. Med. *138*:1077, 1973.
21. Kaliner, M. A., Orange, R. P., and Austen, K. F.: J. Exp. Med. *136*:556, 1972.
22. Kaliner, M. A., Wasserman, S. I., and Austen, K. F.: N. Engl. J. Med. *289*:277, 1973.
23. Kay, A. B., and Austen, K. F.: J. Immunol. *107*:899, 1971.
24. Kellaway, C. H., and Trethewie, E. R.: Q. J. Exp. Physiol. *30*:121, 1940.
25. Kulczycki, A., Isersky, C., and Metzger, H.: J. Exp. Med. *139*:600, 1974.
26. Lewis, R. A., Wasserman, S. I., Goetzl, E. J., and Austen, K. F.: Clin. Res. *22*:422A, 1974.
27. Lichtenstein, L. M., and Osler, A. G.: Proc. Soc. Exp. Biol. Med. *121*:808, 1966.
28. Norman, P. S., Lichtenstein, L. M., and Ishizaka, K.: J. Allergy Clin. Immunol. *52*:210, 1973.
29. Orange, R. P., and Austen, K. F.: Adv. Immunol. *10*:105, 1969.
30. Orange, R. P., and Austen, K. F.: In "Progress in Immunology." Academic Press, New York, 1971, p. 173.
31. Orange, R. P., and Austen, K. F.: In "The Biological Role of the Immunoglobulin E System," K. Ishizaka and D. H. Dayton, eds. US Government Printing Office, Washington, D. C., 1974, p. 151.
32. Orange, R. P., Austen, W. G., and Austen, K. F.: J. Exp. Med. *134*:136S, 1971.
33. Orange, R. P., Kaliner, M. A., La Raia, P. J., and Austen, K. F.: Fed. Proc. *30*:1725, 1971.
34. Orange, R. P., Murphy, R. C., Karnovsky, M. D., and Austen, K. F.: J. Immunol. *110*:760, 1973.
35. Orange, R. P., Stechschulte, D. J., and Austen, K. F.: Fed. Proc. *28*:1710, 1969.
36. Orange, R. P., Stechschulte, D. J., and Austen, K. F.: J. Immunol. *105*: 1087, 1970.
37. Orange, R. P., Valentine, M. D., and Austen, K. F.: J. Exp. Med. *127*:767, 1968.
38. Parish, W. E.: Nature *215*:738, 1967.
39. Parish, W. E.: In "Asthma: Physiology, Immunopharmacology and Treatment," K. F. Austen and L. M. Lichtenstein, eds. Academic Press, New York, 1973, p. 71.
40. Paton, W. D. M.: Br. J. Pharmacol. *6*:499, 1951.
41. Riley, J. F., and West, G. B.: J. Physiol. (Lond.) *120*:528, 1953.
42. Roy, A. C., and Warren, B. T.: Biochem. Pharmacol. *23*:917, 1974.
43. Schild, H. O.: Q. J. Exp. Physiol. *26*:165, 1936.
44. Sheard, P., and Blair, A. M.: Int. Arch. Allergy Appl. Immunol. *38*:217, 1970.
45. Sheard, P., Killingback, P. G., and Blair, A. M.: Nature *216*:283, 1967.
46. Stechschulte, D. J., Orange, R. P., and Austen, K. F.: In "Proceedings of the 7th International Congress of Allergology," Exerpta Medica, Amsterdam, 1970, p. 245.
47. Stoner, J., Manganiello, V. C., and Vaughan, M.: Proc. Nat. Acad. Sci. USA *70*:3830, 1973.

48. Strandberg, K.: Acta Physiol. Scand. *82*:47, 1971.
49. Strandberg, K.: Acta Physiol. Scand. *82*:509, 1971.
50. Strandberg, K., and Uvnäs, B.: Acta Physiol. Scand. *82*:358, 1971.
51. Sullivan, A. L., Grimley, P. M., and Metzger, H.: J. Exp. Med. *134*:1403, 1971.
52. Tauber, A. I., Kaliner, M., Stechschulte, D. J., and Austen, K. F.: J. Immunol. *111*:27, 1973.
53. Tuft, L., and Brodsby, M.: J. Allergy *7*:238, 1936.
54. Vogt, W.: J. Physiol. (Lond.) *136*:131, 1957.
55. Vogt, W.: In "Cellular and Humoral Mechanisms of Anaphylaxis and Allergy," H. Z. Movat, ed. Karger, New York, 1969, p. 197.
56. Walker, J. L.: Adv. Biosci. *9*:235, 1973.
57. Wasserman, S. I., Goetze, E. J., Kaliner, M. A., and Austen, K. F.: Immunology *26*:677, 1974.

Chapter 8

Lysosomal Inflammatory Materials

Originally described in rat liver (28), lysosomes constitute a probably heterogenous class (95,101) of subcellular organelles containing various hydrolytic enzymes, with predominantly acid pH optima, bound in latent form within a relatively impermeable membrane. The isolation and characterization of lysosomes from rabbit (23) and human (45) polymorphonuclear leukocytes opened an era of intensive research, leading to the elucidation of the origin, composition and function of these organelles (9,10,11,33,34,79,106) and the description of a series of their enzymes (10,12).

It is apparent that lysosomes of polymorphonuclear leukocytes contain hydrolytic enzymes capable of digesting a variety of intracellular and extracellular macromolecules. These enzymes, together with other nonenzymatic lysosomal and nonlysosomal substances, provide polymorphonuclear leukocytes with the machinery necessary to set in motion virtually all of the processes involved in the acute inflammatory response. Considerable experimental evidence

TABLE 9. Tasks performed by lysosomal enzymes

Degradation of collagen
Degradation of elastin
Break-down of cartilage proteoglycan
Break-down of arterial wall and basement membrane
Depolymerization of hyaluronate
Digestion of nucleic acids
Splitting of lipids
Cleavage of complex sugars
Inactivation of phosphate esters

has accumulated to support the concept that these cells and certain of their components play a critical role, in vivo, in producing inflammation and tissue injury (Table 9).

1. LYSOSOMES AS MEDIATORS OF TISSUE INJURY AND INFLAMMATION

The vasculitis of Arthus phenomenon was the first experimentally produced lesion found to depend on polymorphonuclear leukocytes. Specific removal of these cells inhibited this reaction in several species (22,29,47,87). Similarly, necrotizing arteritis of experimental serum sickness in rabbits (57) and proteinuria associated with acute nephrotoxic nephritis in rats and rabbits (21) could be prevented by depletion of polymorphonuclear leukocytes in these animals. More recent studies (43) have confirmed these findings.

Two major categories of studies implicating leukocyte lysosomes as mediators of tissue injury and inflammation were carried out. In the first, the activities of lysosomal enzymes were measured at the site of inflammation and, in the second, lysosomal lysates were tested for their capacity to produce tissue damage.

Increased activity of lysosomal enzymes has been reported in human rheumatoid synovial fluid and synovial membrane (14,42, 56,62,66,86). Morphological evidence of lysosomal enzymes has been found in synovial specimens from patients with variety of pathological conditions, including gouty and rheumatoid arthritis (13,43,84, 105).

In the exudates obtained from different models of experimental inflammations or at the site of different types of tissue injury, augmented activity of lysosomal enzymes has been demonstrated as well (1,2,3,5,24,90).

Intradermal injection of polymorphonuclear leukocyte granules, followed by intravenous injection of endotoxin into normal rabbits, results in hemorragic necrosis resembling the localized Schwartzman reaction (15). Lysosomal lysates from homologous polymorphonuclear leukocytes produce acute inflammatory changes when injected into the joint of rabbits; moreover, repeated intra-articular injections cause hypertrophy and hyperplasia of synovial lining cells, round cell infiltration, pannus formation, and cartilage degradation (98,99). Glomerular injury, proteinuria, and ultra-structural changes in the glomerular basement membrane were produced by lysosomal lysates (67). In vitro, the same material has been found to cause cellular detachment and digestion of rabbit corneal endothelial cells (8). Human polymorphonuclear leukocytes exposed to rabbit lysosomes undergo a series of changes culminating in cell death (46).

In addition, certain indirect evidence supports the concept that the release of lysosomal enzymes plays a primary role in the development of inflammatory reactions. This evidence includes the fact that many lysosomal labilizing agents, like polyene antibiotics (5,6,37,97), streptolysin S (96), digitonin (4,37) urate crystals (75) and calcium pyrophosphate crystals (75,104), can trigger an inflammatory response when injected subcutaneously or intra-articularly.

2. ACID AND NEUTRAL PROTEASES

The acid proteases, obtained from rabbit polymorphonuclear leukocyte granules, were among the first lysosomal enzymes to be isolated and considered as important mediators of inflammation. The above enzymes were also found to have properties similar to those of cathepsin D and E (20,23,59,94). It has been recently demonstrated (30) that cathepsin D plays a major role in the intracellular digestion of certain proteins in viable cells. Immunoinhibition of this enzyme has been successfully attempted in rabbit alveolar macrophages (30). Both cathepsins are capable of disintegrating glomerular basement membrane in vitro at acid pH; in animal experiments, however, they failed to produce vascular injury (20). This was undoubtedly due to the fact that the in vivo pH was unfavorable for their activities. In fact, the pathophysiological pH in acute tissue injury is between 6.5 and 7.5. Measurements of the sequential changes in pH in sterile inflammatory exudates in rabbits indicate a lowest value of 7.04 (31), far above the range in which the acid cathepsins can function.

A simple question arising here is: how could enzymes with optimum catalytic activity at pH 3-5 and little or none above pH 6 contribute significantly to the degradation of a variety of connective tissue macromolecules—a characteristic feature of tissue injury resulting from acute and chronic inflammation? The key finding of relevance here is that proteolytic activities at neutral or alkaline pH are indeed present in extracts of polymorphonuclear leukocytes (48,53,54,60,74,88). An enzyme isolated from human granulocytes digests hemoglobin at neutral pH. When injected into normal rabbits, it induces lesions similar to those caused by the Arthus reaction (54). An elastase-like esterase with optimum pH between 6.5-8.0 was localized in the lysosome granule fraction of human granulocytes (53,60). In vivo, it produces changes in canine aortas—alterations in staining properties of the elastica and fragmentation of the internal elastica lamina—resembling those observed in in vitro experiments with frozen sections of human kidney and strips of renal artery (49). A similar enzyme preparation releases protein from rabbit articular cartilage (51) and from insoluble connective tissue fractions of human lung (52), and digests vascular basement membrane (54). This elastase-like enzyme is inhibited by a factor present in the cytosol fraction (51), by a_1-antitrypsin (50,64), and, to a lesser extent, by a_2-macroglobulin (50). A specific collagenase, active at neutral or alkaline pH, and found in granule fraction of human polymorphonuclear leukocytes (60), is able to cleave the native collagen molecule into two fragments and produce extensive lysis of fibrils (60,61). The noncollagenous proteoglycan matrix of hyaline cartilage is degraded at neutral pH by an enzymatic activity present in the lysosomes of human polymorphonuclear leuqocytes (48) (Table 10).

Despite earlier reports to the contrary (20,23), a neutral protease from lysosomes of rabbit polymorphonuclear leukocytes has been isolated and characterized (26,27). This enzyme has relatively little effect upon hemoglobin but does act on calf thymus histone and hydrolyzes proteoglycans (27).

It has also been suggested recently that this histonase-like enzyme could resemble trypsin in augmenting the template activity of the nuclei, exposing sites otherwise unavailable for transcription by RNA polymerase (100). It will be important to determine

TABLE 10. Lysosomal enzymes of human polymorphonuclear leukocyte

Acid phosphatase
α-Amylase
Dextranase
α-Glucosidase
β-Glucosidase
β-Galactosidase
α-Mannosidase
β-Glucuronidase
Cathepsins (acid protease)
Neutral protease(s)
Elastase
Collagenase
Aryl sulphatase
β-N-Acetylglucosaminidase
Aminodipeptidase
Lysozyme

whether, in pathological states, material extruded from leukocyte lysosomes can gain free access to the cytoplasm and/or the nucleus of, as yet, uninvolved cells.

Macrophages also have been proved able to secrete neutral collagenase and elastase (102,103) when stimulated in vitro or in vivo. Kupffer cells and other mononuclear phagocytes may contain collagenolytic activity (35,82). Collagenase formation is also induced in macrophages by products of stimulated lymphocytes (91). It appears, therefore, that like polymorphonuclear leukocytes, these cells are also a rich source of neutral proteases.

The existence of many potential substrates for neutral proteases (Table 11) makes these enzymes excellent candidates for being important mediators of tissue injury and inflammation. The elevated lysosomal content, such as neutral and acid proteases and other nonenzymatic lysosomal materials, in synovial fluid from rheumatoid patients is clearly documented (14,41,42,51,56,62,66,86) and has been mentioned above. In addition, it should be pointed out here that ample experimental evidence has also been amassed to seriously implicate lysosomal neutral proteases as important pathogenetic factors in lung emphysema (36,63,68,69).

TABLE 11. Tissue substrate of leukocyte lysosomal enzymes

Enzymes	Substrate
Acid protease Neutral protease Elastase	Glomerular basement membrane
Acid protease Neutral protease Elastase	Vascular wall
Neutral protease Elastase Collagenase	Cartilage
Neutral protease Elastase	Lung connective tissue
Neutral protease Collagenase	Collagen

3. NONENZYMATIC LYSOSOMAL CONTENT

Among the inflammatory mediators contained in polymorphonuclear leukocytes are a number of substances without known
enzymatic activity (Table 12).

A heterogenous group of *cationic proteins* is capable, either directly or indirectly, to produce tissue damage and inflammation.
They cause adhesion and extravascular emigration of leukocytes
and leukocytes and petechial hemorrages in the microcirculation of
the rat and rabbit mesentery (55), and an acute inflammatory response in rabbit skin (40). These proteins are also able to induce
histamine release from mast cells (77,83,85) and an histamine-
independent increase in vascular permeability (77). More recently
(71,72), two substances with chemical properties similar to those
of hydroxyacids have been described in rabbit polymorphonuclear
leukocytes. They are released upon contact with antigen-antibody
precipitates, causing increase of vascular permeability and histamine release from mast cells.

Among the nonenzymatic inflammatory mediators contained in
leukocytes is the potent vasoactive amine, *histamine*, which was already discussed in detail in Chapter 2. It should, however, be men-

TABLE 12. Biological activity of lysosomal cationic proteins

Chemotactic
Histamine release from mast cells
Pyrogenic
Enhancement of vascular permeability
Anticoagulant
Coagulant
Antiheparin
Antibacterial

tioned here that, in human leukocytes, it is granule associated and has a similar but not identical subcellular distribution as β-glucuronidase (70,76). A *pyrogen* has also been described as being present in human and rabbit leukocytes (17,18). It seems that its release requires the synthesis of new cellular protein (73).

Apart from agents directly capable of producing tissue damage, there exist certain cell-derived substances (mostly enzymes) that do not affect tissues directly but interact with other inflammatory mediator systems through their effects on circulating substrates, thus propagating and amplifying the inflammatory response.

Substances contained in leukocytes either possess *chemotactic activity* or are capable of generating it. Cell-derived, serum-independent chemotactic activity localized in leukocyte lysosomal fractions has been described repeatedly (19,25,92). A chemotactic factor released by human leukocytes, when incubated with non phagocytosable, aggregated γ-globulin, has also been reported (108). Enzymes, acting at neutral pH, which cleave complement components C3 and C5 into chemotactically active fragments, have been identified in human and rabbit leukocyte lysosomes (44,89,93). One of these fragments, namely C5a, has recently been shown to also be capable of mediating lysosomal enzyme release from human polymorphonuclear leukocytes (38).

In addition, polymorphonuclear leukocytes exert *coagulant and fibrinolytic action.* Coagulant activity was found in human, rabbit and dog leukocytes (32,65,78,81). This thromboplastin-like effect is, perhaps, granule associated (58,81). Numerous reports describe a protease able to digest coagulated blood and fibrin (7,16), and a plasminogen present in leukocytes (16,39,80). The plasminogen was also identified in a lysosomal cationic protein fraction (80).

The role of leukocytes in the generation of *kinin activity* is discussed in Chapter 4. Since the conditions necessary for the functioning of the leukokinin system may prevail at the sites of tissue injury, the leukokinins may conceivably be biologically significant inflammatory mediators.

REFERENCES

1. Anderson, A. J.: Ann. Rheum. Dis. *29*:307, 1970.
2. Anderson, A. J., Brocklehurst, W. E., and Willis, A. L.: Pharmacol. Res. Commun. *3*:13, 1971.
3. Arrigoni-Martelli, E., Bramm, E., and Binderup, L.: Pharmacology *14*: 405, 1976.
4. Arrigoni-Martelli, E., Corsico, N., and Fogagnolo, E.: In "Inflammation Biochemistry and Drug Interaction," A. Bertelli and J. C. Houck, eds. Excerpta Medica, Amsterdam, 1969, p. 185.
5. Arrigoni-Martelli, E., and Restelli, A.: Eur. J. Pharmacol. *19*:191, 1972.
6. Arrigoni-Martelli, E., Schiatti, P. F., and Selva, D.: Pharmacology *5*:215, 1971.
7. Astrup, T., Henrichsen, J., and Kwaan, H. C.: Blood *29*:134, 1967.
8. Arya, D. V., Mannagh, J., and Irvine, A. R., Jr.:Invest. Ophtalmol. *11*: 662, 1972.
9. Avila, J. L., and Convit, J.: Clin. Chim. Acta *44*:21, 1973.
10. Avila, J. L., and Convit, J.: Biochim. Biophys. Acta *293*:397, 1973.
11. Avila, J. L., and Convit, J.: Biochim. Biophys. Acta *293*:409, 1973.
12. Baggiolini, M.: Enzyme *13*:132, 1972.
13. Barland, P., Janis, R., and Sandson, J.: Ann. Rheum. Dis. *25*:156, 1966.
14. Barland, P., Novikoff, A. B., and Hamerman, D.: Trans. Assoc. Am. Physicians *77*:239, 1964.
15. Barnhart, M. I., Quintana, C., Lenon, H. L., Bluhm, G. B., and Riddle, J. M.: Ann. N. Y. Acad. Sci. *146*:527, 1968.
16. Barnhart, M. I.: Biochem. Pharmacol. *17* (Suppl.) :205, 1968.
17. Bennett, I. L., Jr., and Beeson, P. B.: J. Exp. Med. *98*:493, 1953.
18. Bodel, P.: Yale J. Biol. Med. *43*:145, 1970.
19. Borel, J. F., Keller, H. U., and Sorkin, E.: Int. Arch. Allergy Appl. Immunol. *35*:194, 1969.
20. Cochrane, C. G., and Aiken, B. S.: J. Exp. Med. *124*:733, 1966.
21. Cochrane, C. G., Unanue, E. R., and Dixon, F. J.: J. Exp. Med. *122*:99, 1965.
22. Cochrane, C. G., Weigle, W. O., and Dixon, F. J.: J. Exp. Med. *110*:481, 1959.
23. Cohn, Z. A., and Hirsch, J. G.: J. Exp. Med. *112*:983, 1960.
24. Coppi, G., and Bonardi, G.: J. Pharm. Pharmacol. *20*:661, 1968.
25. Cornely, H. P.: Proc. Soc. Exp. Biol. Med. *122*:831, 1966.
26. Davies, P., Krakauer, K., and Weissmann, G.: Anal. Biochem. *45*:428, 1972.
27. Davies, P., Rita, G. A., Krakauer, K., and Weissmann, G.: Biochem. J. *123*:559, 1971.

28. de Duve, C., Pressman, B. C., Gianetto, R., Wattiaux, R., and Appelmans, F.: Biochem. J. *60*:604, 1955.
29. DeShazo, C. U., McGrade, M. T., Henson, P. M., and Cochrane, C. G.: J. Immunol. *108*:1414, 1972.
30. Dingle, F. T., Poole, A. R., Lazarus, G. L., and Barrett, A. J.: J. Exp. Med. *137*:1124, 1973.
31. Edlow, D. W., and Sheldon, W. H.: Proc. Soc. Exp. Biol. Med. *137*:1328, 1971.
32. Erdogan, G.: Blut *17*:276, 1968.
33. Farquhar, M. G., Bainton, D. F., Baggiolini, M., and de Duve, C.: J. Cell Biol. *54*:141, 1972.
34. Folds, J. D., Walsh, J. R., and Spitznagel, J. K.: Proc. Soc. Exp. Biol. Med. *139*:461, 1972.
35. Fujuwara, J., Sakai, T., Oda, R., and Igarashi, S.: Biochem. Biophys. Res. Commun. *54*:531, 1973.
36. Galdston, M., Janoff, A., and Davis, A. L.: Am. Rev. Respir. Dis. *107*:718, 1973.
37. Glenn, E. M., Bowman, B. J., and Koslowski, T. C.: Biochem. Pharmacol. *17*:(Suppl.):27, 1968.
38. Goldstein, I. M., Brai, M., Osler, A. G., and Weissman, G.: J. Immunol. *111*:33, 1973.
39. Goldstein, I. M., Wunschmann, B., Astrup, T., and Henderson, E. S.: Blood *37*:447, 1971.
40. Golub, E. S., and Spitznagel, J. K.: J. Immunol. *95*:1060, 1966.
41. Harris, E. D., Jr., Di Bona, P. R., and Krane, S. M.: J. Clin. Invest. *48*:2104, 1969.
42. Hendry, N. G. C., and Carr, A. J.: Nature *199*:392, 1963.
43. Henson, P. M.: Am. J. Pathol. *68*:593, 1972.
44. Hill, J. H., and Ward, P. A.: J. Exp. Med. *133*:885, 1971.
45. Hirschorn, R., and Weissmann, G.: Proc. Soc. Exp. Biol. Med. *119*:36, 1965.
46. Hirschorn, R., and Weissmann, G.: Nature *214*:892, 1967.
47. Humphrey, J. H.: Br. J. Exp. Path. *36*:268, 1955.
48. Ignarro, L. J., Oronsky, A. L., and Perper, R. J.: Clin. Immunol. Immunopathol. *2*:36, 1973.
49. Janoff, A.: Lab. Invest. *22*:228, 1970.
50. Janoff, A.: Am. Rev. Respir. Dis. *105*:121, 1972.
51. Janoff, A., and Blondin, J.: Proc. Soc. Exp. Biol. Med. *135*:302, 1970.
52. Janoff, A., Sandhaus, R. A., Hospelhorn, V. D., and Rosenberg, R.: Proc. Soc. Exp. Biol. Med. *140*:516, 1972.
53. Janoff, A., and Scherer, J.: J. Exp. Med. *128*:1137, 1968.
54. Janoff, A., and Zeligs, J. D.: Science *161*:702, 1968.
55. Janoff, A., and Zweifach, B. W.: Science *144*:1465, 1964.
56. Kerby, G. P., and Haylor, S. M.: Proc. Soc. Exp. Biol. Med. *126*:865, 1967.
57. Kniker, W. T., and Cochrane, C. G.: J. Exp. Med. *122*:83, 1965.
58. Kociba, G. J., Loeb, W. F., and Wall, R. L.: J. Lab. Clin. Med. *79*:778, 1972.
59. Lapresle, C., and Webb, T.: Biochem. J. *84*:455, 1962.
60. Lazarus, G. S., Daniels, J. R., Brown, R. S., Bladen, H. A., and Fullmer, H. M.: J. Clin. Invest. *47*:2622, 1968.

61. Lazarus, G. S., Daniels, J. R., Lian, J., and Burleigh, M. C.: Am. J. Pathol. *68*:565, 1972.
62. Lehman, M. A., Kream, J., and Brogna, D.: J. Bone Joint Surg. *46A*: 1732, 1964.
63. Lieberman, J., and Gawal, M.: J. Lab. Clin. Med. *77*:713, 1971.
64. Lieberman, J., and Kaneshiro, W.: J. Lab. Clin. Med. *80*:88, 1972.
65. Lerner, R. G., Goldstein, R., and Cummings, G.: Proc. Soc. Exp. Biol. Med. *138*:145, 1971.
66. Luscombe, M.: Nature *197*:1010, 1963.
67. Manaligod, J. R., Krakower, C. A., and Greenspon, S. A.: Am. J. Pathol. *56*:533, 1969.
68. Marco, V., Mass, B., Meranze, D., Weinbaum, G., and Kimbel, P.: Ann. Rev. Respir. Dis. *104*:595, 1971.
69. Mass, B., Ikeda, T., Meranze, D., Weinbaum, G., and Kimbel, P.: Am. Rev. Respir. Dis. *106*:385, 1972.
70. May, C. C., Levine, B., and Weissmann, G.: Proc. Soc. Exp. Biol. Med. *133*:758, 1970.
71. Movat, H. Z., Macmorine, D. R. L., and Takeuchi, Y.: Int. Arch. Allergy *40*:218, 1971.
72. Movat, H. Z., Uriuhava, T., Takeuchi, Y., and Macmorine, D. R. L.: Int. Arch. Allergy *40*:197, 1971.
73. Moore, D. M., Murphy, P. A., Chesney, P. J., and Wood, W. B., Jr.: J. Exp. Med. *137*:1263, 1973.
74. Mounter, L. A., and Atiyeh, W.: Blood *15*:52, 1960.
75. Phelps, P., and McCarty, D. J.: J. Exp. Med. *124*:115, 1966.
76. Pruzansky, J. J., and Patterson, R.: Proc. Soc. Exp. Biol. Med. *124*:56, 1967.
77. Ranadive, N. S., and Cochrane, C. G.: J. Exp. Med. *128*:605, 1968.
78. Rapaport, S. I., and Hjort, P. F.: Thromb. Diath. Haemorrh. *17*:222, 1967.
79. Robertson, P. B., Ryel, R. B., Taylor, R. E., Shyn, K. W., and Fullmer, H. M.: Science *177*:64, 1972.
80. Saba, H. I., Herison, J. C., and Roberts, H. R.: Blood *34*:835, 1969.
81. Saba, H. I., Herison, J. C., Walker, R. I., and Roberts, H. R.: Proc. Soc. Exp. Biol. Med. *142*:614, 1973.
82. Salthouse, T. N., and Malaga, B. F.: Experientia *28*:326, 1972.
83. Scherer, J., and Janoff, A.: Lab. Invest. *18*:196, 1968.
84. Schumacher, H. R., and Agudelo, C. A.: Science *175*:1139, 1972.
85. Seegers, W., and Janoff, A.: J. Exp. Med. *124*:833, 1966.
86. Smith, C., and Hamermann, D.: Arthritis Rheum. *5*:411, 1962.
87. Stetson, C. A.: J. Exp. Med. *94*:347, 1957.
88. Stiles, M., and Fraenkel-Conrat, J.: Blood *32*:119, 1968.
89. Taubman, S. B., Goldschmidt, P. R., and Lepow, I. H.: Fed. Proc. *29*:434, 1970.
90. Thomas, L.: Proc. Soc. Exp. Biol. Med. *115*:235, 1964.
91. Wahl, L. M., Wahl, S. M., Mergenhagen, S. E., and Martin, G. R.: Science *187*:261, 1975.
92. Ward, P. A.: J. Exp. Med. *128*:1201, 1968.
93. Ward, P. A., and Hill, H. J.: J. Immunol. *104*:535, 1970.
94. Wasi, S., Murray, R. K., Macmorine, D. R. L., and Movat, H. Z.: Br. J. Exp. Path. *47*:411, 1966.

95. Watanabe, I., Donahue, S., and Hoggat, N.: J. Ultrastruct. Res. *20*:366, 1967.
96. Weissmann, G., Becher, B., Wiedermann, G., and Bernheimer, A. W.: Am. J. Pathol. *46*:129, 1965.
97. Weissmann, G., Pras, M., and Rosenberg, L.: Arthritis Rheum. *10*:325, 1967.
98. Weissmann, G., and Spilberg, I.: Arthritis Rheum. *9*:162, 1968.
99. Weissmann, G., Spilberg, I., and Krakauer, K.: Arthritis Rheum. *12*:103, 1969.
100. Weissmann, G., Zurier, R. B., and Hoffstein, S.: Am. J. Pathol. *68*:539, 1972.
101. Welsh, I. R. H., and Spitznagel, J. K.: Infect. Immun. *4*:97, 1971.
102. Werb, Z., and Gordon, S.: J. Exp. Med. *142*:346, 1975.
103. Werb, Z., and Gordon, S.: J. Exp. Med. *142*:361, 1975.
104. Willoughby, D. A., Dunn, C. J., Yamamoto, S., Capasso, F., Deporter, D. A., and Giroud, J. P.: Agents Actions *5*:35, 1975.
105. Wyllie, J. C., Haust, M. D., and More, R. H.: Lab. Invest. *15*:519, 1966.
106. Zeya, H. I., and Spitznagel, J. K.: Lab. Invest. *24*:229, 1971.
107. Ziff, M., Gribetz, H. J., and LoSpalluto, J.: J. Clin. Invest. *39*:405, 1960.
108. Zigmond, S. H., and Hirsch, J. G.: J. Exp. Med. *137*:387, 1973.

Chapter 9

Cyclic Nucleotides: Modulators of Inflammation

During the past decade, cyclic nucleotides (cAMP and cGMP) have been identified as key intermediates in the reaction of cells to exogenous stimuli. The nature of the immune and inflammatory response with its requirement for specific cellular recognition, cell proliferation and differentiation, secretion of antibodies and non-specific mediators makes the involvement of cyclic nucleotides very likely. It has been recognized that diverse systems of inflammation of either immunological or other origin are modulated by the intra-cellular concentrations (and by factors and agents affecting intra-cellular concentrations) of cyclic nucleotides. The first step in the immune response, which ultimately results in an immunologic in-flammation, is the activation of lymphocytes of either the B (bone-marrow-derived) or T (thymus-derived) type. The former are the effector cells in humoral immunity, the latter—in cellular immunity. Upon the encounter of antibodies or sensitized cells with soluble or cellular antigens, mediators are released or processes considered typical of cell-mediated immunologic reactions are initiated. The role of cyclic nucleotides in inflammation will be discussed in relation to the activation of lymphocytes, release of mediators and cellular immunity.

1. CYCLIC NUCLEOTIDES AND LYMPHOCYTE ACTIVATION

The immune response is initiated by the binding of antigen to receptors on the surface of immunocompetent lymphocytes (68). This binding triggers a complex series of biochemical events culminating in lymphocyte proliferation and maturation into either the antibody-forming B cells, or the T cells involved in cellular immunity (79). Since the percentage of lymphocytes capable of responding to a single antigenic stimulus is very low even in previously immunized animals (1,76), another lymphocyte activation system was chosen to study this aspect of immune response and the concomitant biochemical events. A variety of plant lectins have been shown to induce a blastogenic reaction where a substantial percentage of lymphocytes was found to respond (39,103). Of these lectins, phytohemoagglutinin (PHA) and concanavalin A (con A) have been investigated more extensively. The mitogenic lectins initiate a series of biochemical events resulting in striking alterations in cell morphology and mitosis.

The biochemical changes include augmented incorporation of labeled phosphate, choline, and fatty acids (25,26,97); a selective increase in uptake of some amino acids (74), and transport of sugars and nucleosides (90,91); and an higher rate of K^+ and Ca^{2+} entry into the cell (4,6).

At the nuclear level, there is a considerable increase in uridine and thymidine uptake, with a concomitant rise in RNA, DNA and nucleic acid turnover (32,53,99,100).

These biochemical changes are followed by morphological modifications, including capping (96), increased pinocytosis (3), altered chromatin staining (37) and mitosis.

Thymidine uptake is the accepted method for evaluating lectin-induced mitogenesis and—for most purposes—it probably provides a good approximation. However, this technique has certain limitations because of both the recently observed lack of direct correlation between changes in DNA content and thymidine uptake, and the possibility that not every cell stimulated by mitogen undergoes a qualitatively similar response (77,99,112).

The conjecture that *cAMP plays a specific role in lymphocyte transformation* is based on the complex nature of the transformation response and the flexibility of cAMP as a regulatory agent. During lymphocyte transformation, there is a need for a substance with the ability to coordinate diverse biochemical events in different parts of the cell (70). Considering the large number of biochemical reactions that it modulates, cAMP seems uniquely suited for this role.

The stimulation of mitogenesis involves an action of lectins at the lymphocyte surface (29,66,81) and cAMP is known to be an intracellular messenger for hormones which interact with plasma membranes. Many of the very early changes in membrane functions of lectin-stimulated cells are mimicked by cAMP in nonlymphocytic tissues (2,78,98,117); thus, for example, in the acinar cells of salivary glands, the rise in cAMP due to isoproterenol results in increased DNA formation (30). Moreover, cAMP is known to act at the transcriptional and/or translational level to induce specific enzyme synthesis in prokariotic and eukariotic cells (49,50,72,75); it seems likely that extensive gene activation is required during lymphocyte transformation which converts a resting population of cells to one with greatly increased metabolic activity.

Studies carried out in a number of laboratories indicate that peripheral lymphocytes contain cAMP and possess active adenylate cyclase and phosphodiesterase, enzymes providing the same possibilities for modulating cellular function as are inherent in other tissues (11,27,54,69,80,105). The intracellular level of cAMP in human lymphocytes—approximately 25 pmoles/10^7 cells (88)—is increased up to 30 fold by prostaglandins (86). Adrenergic stimulation (86,105), acetylcholine (87) and histamine (12) also induce a rise in the intracellular levels of cAMP. Recent observations (116) suggest that heterogeneity exists among the lymphocytes in this respect. Adenylate cyclase (105) and cAMP phosphodiesterase (58) have also been demonstrated in homogenates of human lymphocytes.

Extensive investigations on the *effects of lectins on lymphocyte cAMP concentrations* have been performed (89,105,106,113). Few minutes after the addition of phytohemoagglutinin, a rise in intracellular cAMP occurs. There is a subsequent decline to control levels and, after approximately 12 hours, the phytohemoagglutinin-treated cells contain significantly less cAMP than do control cells. Though there is still some uncertainty about this, the evaluation of lectin action on adenylate cyclase was substantially in agreement with the above observations (69,121,122). It appears, however, that the effects on lymphocyte cAMP accumulation exerted by lectin depend on its concentration, cell density, relative number of T and B lymphocytes, medium and time of incubation, and the presence or absence of nonlymphocytic cells.

Attempts to obtain convincing evidence that the action of lectin can be fully duplicated by manipulating cAMP concentrations inside the lymphocytes were substantially unsuccessful. Cyclic AMP, its butyryl derivative, ATP, and adenosine, at concentrations between $10^{-4} - 10^{-5}$M, inhibit DNA, RNA and protein synthesis (104,106). These substances and theophylline also suppress DNA formation—a response to phytohemoagglutinins (38). It has been suggested, that cAMP could have both a stimulatory and inhibitory effect. Thus, low concentrations (10^{-7}M) of dibutyryl cAMP and of cAMP itself enhance the response to lectins whereas higher levels suppress it strongly (21,28,38,106). These observations, however, have not been confirmed by other investigations (73).

It might be argued that the delayed drop in cAMP is more important than its initial increase. However, this rise is the first measurable biochemical event in lectin-stimulated cells; furthermore, in other cells, cAMP has been shown to modulate many of the early biochemical changes occurring in lectin-stimulated cells. There is evidence which indicates that changes in cAMP occur in discrete areas of the lymphocytes, where the local increase in cAMP may be considerably high (9,10,105,113,114). These studies also revealed that the pattern of intracellular cAMP accumulation varies, depending on the agent used to stimulate the latter. Thus, phytohemoagglutinins induce accumulation within or near the external plasma membrane, which is noteworthy since the activation of DNA synthesis by phytohemoagglutinin is a surface phenomenon (29). In contrast, prostaglandin E_1 stimulated cAMP increase in cytoplasm, while isoproterenol did so mainly in the nucleus. Selective hormonal and mitogen activation of adenylate cyclase has been demonstrated in appropriate isolated subcellular fractions (113, 115).

The possibility that cGMP plays a role in lymphocyte activation cannot be ruled out since there is increasing evidence that this cyclic nucleotide can serve as a second messenger for extracellular hormonal stimuli (33,57,59). In addition, it has recently been shown that, in lectin-stimulated human lymphocytes, there is a rise up to 50 fold in cGMP concentrations (31).

To evaluate the role of cyclic nucleotides in the immune response more closely, the effects of modifying intralymphocytic cAMP concentration in regard to the production of antibodies or cellular immunity have been examined. These studies were carried out under a number of different conditions (17,18,44,45). It is apparent from the above investigations that the increase in cAMP (or adenylate cyclase) concentrations amplified the response of immunocompetent cells. Moreover, it has been shown in in vivo experiments that a rapid, transient increase in cAMP levels occurs in antigen-stimulated mouse spleen (94,124), followed by a return to or below the control values. A rise in cGMP levels, persisting for several days, has also been reported (125).

2. CYCLIC NUCLEOTIDES AND MEDIATORS RELEASE

The modulatory role of cyclic nucleotides on the release of different mediators has been already discussed in preceding chapters. Due to the particular interest of this topic, it will be re-examined here more comprehensively.

The release of lysosomal enzymes from phagocytic cells—macrophages, polymorphonuclear leukocytes and fixed-tissue histiocytes —is thought to involve granule movement and the direct discharge of lysosomal contents into phagocytic vesicles not completely occluded by plasma membranes (119). Phagocytic cells participate in immunologic inflammation by ingesting and degrading antigen-antibody complexes and cell debris, and by serving as a source of proteolytic enzymes which act outside the cell. The cyclic nucleotides can be involved in the perception of phagocytic stimulus, in the degradation and interiorization of the foreign materials and in the release of lysosomal enzymes. The evidence concerning the possible role of cyclic nucleotides in the transmission of phagocytic stimuli is scanty and somewhat contradictory. In mixed human leukocytes exposed to latex particles, an increase in cAMP has been reported (85) but this finding has not been confirmed in purified polymorphonuclear preparations (67).

The effects of cyclic nucleotides on lysosomal enzyme release have been demonstrated in different cells from various animal species (42,43,118). (Table 13 and 14) Cyclic AMP, cGMP and dibutyryl cAMP, at a concentration of 5mM, inhibit lysosomal enzyme release from mouse macrophages exposed to zymosan particles (118). In human neutrophils, cAMP alone has no effect but suppresses enzyme release in combination with theophylline (118). In mixed human leukocyte preparations, epinephrine has a blocking

TABLE 13. Effect of catecholamines, cyclic 3,5-adenosine monophosphate, and analogs on release of β-glucuronidase
from human neutrophils

Agent Tested	% Inhibition of β-Glucuronidase Release (Molar conc. of agent 10^{-5})
Epinephrine (E)	61 ± 6.2
Isoproterenol	50 ± 4.2
Theophylline	28 ± 1.7
E + theophylline (10^{-6}M)	94 ± 7.5
E + propranolol (10^{-5}M)	8 ± 0.8
E + phentolamine (10^{-5}M)	67 ± 4.6
Cyclic AMP + theophylline (10^{-6}M)	44 ± 2.7
Dibutyryl cyclic AMP	49 ± 2.6
Dibutyryl cyclic AMP + propranolol (10^{-5}M)	45 ± 3.1
8-Bromo cyclic AMP	60 ± 4.3
AMP	0

action which is potentiated by theophylline but antagonized by pro-
pranolol (40). In human leukocytes pretreated with cytochalasin B
and exposed to phagocytic stimulus, both cAMP and its dibutyryl
derivative markedly inhibit release (127). In addition, it has been
shown in the same preparation that epinephrine and isoproterenol
suppress release while carbamylcholine—a cholinergic stimulator—
or cGMP enhance it (41,127). PGE_1 PGE_2 and $PGF_{2}\alpha$, known to
activate adenylate cyclase in human mixed leukocytes (95) and to
raise the level of intracellular cAMP (15), inhibit discharge of lysosomal enzymes from both phagocytosing and non-phagocytosing
leukocytes (120,126). Thus, it seems that a β-adrenergic stimulus
and cAMP inhibit release while cholinergic stimulus and cGMP enhance it. These observations have been confirmed and extended in
isolated lysosomes from guinea-pig polymorphonuclear leukocytes
and rat liver (42,43), thus suggesting that similar effects can be
obtained in a variety of tissues.

A finding difficult to reconcile with the alleged inhibitory effect

TABLE 14. Effect of catecholamines, cyclic 3,5-guanosine monophosphate, and analogs on release of β-glucuronidase
from human neutrophils

Agent Tested	% Increase of β-Glucuronidase Release (Molar conc. of agent 10^{-5})
Acetylcholine (Ach)	176 ± 16
Acetyl β-methylcholine	202 ± 17
Ach + atropine $(10^{-5}M)$	21 ± 1.5
Ach + hexamethonium $(10^{-5}M)$	168 ± 12
Cyclic GMP	84 ± 7.0
Cyclic GMP + atropine $(10^{-5}M)$	91 ± 8.2
Dibutyryl cyclic GMP	99 ± 8.3
8-Bromo cyclic GMP	110 ± 10
GMP	7 ± 0.2

of cAMP on lysosomal enzyme release is that cholera toxin, an agent
which causes a delayed but substantial increase in cAMP in many
different tissues, does not inhibit the release of lysosomal enzyme
from human leukocytes exposed to phagocytic stimulus (12). It cannot be excluded, however, that this apparent discrepancy depends
upon a subcellular compartmentalization of cAMP.

Adenylate cyclase and cAMP may possibly play a role in the
release of histamine and other mediators of the immediate hypersensitivity reaction; this hypothesis is based on the apparent localization of the initial stimulatory event at the cell surface (110) and
the rapidity with which histamine appears in the medium (8).
Pharmacological agents known to operate through cAMP were demonstrated to exert a potent effect on histamine release long before
the existence of cAMP was even suspectd (102). Various adrenergic
drugs (71,84,109), methylxanthines (65,82), dibutyryl cAMP (65,
82), and prostaglandins (111), which increase cAMP concentrations in the leukocyte population as a whole inhibit the immunologic
release of chemical mediators. Exogenous histamine can also increase intracellular levels of cAMP and prevent antigen-induced
release of endogenous histamine (61).

There is evidence that H_2-receptors are involved in this phenomenon (64). The response of the human leukocyte system to antigen can be divided into two phases: the first, calcium-independent, during which antigen is bound and activates the cell, and the second, calcium-dependent, when the release of mediators occurs (60). Prostaglandin E_1, methylxanthines, β-agonists and dibutyryl cAMP inhibit only the calcium-independent phase (13).

Studies on human, primate and guinea-pig models confirmed the results obtained with mixed leukocytes. Release of histamine and slow-reacting substance of anaphylaxis from human, primate, and guinea-pig sensitized lungs is blocked by β-agonists, methylxanthines and dibutyryl cAMP (5,46). The inhibitory potency of these agents and prostaglandin E_1 correlates with their ability to increase the total tissue content of cAMP. Interestingly, this potency is several orders of magnitude higher in sensitized lungs than in the peripheral leukocyte system (83).

Cholinergic or α-adrenergic agents enhance antigen-mediated release from human lung, suggesting that the stimulus for the release might be a decline in cAMP, or a rise in cGMP, or both (51, 52).

Inhibition of mediator release by agents which raise tissue cAMP concentrations has also been reported in other complex in vitro systems; moreover, similar effects have been observed in vivo in human beings, monkeys, mice, guinea pigs, and rats (13,92). In heterogenous tissues, however, pharmacological action on mediator release may be indirect, occurring through other cells present in the cell mixture. Thus, epinephrine is apparently unable to suppress release from a highly purified mast cell preparation at concentrations producing a significant rise in cAMP, although the same agents block release in unpurified cell mixtures (47,108).

Because of several unsolved technical problems, the role of cAMP in mediator release from purified mast cells is still subject to considerable controversy (48,108). There is good evidence to indicate that a fall in cAMP is part of the critical early stimulus but it could be argued that the effects of pharmacological agents which enhance or inhibit the response are not completely consistent with this simple conclusion.

Many of the problems in the design and interpretation of experiments with mast cells also exist in respect to platelets. Information currently available (20,23,34,101,123) supports the concept that an overall increase in platelet cAMP is associated with inhibition of aggregation and mediator release; it also seems that a decrease in cAMP content initiates aggregation.

3. CYCLIC NUCLEOTIDES AND CELLULAR IMMUNITY

Cell-mediated immune responses, typified by delayed hypersensitivity reaction and homograft rejection, are thought to reflect the activities of T lymphocytes (7). These activities include the capacity to destroy other cells when they are antigens (19), to release a spectrum of nonspecific soluble mediators (lymphokines) which affect other host cells as well as target cells (22), and to give off large molecular weight substances possessing certain of the specificity characteristic of antibody (24).

It has been found that diverse pharmacological agents—isoproterenol, prostaglandins E_1 and E_2, histamine, theophylline, cholera toxin—able to induce an increase in cAMP concentration block T-cell mediated cytolysis, and that exogenous cAMP and its dibutyryl derivative are equally effective inhibitors (35,36,62,63,107). The suppression of cytolysis appears correlated with cAMP increase. The inhibition produced by isoproterenol is maximal after few minutes of incubation when there is a 5-fold increase in cAMP, whereas inhibition by cholera toxin does not occur until after a lag of several hours; such lag would be expected because of the induction period needed for the cAMP response of lymphocytes (35,36, 62).

There is little information concerning the ability of cyclic nucleotides to modulate the release of the nonspecific and specific mediators of cellular immunity. It has been observed, however, that theophylline and isoproterenol did inhibit the effect of MIF (migration inhibitory factor) on macrophage migration (55,56), and that the production of interferon is prevented by exposure of activated lymphocytes to cholera toxin and other cAMP-active substances (14). More recently, it has been shown that the formation of MIF by antigen-stimulated sentized guinea-pig lymph-node cells is suppressed by theophylline and dibutyryl cAMP (93).

There is also some preliminary evidence suggesting a role for cGMP in the cytolytic response. Carbamylcholine and acetylcholine, which raise the concentration of cGMP in other tissues (57), can stimulate the cytolytic response to a modest extent (107).

4. COMMENTS

Despite the indirect character of much of the experimental studies and the problems inherent in interpreting existing data, it seems that the cyclic nucleotides exert vital control at virtually every level of the immune response. In general, the effect of high intracellular cAMP concentrations is to reduce the immunological (and inflammatory) effects of leukocytes, thus inhibiting cell proliferation, chemotaxis and mediator release. However, lymphocyte transformation and B-cell proliferation, also provide evidence that cAMP has a stimulatory function. If the tentative formulation of cAMP compartmentalization could be verified, the model would provide a plausible mechanism for cAMP action. It is noteworthy that the possibility of higher gradients of cAMP existing in locally perturbed areas of phagocytic cells has been suggested to explain translocation of lysosomes to phagosomes (119). Because histamine and other mediators of inflammation markedly stimulate cAMP formation, a negative feedback response has been proposed (14,16). According to this hypothesis, the increase in cAMP following mediator release would, in turn, limit further release which would otherwise extend or intensify the inflammatory reaction.

REFERENCES

1. Ada, G. L.: Transplant. Rev. *5*:105, 1970.
2. Adamson, L. F.: Biochim. Biophys. Acta *201*:446, 1970.
3. Adler, W. H., Osunkoya, B. O., Takiguchi, T., and Smith, R. T.: Cell. Immunol. *3*:590, 1972.
4. Allwood, G., Asherson, G. L., Davey, M. J., and Goodford, P. J.: Immunology *21*:509, 1971.
5. Assen, E. S. K., and Schild, M. O.: Int. Arch. Allergy Appl. Immunol. *40*: 576, 1971.
6. Averdunk, R.: Hoppe-Seyler's Z. Physiol. Chem. *353*:79, 1972.
7. Bloom, B. R.: Adv. Immunol. *13*:101, 1971.
8. Bloom, G. D., and Chakravarty, N.: Acta Physiol. Scand. *78*:410, 1970.
9. Bloom, F. E., Hoffer, B. J., Battenberg, E. R., Siggins, G. R., Steiner, A. L., Parker, C. W., and Wedner, H. J.: Science *177*:436, 1972.
10. Bloom, F. E., Wedner, H. J., and Parker, C. W.: Pharmacol. Rev. *25*:343, 1973.
11. Bourne, H. R., Lehrer, R. I., Cline, M. J., and Melmon, K. L.: J. Clin. Invest. *50*:920, 1971.
12. Bourne, H. R., Lehrer, R. I., Lichtenstein, L. M., Weissmann, G., and Zurier, R. B.: J. Clin. Invest. *52*:698, 1973.
13. Bourne, H. R., Lichtenstein, L. M., and Melmon, K. L.: J. Immunol. *108*: 695, 1972.
14. Bourne, H. R., Lichtenstein, L. M., Melmon, K. L., Henney, C. S., Weinstein, Y., and Shearer, G. M.: Science *184*:19, 1974.
15. Bourne, H. R., and Melmon, K. L.: J. Pharmacol. Exp. Ther. *178*:1, 1971.
16. Bourne, M. R., Melmon, K. L., and Lichtenstein, L. M.: Science *173*:743, 1971.
17. Braun, W., and Ishizuka, M.: J. Immunol. *107*:1037, 1971.

18. Braun, W., Ishizuka, M., Winchurch, R., and Webb, D.: Ann. N. Y. Acad. Sci. *185*:417, 1971.
19. Cerottini, J. C., Nordin, A. A., and Brunner, K. T.: Nature *228*:1308, 1972.
20. Cole, B., Robinson, G. A., and Hartmann, R. C.: Ann. N. Y. Acad. Sci. *185*:477, 1971.
21. Cross, M. E., and Ord, M. G.: Biochem. J. *124*:241, 1971.
22. David, J. R.: Prog. Allergy *16*:300, 1972.
23. Droller, M. J., and Wolfe, S. M.: N. Engl. J. Med. *286*:948, 1972.
24. Evans, R., Grant, C. K., Cox, H., Steele, K., and Alexander, P.: J. Exp. Med. *136*:1318, 1972.
25. Fisher, D. B., and Mueller, G. C.: Proc. Natl. Acad. Sci. USA *60*:1396, 1968.
26. Fisher, D. B., and Mueller, G. C.: Biochim. Biophys. Acta *248*:434, 1971.
27. Franks, D. I., and MacManus, J. P.: Biochem. Biophys. Res. Commun. *42*:844, 1971.
28. Gallo, R. C., and Whang-Peng, J.: J. Natl. Cancer Inst. *47*:91, 1971.
29. Greaves, M. F., and Bauminger, S.: Nature (New Biol.) *235*:67, 1972.
30. Guidotti, A., Weiss, B., and Costa, E.: Mol. Pharmacol. *8*:521, 1972.
31. Hadden, J. W., Hadden, E. M., Haddox, M. K., and Goldberg, N. G.: Proc. Natl. Acad. Sci. USA *69*:3024, 1972.
32. Hansen, P., Stein, H., and Peters, H.: Eur. J. Biochem. *9*:542, 1969.
33. Hardman, J. G., Robinson, G. A., and Sutherland, E. W.: Ann. Rev. Physiol. *33*:311, 1971.
34. Haslam, R. J., and Taylor, A.: Biochem. J. *125*:377, 1971.
35. Henney, C. S., Bourne, H. R., and Lichtenstein, C. M.: J. Immunol. *108*:1526, 1972.
36. Henney, C. S., and Lichtenstein, L. M.: J. Immunol. *107*:610, 1971.
37. Hirschhorn, R., Decsi, M. I., and Troll, I. M.: Cell. Immunol. *2*:696, 1971.
38. Hirschhorn, R., Grossman, J., and Weissmann, G.: Proc. Soc. Exp. Biol. Med. *133*:1361, 1970.
39. Hossaini, A. A.: Vox Sang. *15*:410, 1968.
40. Ignarro, L. J.: Nature (New Biol.) *245*:151, 1973.
41. Ignarro, L. J.: J. Immunol. *112*:210, 1974.
42. Ignarro, L. J., and Colombo, C.: Science *180*:1181, 1973.
43. Ignarro, L. J., Krassikoff, N., and Slywka, J.: Life Sci. *11*:317, 322.
44. Ishizuka, M., Braun, W., and Matsumoto, T.: J. Immunol. *107*:1027, 1971.
45. Ishizuka, M., Gafin, M., and Braun, W.: Proc. Soc. Exp. Biol. Med. *134*:963, 1970.
46. Ishizaka, T., Ishizaka, K., Orange, R. P., and Austen, K. F.: Fed. Proc. *29*:575, 1970.
47. Johnson, A. R., and Moran, N. C.: J. Pharmacol. Exp. Ther. *175*:632, 1970.
48. Johnson, A. R., Moran, N. C., and Mayer, S. E.: Fed. Proc. *32*:744, 1973.
49. Jost, J. P., Hsie, A., Hughes, S. D., and Ryan, L.: J. Biol. Chem. *245*:351, 1970.
50. Jost, J. P., and Sahib, M. K.: J. Biol. Chem. *246*:1623, 1971.
51. Kaliner, M., Orange, R. P., and Austen, K. F.: J. Exp. Med. *136*:556, 1972.
52. Kaliner, M., Orange, R. P., La Raia, P. J., and Austen, K. F.: Fed. Proc. *31*:748, 1972.
53. Kay, J. E., and Cooper, H. L.: Biochim. Biophys. Acta *186*:62, 1969.

54. Klainer, L. M., Chi, Y. M., Freidberg, S. L., Rall, T. W., and Sutherland, E. W.: J. Biol. Chem. *327*:1239, 1962.

55. Koopman, W. J., and David, J. R.: In "Inflammation, Mechanism and Control," I. Lepow and P. Ward, eds. Academic Press, New York, 1972, p. 151.

56. Koopman, W. J., Gillis, M. H., and David, J. R.: J. Immunol. *110*:1609, 1973.

57. Kuo, J. F., Lee, T. P., Reyes, P. L., Walton, K. G., Connelly, T. E., and Greengard, P.: J. Biol. Chem. *247*:16, 1972.

58. Lagarde, A., and Colobert, L.: Biochim. Biophys. Acta *276*:444, 1972.

59. Lee, T. P., Kuo, J. F., and Greengard, P.: Proc. Natl. Acad. Sci. USA *69*: 3287, 1972.

60. Lichtenstein, L. M.: J. Immunol. *107*:1122, 1971.

61. Lichtenstein, L. M.: In "Clinical Immunobiology," Vol. 1, F. H. Bach and R. A. Good, eds. Academic Press, New York, 1972, p. 243.

62. Lichtenstein, L. M., Bourne, H. R., Henney, C. S., and Greenough, W. B., III. J. Clin. Invest. *52*:691, 1973.

63. Lichtenstein, L. M., Gillespie, E., Bourne, H. R., and Henney, C. S.: Prostaglandins *2*:519, 1972.

64. Lichtenstein, L. M., and Gillespie, E.: Nature *244*:287, 1973.

65. Lichtenstein, L. M., and Margolis, S.: Science *161*:902, 1968.

66. Lindahl-Kiesseling, K.: Exp. Cell Res. *70*:17, 1972.

67. Manganiello, V., Evans, W. H., Stossel, T. P., Mason, R. J., and Vaughan, M.: J. Clin. Invest. *50*:2741, 1971.

68. Makela, O.: Transpl. Rev. *5*:1, 1970.

69. Makman, M. H.: Proc. Natl. Acad. Sci. USA *68*:885, 1971.

70. Mamont, P., Hershko, A., Kram, R., Schachter, L., Lust, J., Tomkins, G. M.: Biochem. Biophys. Res. Commun. *48*:1378, 1972.

71. Mannaioni, P. F., Zilletti, L., Guidotti, A., Giotti, A.: Life Sci. *3*:347, 1964.

72. Martin, P. W. Jr., Tompkins, G. M., Presler, M. A.: Proc. Natl. Acad. Sci. USA *63*:842, 1969.

73. Mendlesohn, J., Multer, M. M., Boone, R. F.: J. Clin. Invest. *52*:2129, 1973.

74. Mendlesohn, J., Skinner, A., Kornfeld, S.: J. Clin. Invest. *50*:818, 1971.

75. Miller, S., Varmus, H. E., Parks, J. S., Perlman, R. L., Pastan, I.: J. Biol. Chem. *246*:2898, 1971.

76. Moller, G., Michael, G.: Cell. Immunol. *2*:309, 1971.

77. Monjardino, J. P., Mac Gillivray, A. J.: Exp. Cell. Res. *60*:1, 1970.

78. Nayler, W. G., Mc Innes, I., Chipperfield, D., Carson, V., Doile, P.: J. Pharmacol. Exp. Ther. *171*:265, 1970.

79. Nossal, G. S.: Harvey Lect. *63*:179, 1969.

80. Novogrodsky, A., Katchalski, E.: Biochim. Biophys. Acta *215*:291, 1970.

81. Ono, T., Terayama, H., Takaku, F., Nakao, K.: Life Sci. *9*:1217, 1970.

82. Orange, R. P., Austen, W. G., Austen, K. F.: J. Exp. Med. *134*:136S, 1971.

83. Orange, R. P., Austen, W. G., and Austen, K. F.: J. Exp. Med. *134*: Suppl. 1365, 1971.

84. Orange, R. P., Kaliner, M. A., La Raia, P. J., and Austen, K. F.: Fed. Proc. *30*:1725, 1971.

85. Park, B. H., Good, R. A., Beck, N. P., and Davis, B. B.: Nature (New Biol.) *229*:27, 1971.

86. Parker, C. W., Baumann, M. L., and Huber, M. G.: J. Clin. Invest. *52*: 1336, 1973.
87. Parker, C. W., and Morse, S. J.: J. Exp. Med. *137*:1078, 1973.
88. Parker, C. W., and Smith, J. W.: J. Clin. Invest. *52*:48, 1973.
89. Parker, C. W., Smith, J. W., and Steiner, A. L.: Int. Arch. Allergy. Appl. Immunol. *41*:40, 1971.
90. Peters, J. H., and Hausen, P.: Eur. J. Biochem. *19*:502, 1971.
91. Peters, J. H., and Hausen, P.: Eur. J. Biochem. *19*:509, 1971.
92. Perper, R. J., Sanda, M., and Lichtenstein, L. M.: Int. Arch. Allergy Appl. Immunol. *43*:837, 1972.
93. Pick, E.: Immunology *26*:649, 1974.
94. Plescia, O. J., Yamamoto, I., Shimamura, T., and Feit, C.: Ann. N. Y. Acad. Sci. *249*:362, 1975.
95. Polgar, P., Vera, J. C., Kelley, P. R., and Rutenburg, A. M.: Biochim. Biophys. Acta *297*:378, 1973.
96. Raff, M. C., and De Petris, S.: Fed. Proc. *32*:48, 1973.
97. Resch, K., and Ferber, E.: Eur. J. Biochem. *27*:153, 1972.
98. Riddick, D. H., Kregenow, F., and Orloff, I.: Fed. Proc. *28*:339, 1969.
99. Rogers, J. C., Boldt, D., Kornefeld, S., Skinner, A., and Valeri, C. R.: Proc. Natl. Acad. Sci. USA *69*:1685, 1972.
100. Rosenfeld, M. C., Abrass, I. B., Mendelsohn, J., Roos, B. A., Boone, R. F., and Garren, L. D.: Proc. Natl. Acad. Sci. USA *69*:2306, 1972.
101. Salzman, E. W.: N. Engl. J. Med. *286*:358, 1972.
102. Schild, H. O.: Q. J. Exp. Physiol. *26*:165, 1936.
103. Sharon, N., and Lis, H.: Science *177*:949, 1972.
104. Smith, J. W., Steiner, A., Newberry, W. M., Jr., and Parker, C. W.: Fed. Proc. *28*:566(Abstr.) 1969.
105. Smith, J. W., Steiner, A., Newberry, W. M., Jr., and Parker, C. W.: J. Clin. Invest. *50*:432, 1971.
106. Smith, J. W., Steiner, A., and Parker, C. W.: J. Clin. Invest. *50*:442, 1971.
107. Strom, T. B., Deisseroth, A., Morganroth, J., Carpenter, C. B., and Merrill, G. P.: Proc. Natl. Acad. Sci. USA *69*:2995, 1972.
108. Sullivan, T., Parker, K., Stenson, W., Eisen, S. A., and Parker, C. W.: Clin. Res. *20*:797, 1972.
109. Tabachnick, I. I. A., Gulgenkian, A., and Schobert, L. J.: Biochem. Pharmacol. *14*:1283, 1965.
110. Tasaka, K., Ende, K., and Yamasaki, M.: Jpn. J. Pharmacol. *22*:89, 1972.
111. Tauber, A. I., Kaliner, M., Stechschulte, D. J., and Austen, K. F.: J. Immunol. *111*:27, 1973.
112. Wallen, W. C., Dean, J. H., and Lucas, D. O.: Cell. Immunol. *6*:110, 1973.
113. Wedner, H. J., Bloom, F. E., and Parker, C. W.: Clin. Res. *20*:798, 1972.
114. Wedner, H. J., Hoffer, B. W., Battenberg, E., Steiner, A. L., and Parker, C. W.: J. Histochem. Cytochem. *20*:293, 1972.
115. Wedner, M. J., Hoffer, B. W., Bloom, F. E., and Parker, C. W.: Fed. Proc. *32*:744, 1973.
116. Weinstein, Y., Melmon, K., Bourne, H. R., and Sela, M.: J. Clin. Invest. *52*:1349, 1973.
117. Weiss, I. W., Morgan, K., and Phang, I. M.: J. Biol. Chem. *247*:760, 1972.
118. Weissmann, G., Dukor, P., and Zurier, R. B.: Nature (New Biol.) *231*:

131, 1971.
119. Weissmann, G., Zurier, R. B., and Hoffstein, S.: Am. J. Pathol. *68*:539, 1972.
120. Weissmann, G., Zurier, R. B., Spjeler, P. J., and Goldstein, I. M.: J. Exp. Med. *134*:149S, 1971.
121. Winchurch, R., and Actor, P.: J. Immunol. *108*:1305, 1972.
122. Winchurch, R., Ishizuka, M., Webb, D., and Braun, W.: J. Immunol. *106*: 1399, 1971.
123. Wolfe, S. M., and Shulman, N. R.: Biochem. Biophys. Res. Commun. *41*: 128, 1970.
124. Yamamoto, I., Shimamura, T., and Plescia, O. J.: Fed. Proc. *33*:794, 1974.
125. Yamamoto, I., and Webb, D. R.: Proc. Natl. Acad. Sci. USA *72*:2320, 1975.
126. Zurier, R. B., Hoffstein, S., and Weissmann, G.: J. Cell. Biol. *58*:27, 1973.
127. Zurier, R. B., Tynant, N., and Weissmann, G.: Fed. Proc. *32*:744, 1973.

Chapter 10

Non-Antibody Lymphocyte Activation Products (Lymphokines)

When a thymus-derived lymphocyte (T cell) encounters a specific antigen, it is triggered to release soluble non-antibody proteins known as lymphokines. Lymphokines exhibit a number of biological activities and can be distinguished from classical immunoglobulins by several physicochemical criteria. Their biological activity is retained after removal of the antigen that stimulated their formation and does not require further supplementation of specific antigen at the time of test (23).

Current interest in lymphokines arises from the proposition that they may act as molecular mediators of cellular immune response.

1. LYMPHOKINES AS MEDIATORS OF CELLULAR IMMUNE RESPONSE

The biological and clinical significance of the cellular immune response derives from its important role in the following processes: resistance to facultative and obligate intracellular infections, delayed hypersensitivity and allograft rejection, autoimmune disease, tumor growth control, and enhancement of antibody production. Available evidence indicates no mandatory participation of classical humoral antibodies in these phenomena which result, it seems, from a direct interaction between sensitized T cells and antigen present in the local biological environment (10,21,23,55). Thus, it appears that the cell-mediated immune response can be considered in terms of the inflammatory, surveillant and adjuvant functions of the T cell, mobilized by the above interaction.

However, during the past few years, it has become evident that T lymphocytes can also perform their functions through an indirect pathway involving lymphokine formation (33). This was first proved by the demonstration that cell-free leukocyte extracts can transfer delayed hypersensitivity in man (31) and that products of antigen-lymphocyte interaction in guinea pig were able to inhibit the migration of guinea-pig macrophages in vitro (8,12,16).

Experimental analysis of cell-mediated immune phenomena points to the role of cellular interactions between a few specifically sensitized lymphocytes and the majority of other host cells participating in these responses (other lymphocytes, macrophages, polymorphs). The transfer of delayed hypersensitivity occurs when sensitized donor lymphocytes cooperate with unsensitized recipient lymphoid cells but a minority of donor cells is present at the site of recipient's reaction (56). High cellular response, observable on clonal view of lymphocyte sensitization, has been demonstrated in lymphocyte transformation by antigen (34), suggesting the same type of lymphocyte cooperation. This phenomenon is also likely to occur during the cellular response in lymph nodes involved in the development of delayed hypersensitivity when considerable paracortical hyperplasia is evident on clonal view alone (56). The inhibition of macrophage migration by antigen does not occur if lymphocytes are removed (8,52), thus suggesting a cooperation between sensitized lymphocytes and macrophages. A number of other recent experimental reports (19,24,37,48,57,58) indicate that certain macrophage functions may be performed efficiently or may be modulated by effects of lymphokines in a microenvironment. These observations are consistent with the hypothesis that lymphokines could serve as mediators of cellular immunity, facilitating cellular interactions, which reproduce—at least partially—some of the features of delayed hypersensitivity and, therefore, play an important role in both the manifestations and regulation of cellular immune response. It must be stressed, however, that lymphokines have not yet been proved to meet all the classical criteria needed to qualify them as chemical mediators. Thus, for instance, it has yet to be shown that they are present in vivo at the site of the cell-mediated immune reaction and that agents which specifically block lymphokine action would also suppress the induction or manifestation of cellular immune response in vivo (7).

When lymphocytes from suitably sensitized animals or man are cultured with the sensitizing antigen, culture supernatants develop a number of biological activities for which the generic term of lymphokines was coined (23). Similar biological phenomena occur during lymphocyte activation by certain phytomitogen lectins (35,42, 44). Several different biological activities have been described; the principal ones are listed in Table 15 which also enumerates the biological reactions revealing these activities and the features of cellular immune response which may involve the action of individual lymphokines. Although current biochemical evidence suggests that the latter consist of anionic proteins or glycoproteins and are partially separable (14), the extent of their heterogeneity has not been established. In support of the relevance of lymphokines to the cellular immune response, simple biochemical fractionations indicate that some of their activities are concentrated in chromatographic and electrophoretic fractions, which is not where, for instance, classical immunoglobulins are found (18,22,23,44,46,47). For purposes of a working classification of the non-antibody lymphocyte activation products, it was suggested (19) that they consist of two components: lymphokines and transfer (or transfer-like) factors. When the antigen responsible for their formation is removed, lymphokines still retain their activity which persists without further specific antigen being added at the time of test. The transfer (or transfer-like) factors are dialysable or undialysable moieties extracted from sensitized lymphoid cells or released by short-term lymphocyte culture containing specific antigen. As opposed to lymphokines, these factors are antigen-dependent since specific sensitizing antigen must be introduced into the test system for their activity to be maintained (1,51,59). Recent evidence suggests that this activity resides entirely or partly in a species of double-stranded RNA low molecular weight (15) (Table 15).

TABLE 15. Biological activities of non-antibody lymphocyte activation products

Name	Method Revealing Biological Activity	Aspects of Cellular Immune Response Involving Given Factor	References
Lymphocyte-mitogenic factor	Enhancement of DNA synthesis	Lymphocyte transformation; recruitment of non-committed lymphocytes into metabolic activity at effector site	14, 18, 23, 29, 36, 59, 62
Skin-reactive factor	Assay of inflammatory response to intradermal injection	Increased vascular permeability and cellular immigration in delayed hypersensitivity	14, 18, 23, 38
Migration-inhibition factor	Inhibition of polymorphs and macrophage migration from cell explants in capillary tubes	Retention of emigrated cells at effector site	8, 12, 14, 16, 52, 53
Chemotactic factor	Accelerated passage of polymorphs and macrophages through millipore membrane	Enhancement of cell migration to effector sites	14, 61

Macrophage-activating factor	Enhancement of metabolic, phagocytic and microbicidal capacity of cultured macrophages	Increase in acquired cellular resistance of macrophages	4, 14, 25, 40
Lymph-node-activating factor	Intralymphatic injection increases weight and paracortical cellularity of lymph nodes	Facilitation of lymphocyte trapping and activation	17, 20, 30
Transfer factor(s)	Mitogenic, migration inhibition, inflammatory, "transfer" of delayed hypersensitivity	Mediators of adoptive sensitization for T-cell responses	1, 5, 9, 13, 15, 51, 54, 59
Interferon-like factors	Interference with virus pathogenicity in cell culture	Non-specific resistance to viral infection	14, 27

TABLE 16. Possible biological significance of lymphokines

Cellular Immune Responses in Vivo	Possible Lymphokines Involved
Inflammatory response: delayed hypersensitivity, graft versus host reactions, allograft rejection, granuloma formation	Skin reactive factor, chemotactic factor, lymphocyte-mitogenic factor, macrophage-activating factor
Surveillance response: restriction of parasite multiplication and tumor growth, destruction of parasitized host cells	Macrophage-activating factor, migration-inhibition factor, interferon-like factor
Adjuvant response: potentiation of cell-mediated immune response, promotion of autoimmune response, enhancement of antibody production	Lymphocyte-mitogenic factor, lymph-node-activating factor, macrophage-activating factor

2. BIOLOGICAL SIGNIFICANCE OF LYMPHOKINES

It may be proposed that in the presence of specific antigen, transfer factor and related, antigen-dependent materials induce non-committed T cells to generate lymphokines which—produced by adoptively and actively sensitized lymphocytes—act to amplify and regulate the inflammatory, surveillant and adjuvant manifestations of cellular immune response (1,3,5,9,13,15,51,54,59) (Table 16).

As mentioned before, at present there is only indirect evidence available that non-antibody lymphocyte activation products obtained under in vitro conditions are the actual mediators of cellular immune reactions in vivo. In absence of definite proof, the role of lymphokines in vivo is, nevertheless, suggested by several experimental observations.

Intralymphatic injection of purified lymphokines causes an increase in the weight and cellular content of draining lymph nodes (30). Highly purified migration inhibition factor is able to prevent the growth of a transplantable tumor in an otherwise susceptible host (6). Overwhelming evidence indicates that lymphokines stimulate several macrophage functions (5,8,26,39,40,41,43,45) and the important role played by these cells in delayed hypersensitivity and other chronic inflammatory lesions is well known. Furthermore, there is direct proof that lymphokines mediate the interaction between lymphocytes and macrophages in immune reactions (19,24, 57, 58). Lymphokine-like materials have been found in synovial fluids and in supernatants of explants from inflamed synovial tissues in patients with arthritis (49,50). Lymphokine production in vivo has been demonstrated in the following: lymph nodes of sensitized sheep injected with purified protein derivative (PPD) (28), extracts of delayed hypersensitivity skin-reaction sites (11), and synovial membrane cultures of joints from rabbit with antigen-induced arthritis (50). Lymphokine-rich supernatants caused synovitis when injected into rabbit joints (2) and an inflammatory reaction when injected into the skin of guinea pigs (43).

It could be suggested that the lymphokine system plays a role —even if as yet not completely defined—in several manifestations of cellular immune response, which are expressed in vivo as the inflammatory, surveillant and adjuvant effects of activated T lymphocytes.

REFERENCES

1. Amos, H. and Lachmann, P. J.: Immunology *18*:415, 1970.
2. Andries, M., Stastny, P., and Ziff, M.: Arthritis Rheum. *17*:537, 1974.
3. Baram, P., and Condoulis, W.: J. Immunol. *104*:769, 1970.
4. Barnet, K., Pekarek, J., and Hohanovsky, J.: Experientia *27*:948, 1968.
5. Bennett, B., and Bloom, B. R.: Proc. Natl. Acad. Sci. USA *59*:756, 1968.
6. Bernstein, I. D., Thor, D. E., Zhar, B., and Rapp, H. L.: Science *172*:729, 1971.
7. Bloom, B. R.: Adv. Immunol. *14*:340, 1971.
8. Bloom, B. R., and Bennett, B.: Science *153*:80, 1966.
9. Burnet, F. M.: J. Allergy, Clin. Immunol. *54*:1, 1974.
10. Cerottine, J. C., and Dumonde, D. C.: In "Progress in Immunology," B. Amos, ed. Academic Press, New York, 1971, p. 1459.
11. Cohen, S., Ward, P. A.,Yoshida, T., and Burek, C. L.: Immunol. *9*:363, 1973.
12. David, J. R.: Proc. Natl. Acad. Sci USA *56*:72, 1966.
13. David, J. R.: N. Engl. J. Med *288*:143, 1973.
14. David, J. R., and David, R. R.: Prog. Allergy *16*:300, 1972.
15. Dressler, D., and Rosenfeld, S.: Proc. Natl. Acad. Sci USA *71*:4429, 1974.
16. Dumonde, R. C.: Br. Med. Bull. *23*:9, 1967.
17. Dumonde, D. C.: In "Sixth International Symposium on Immunopathology," P. A. Miescher, ed. Schwabe, Basel, 1971, p. 289.
18. Dumonde, D. C., Howson, W. T., and Wolstencroft, R. A.: In "Immunopathology: 5th International Symposium," P. A. Miescher and P. Grabar, eds. Schwabe, Basel, 1968, p. 263.
19. Dumonde, D. C., Kelly, R. H., Preston, P. M., and Wolstencroft, R. A.: in "Mononuclear Phagocytes in Immunity, Infection and Pathology," R. Van Furth, ed. Blackwell, Oxford, 1975, p. 675.

20. Dumonde, D. C., Kelly, R. H., and Wolstencroft, R. A.: In "Microenvironmental Aspects of Immunity," B. D. Jankovic and K. Isakovic, eds Plenum Press, 1973, p. 705.
21. Dumonde, D. C., and Maini, R. N.: Clin. Allergy 1:123, 1971.
22. Dumonde, D. C., Page, D. A., Matthew, M., and Wolstencroft, R. A.: Clin. Exp. Immunol. 10:25, 1972.
23. Dumonde, D. C., Wolstencroft, R. A., Panayi, G. S., Matthew, M., Morley, J., and Howson, W. T.: Nature 224:38, 1969.
24. Feldmann, M., Schrader, J. W., and Bolyston, A.: in "Mononuclear Phagocytes in Immunity, Infection and Pathology," R. Van Furth, ed. Blackwell, Oxford, 1975, p. 779.
25. Godal, T., Rees, R. J. W., and Lamvik, J. O.: Clin. Exp. Immunol. 8:625, 1971.
26. Granger, G. A., and Kolb, W. P.: J. Immunol. 101:111, 1968.
27. Green, J. A., Cooperband, S. R., Rutstein, J. A., and Kibrick, S.: J. Immunol. 105:48, 1970.
28. Hay, J. D., Lachman, P. J., and Traka, S.: Eur. J. Immunol. 3:127, 1973.
29. Kasakura, S.: J. Immunol. 105:1162, 1970.
30. Kelly, R. H., Wolstencroft, R. A., Dumonde, D. C., and Balfour, B. M.: Clin. Exp. Immunol. 10:49, 1972.
31. Lawrence H.: In "Ciba Foundation Symposium on Cellular Aspects of Immunity," G. E. W. Wolstenholme, ed. Churchill, London, 1960, p. 243.
32. Lawrence, H. S.:Adv. Immunol. 11:195, 1969.
33. Lawrence, H. S., and Landy, M. (Eds.): "Mediators of Cellular Immunity." Academic Press, New York, 1969.
34. Ling, N. R.: "Lymphocyte Stimulation." North-Holland, Amsterdam, 1968.
35. Mackler, B. F., Wolstencroft, R. A., and Dumonde, D. C.: Nature (New Biol.) 239:139, 1972.
36. Maini, R. N., Bryceson, A. D. M., Wolstencroft, R. A., and Dumonde, D. C.: Nature 224:43, 1969.
37. McGregor, D. D., and Logie, P. S.: In "Mononuclear Phagocytes in Immunity, Infection and Pathology," R. Van Furth, ed. Blackwell, Oxford, 1975, p. 631.
38. Morley, J., and Wolstencroft, R. A.: Br. J. Pharmacol. 44:334, 1973.
39. Nath, J., Poulter, L. W., and Turk, J. L.: Clin. Exp. Immunol. 13:455, 1973.
40. Nathan, C. F., Karnovsky, M. L., and David, J. R.: J. Exp. Med. 133:1356, 1971.
41. Pantalone, R. M., and Page, R. C.: Proc. Natl. Acad. Sci USA 72:2091, 1975.
42. Pick, E., Brostoff, J., Krejci, J., and Turk, J .L.: Cell. Immunol. 1:92, 1970.
43. Pick, E., Krejci, J., Cech, K., and Turk, J. L.: Immunology 17:741, 1969.
44. Pick, E., Krejci, J., and Turk, J. L.: Nature 225:236, 1970.
45. Pick, E., and Turk, J. L.: Clin. Exp. Immunol. 10:1, 1972.
46. Remold, H. G., and David, J. R.: J. Immunol. 107:1090, 1971.
47. Remold, H. G., Katz, A. B., Haber, E., and David, J. R.: Cell. Immunol. 1:133, 1970.
48. Rosenthal, A. S., Lipsky, P. E., and Shevach, E. M.: In "Mononuclear Phagocytes in Immunity, Infection and Pathology," R. Van Furth, ed. Blackwell, Oxford, 1975, p. 813.

49. Rosenthal, M., Stastny, P., and Ziff, M.: J. Rheumatol. *1*: (Suppl): 30, 1974.
50. Stastny, P., Rosenthal, M., Andreis, M., Cooke, D., and Ziff, M.: Ann. N.Y. Acad. Sci. *256*:117, 1975.
51. Svejcar, J., Pekarek, J., and Johanovsky, J.: Immunology *58*:1, 1968.
52. Søborg, M.: Acta Med. Scand. *185*:221, 1969.
53. Søborg, M., and Bendixen, G.: Acta Med. Scand. *181*:247, 1967
54. Thor, D. E., and Dray, S.: Immunol. *101*:469, 1968.
55. Turk, J. L. (Ed.): Br. Med. Bull. *23* (1), 1967.
56. Turk, J. L.: "Delayed Hypersensitivity." North-Holland, Amsterdam, 1967.
57. Turk, J. L., and Poulter, P. W.: In "Mononuclar Phagocytes in Immunity, Infection and Pathology," R. Van Furth, ed. Blackwell, Oxford, 1975, p. 711.
58. Unanue, E. R.: In "Mononuclear Phagocytes in Immunity, Infection and Pathology," R. Van Furth, ed. Blackwell, Oxford, 1975, p. 721.
59. Valentine, F. T., and Lawrence H. S.: Science *165*:1014, 1969.
60. Vladimarsson, H., Holt, L., Riches, H. R. C., and Hobbs, J. R.: Lancet *1*:1259, 1970.
61. Ward, P. A., Remold, H. G., and David, J. R.: Cell. Immunol. *1*:162, 1970.
62. Wolstencroft, R. A., and Dumonde, D. C.: Immunology *18*:599, 1970.

Chapter 11

Experimental Evaluation of Antiinflammatory Agents

The search for efficacious antirheumatic drugs has been hampered by the lack of satisfactory animal models of the disease. Hopefully, as our understanding of the human syndrome improves, an appropriate animal model can be produced to provide a more rational basis for developing and testing new drugs. However, as a corollary of the search for appropriate models of rheumatic disease, numerous methods were devised for detecting compounds with an antiinflammatory action, and we shall devote this chapter to their discussion. A few of the techniques developed have achieved popularity because of their simplicity, economic feasibility, and ability to identify drugs known to afford some benefit in the clinical management of rheumatoid disease. It must be remembered, however, that such traditional antiinflammatory drugs as phenylbutazone, aspirin, cortisone, gold preparations and chloroquine were discovered without the benefit of these screening procedures.

The most popular methods of assay are discussed here in some detail. Additional information can be found in the following references: 58,62,86,87,137,153,194,215,240,241,242,247,254,257,290,300, 318,319.

1. ERYTHEMA

The method most widely used for detecting antiinflammatory agents involves the erythematous response associated with direct injury to epidermal and subjacent structures—like that induced by ultraviolet light irradiation of depilated skin. It is the only generally accepted assay for this type of drugs that utilizes a species other than the rat as test animal. The technique employed today, represents a modification of the original procedure (305,306). Using guinea pigs, circumscribed areas of skin, depilated at least 12 hours earlier, are exposed to an ultraviolet light for approximately 60 seconds. The erythema that develops is subjectively scored 2-4 hours later on a blind basis. Usually, the data are expressed as "yes or no" response according to the completeness of the circle of erythema and not to its intensity (21).

Two subsequent phases of increased vascular permeability caused by skin exposure to ultraviolet light have been described. The first sets in before any erythema is detectable and is susceptible to antihistamines which are ineffective in modifying the intensity of erythema (162). The latter usually appears 1 hour after exposure to ultraviolet light and reaches a maximum after 2-4 hrs. The second phase of increased vascular permeability begins concomitantly with the erythema but persists longer (113,161). Leukocytes rapidly immigrate to the site of injury that subsequently necroses (161).

Non-steroidal antiinflammatory drugs (with the exception of oxyphenbutazone) defer but do not abolish the erythematous reaction even after repeated dosing. Delays in the vascular-permeability response to ultraviolet light have been achieved with doses of 10 mg/kg and 30 mg/kg, respectively, for phenylbutazone and acetylsalicylic acid (149). The steroids are ineffective in this regard (318). Estimates of relative drug potency in this assay are generally similar to those obtained in carrageenin edema. This test seems also quite specific since a different group of otherwise pharmacologically active agents does not influence the appearance of erythema (313).

Other erythema assays utilizing the ear (269) or flank area of the mouse (234) and ultraviolet light have been described. Erythema has also been induced in both man (2,301) and guinea pig (115) by means of an alcoholic solution of tetrahydrofurfuryl nicotinate. In man, it appears sensitive to aspirin (301), ibuprofen and ibufenac (2). The response in guinea pig is inhibited by low doses of phenylbutazone and salicylate (115).

2. EDEMA

Methods based on the inhibition of a swelling induced in rat paw are among the most popular. The general procedure is to inject a small amount of solution or suspension of an edemogen into the plantar tissues of a hind paw of the rat. The amount of swelling is measured by determining the thickness of the paw (32), its weight (173) or, more frequently, the amount of water (276) or mercury (270,321) that it displaces.

Many different substances have been employed to induce edema: formalin (26,90,166,187,162) dextran (9,44,61,103,116,121, 140,192), kaolin (43,279) egg albumen (9,109,150,310), silver nitrate (154,291), proteolytic enzymes (60,135,229,277), brewers yeast (212). Putative humoral mediators of inflammation have also been utilized for this purpose (24,91,150,193,263,272,291).

The most widely used assay in this category, is certainly the *carrageenin-induced edema,* introduced about 15 years ago (321).

Carrageenin is a mixture of polysaccharides composed of sulfated galactose units and is derived from Irish sea moss, Chondrus crispus (237). Certain physicochemical features are essential for edemogenic activity (168,276). As originally described (321), the assay consists of drug administration followed 60 minutes later by the injection of 0.05 ml of a 1% solution of carrageenin into the plantar tissues of one hind paw. The size of the paw is determined at this time and then 3 and/or 5 hours later. Data are most often expressed as percentage of edema inhibition (Fig. 10).

The edema which develops in rat paw after carrageenin injection is a biphasic event (276). The initial phase is attributed to the release of histamine and serotonin, the edema maintained between the first and the second phase—to kinin-like substances, and the second phase—to prostaglandin-like compounds (53,56). The recognition of different mediators in different phases of the edema has important implications for interpreting drug effects. The histamine-serotonin antagonist, cyproheptadine, is inactive in this assay (276, 317). However, the early phase of the edema can be inhibited by depleting histamine stores with compound 48/80 (53) or by the combined administration of cyproheptadine and an antihistamine (53). In rats, kininogen depletion substantially reduces the intensity of the intermediate phase of the edema, while the administration of antiproteases (55,270) suppresses it altogether. The significance of leucocyte immigration for the full development of carrageenin edema has been acknowledged (271,275). It has also been shown recently (205) that, in the early phases of the edema, the dominant cells are polymorphonuclears whereas in the advanced stages mononuclears predominate. The importance of these latter cells in the advanced phase of carrageenin edema (53), their interrelation with prostaglandin activation (53) and the inhibition of their immigration by non-steroidal antiinflammatory drugs (54) have been stressed. Strain, sex and body weight of the rats are not significant variables in the assay (8). Carrageenin edema is also not influenced by changes in ambient temperature or humidity (85). The effects of drug-induced hypothermia or hypotension are a matter of debate (8,85). It seems, however, that the reduction of blood pressure does influence edema formation. Nonspecific inhibition of carrageenin edema can be obtained with such irritants as hypertonic saline, dilute acetic acid, formalin, kaolin and inflammatory exudate (14,85, 141,285).

Carrageenin edema serves to detect useful antiinflammatory substances (8,56,276). The claim that a number of drugs not usually thought of as antiinflammatory inhibit this edema (185,233) can be ruled out since these compounds have been used at doses producing behavioral or autonomic effects (319). What the appropriate time is for administering the test compound has been a subject of discussion (53,256,276) but, as could be expected, no definite conclusions have been reached. It would, in fact, depend on the half-life of the compound, the phase of the edematous reaction it is likely to inhibit, and the mechanism of its antiedemic action. Furthermore, no clear-cut correlation between either compartment concentration of at least one drug, phenylbutazone, and its antiedemic effect has been observed (107). A plot of dose log versus percentage of edema inhibition has yielded linear and parallel regression lines for standard antiinflammatory drugs (220,266,321), so that this method can be used for a comparative bioassay of drugs (317). (Fig. 10) Other investigators did not obtain similar results (107,283), and this failure may be attributed to a variety of causes discussed in part, previously. Notwithstanding these discrepancies, the carrageenin assay is suited for comparative bioassays of antiinflammatory agents and the relative potency estimates obtained for certain

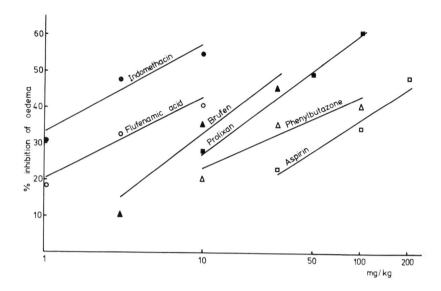

FIG. 10.   Dose-response curves of non-steroidal antiinflammatory drugs in carrageenin edema

drugs seem to reflect clinical experience (Table 17).

Several polyene antibiotics have been reported to induce edema when injected into the plantar tissues of rat paw (12,296). This property supposedly depends on their disrupting the lysosomal membrane (296), which causes release of hydrolytic enzymes contained within the lysosomes. One of these inflammatory reactions— *nystatin-induced edema*—has been described in more detail (10,12). Nystatin (Mycostatin®) is a polyene antifungal antibiotic. When 30.000 I.U. of this agent, in 0.1 ml of sterile saline, are injected into the plantar tissues of rat paws, a long-lasting edema is produced which reaches its peak about 24 hours after the intervention and persists for at least 96 hours (10). The presence of substantial amounts of free lysosomal enzymes in the inflammatory fluid correlates with edema development (10). It seems that immigrated leukocytes (10) are the major source of lysosomal enzymes. Nystatin edema is scarcely susceptible to nonspecific pharmacological effects but is inhibited in dose-dependent manner by steroidal and nonsteroidal antiinflammatory drugs (12). Moreover, it has been

TALE 17. Effect of non-steroidal antiinflammatory drugs in the carrageenin-induced rat-paw edema assay

Drug	Dose mg/kg, p.o.	% Inhibition	Potency* (95% confidence limits)
Phenylbutazone	25.0	27	1
	50.0	39	
	100.0	57	
Acetylsalicylic acid	50.0	23	0.36 (0.13-0.85)
	100.0	32	
	200.0	40	
	400.0	43	
Tolmetin	6.25	38	2.17 (0.82-5.94)
	25.0	40	
	100.0	44	
Naproxen	0.78	16	15.5 (6.6-39.6)
	1.56	40	
	6.25	43	
	25.0	52	
	50.0	60	
Sudoxicam	0.37	7	24.1 (10.2-56.1)
	1.11	30	
	3.33	39	
	10.0	48	
Indomethacin	0.37	29	62.7 (26.1-148.5)
	1.11	38	
	3.33	46	
	10.0	47	

*Weighted linear regression analysis.

found that the administration of antiinflammatory drugs to animals with an already established inflammatory reaction results in a substantial decrease of the edema (227). Nystatin edema is sensitive to the antiinflammatory action of immunosuppressants (12) and gold salts (6). It has been also reported that D-penicillamine has a biphasic effect upon single administration: it inhibits the early phase but enhances the more advanced stage of the edema (6). After repeated administration, it suppresses only the early phase (6) (Fig. 11, 12 and 13).

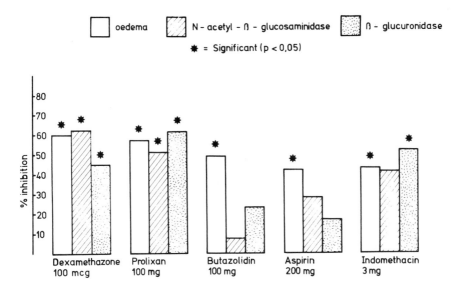

FIG. 11.   Effects of antiinflammatory drugs on nystatin
edema and lysosomal-enzyme content in paw perfusate

3. INFLAMMATORY EXUDATION

The inflammatory exudate has a fluid and a cellular component.
Since leukocyte emigration and plasma-protein leakage do not necessarily take place at the same time and are probably an expression
of different processes, they will be considered separately. *The increase in permeability of small blood vessels* that occurs during an
inflammatory reaction is usually biphasic. The initial phase, which
can be inhibited by antagonists of known endogenous permeability
factors (162), involves primarily the venules, whereas in the delayed prolonged phase capillaries are affected as well (41). In certain types of inflammation, the venules appear to be solely responsible for the delayed phase (122). The latter is generally insensitive
to antagonists of permeability factors. Increased vascular permeability per se and edema formation are, in fact, separate phenomena
(29,42,102,191). Edema can result from a simple elevation of capillary pressure; on the other hand, it should be possible for permeability to augment without producing edema if there is sufficient
circulatory and lymphatic drainage.

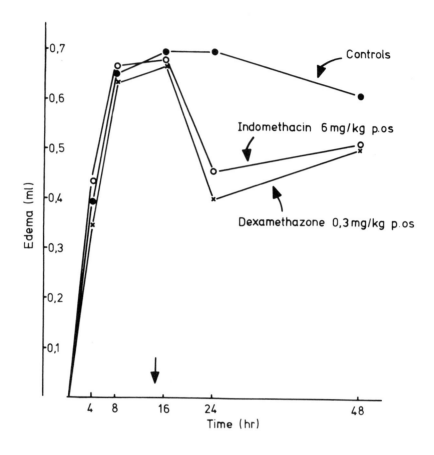

FIG. 12. "Regression" of nystatin edema produced by indomethacin and dexamethazone

The methods most widely used to demonstrate increased vascular permeability are based on the leakage of protein-bound dye into the inflamed area. Azo dyes, such as trypan blue and Evans blue, interact with the basic nitrogens of plasma albumin and, thus, when injected intravenously, are suitable plasma markers for detecting

FIG. 13.   Effects of various agents on nystatin edema
    = inhibition   = enhancement
    O = no effect

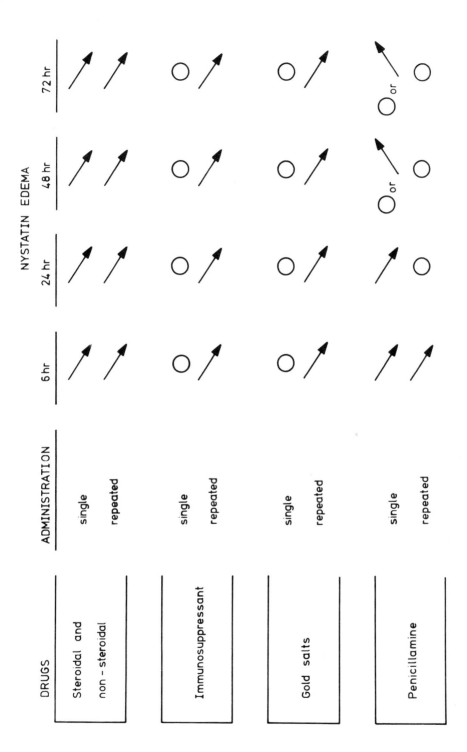

protein leakage into a site of inflammation (325). Methods for extracting dye from its complex with protein are essential for the precise quantification of changes in dye distribution or for measuring its concentration in the inflamed area. Several techniques have been suggested (4,134,142,325) but, for the most part, they are tedious and time consuming. Consequently, many investigators make a semiquantitative assessment of the intensity of blueing of the area or of the size of the surface stained (4,13,249). In addition to vital dyes, plasma protein labeling with [131]I (288) or fluorescein has also been employed (323). When the site of inflammation is located in the peritoneal or pleural cavity, a simple determination of the volume of exudate, especially when combined with protein determination and cell count, can be a satisfactory measure of the degree of inflammation.

Peritoneal and pleural irritation has been achieved with many substances: serotonin, bradykinin, acetic acid, glycogen, carrageenin, formaline, turpentine, silver nitrate, calcium pyrophosphate, and actinomycin D (7,92,96,97,98,99,100,101,102,122,224,225,243, 245,292,311). Extensive examination of turpentine-induced pleurisy in rats has shown that the vascular-permeability response is biphasic, the initial phase being mediated by histamine and inhibited by specific antagonists of this substance. Non-steroidal antiinflammatory drugs seem to be scarcely effective here (282), but antiinflammatory activity of cyclophosphamide, 6-mercaptopurine, methotrexate (253) and antilymphocyte serum (268) has been demonstrated in this model. Inhibition of pleural effusion has been used for a comparative bioassay of antiinflammatory drugs, the irritant employed being a mixture of carrageenin and Evans blue. The relative potency estimates for non-steroidal drugs are in agreement with the data obtained in carrageenin paw edema and adjuvant arthritis (224). The same investigator was able to demonstrate that gold sodium thiomalate is an inhibitor of this experimental pleurisy although at relatively high dosages.

An assessment of increased vascular permeability following intradermal injection of irritants, such as inorganic salts, turpentine or chloroform, or permeability factors, such as kallikrein, bradykinin, histamine, serotonin, prostaglandins or phospholipase A, has been made in many different animal species (5,13,15,37,102, 132,149,155,170,175,206,249,282). This type of assay has not found extensive application in screening antiinflammatory agents which have only a slight or no effect in most of these tests. The application of xylene to mouse ear and subsequent measurement of protein-bound dye has been used with more satisfactory results (29).

The granuloma pouch procedure (52,71,214,230) has been employed to evaluate both the antiexudative and antiproliferative activities of drugs. Subcutaneous injection of a volume of air forms a pouch, usually in the back of rat. Croton oil (230), mycobacterial adjuvant (22), carrageenin (25,83,84), or D-a-tocopherol (96) are then injected into the pouch. The day after, the air is withdrawn and the response is evaluated 4-15 days later, measuring the volume of the fluid and the thickness or weight of the wall of granulomatous tissue. The exudate is not the kind associated with more acute inflammation—it derives primarily from cell destruction. The wall thickness reflects the proliferative component of the response. Steroids appear superior to non-steroids in their action against either component. It should be noted, however, that the weak activity of non-steroidal drugs can be better demonstrated in respect to the proliferative response, whereas the effect of steroids is more evident on the exudative component (64,83,84,133). Similar assays include the carrageenin abscess or hygroma method (18,33,64,100).

As with methods where activity is measured by protein exudation, nearly any inflamed site may be used to determine the degree of *cellular immigration*. This aspect of the inflammatory process has, probably, not received the great attention it deserves as a possible approach to assessing potential antirheumatic activity. Cell counts and types can be determined in peritoneal or pleural exudates (7,54,92,312).

The skin-window technique, which consist of placing a cover slip on an abraded area of skin and determining the number and types of cells that have adhered to it after a specified time, has been used in animals (54,213,278) and in humans (213). This method, apparently, has not been extensively adopted for testing antiinflammatory drugs.

Two other procedures for evaluating the effect of drugs on cellular immigration have been described. The first estimates the number and kinds of cells emigrating into a plastic sponge or cotton pellet implanted subcutaneously in the rat (226,267). Here phenylbutazone, hydrocortisone and immunosuppressives were found active. The second method assesses the degree of cellular immigration into the granuloma pouch as a measure of drug activity (52,131, 274).

Recently, a more sophisticated approach has been described (205,206). Immigration of exogenous ^{51}Cr-labeled neutrophils or mononuclears is determined in amputed, carrageenin-inflamed paw by direct scintillation count. It has been found that steroidal drugs inhibit chemotaxis of both cell types, while non-steroidal drugs suppress that of mononuclears but not of neutrophils.

4. INFLAMMATORY GRANULATION

The repair phase of inflammation—characterized by the proliferation of fibroblasts and multiplication of small blood vessels—typically occurs after the vascular and exudative changes. Several methods for evaluating antiinflammatory activity of compounds, based on preventing the formation of granulation tissue, have been described (1,48,58,63,143,157,171,172,289,317). The *cotton pellet granuloma* inhibition assay (171), subsequently modified (36, 70,172,314,322), is, perhaps, the most widely used method.

The size of the cotton pellet varies from a few milligrams to 50 mg. The amount of granulation tissue has been claimed to depend on the size (322) or surface (20) of the pellet. The site of implantation is, as a rule, the subcutaneous tissue on the back or flanks of the rat. The proliferative phase of the response is well established one week after implantation (46) and the antiinflammatory activity of new compounds is usually assessed at this time by measuring the dry weight of the granulomas.

Three phases of the inflammatory response to subcutaneous implantation of pellets have been described (258). The first, short-lasting phase, of a few hours duration, is characterized by the imbibition of the pellet with fluid of low-protein content. Exudation of fluid containing protein is typical for the second phase which lasts 2-3 days. The last phase is proliferative and is characterized by the appearance of collagen in granuloma, preceded by mucopolysaccharide synthesis, and accompanied by the greatest increase in the number of fibroblasts.

It seems that the cotton pellet granuloma assay is a relatively good test for evaluating the antiinflammatory activity of steroids but is less satisfactory for non-steroidal compounds (63,314,315, 316). Certain immunosuppressive drugs are also capable of inhibiting granuloma formation, apparently by an intrinsic antiinflammatory activity (253,267). The endocrine status of the animals (172), impairment of body growth with catabolic steroids or anorexigens (51) or administration of glycolytic metabolic inhibitors (101) have been found to "nonspecifically" prevent granuloma formation.

The granulations developed after subcutaneous injection of

carrageenin in guinea pigs (17,148) and rats (120,210) have been used to study the biochemical aspects of connective tissue formation. It seems that antiinflammatory steroids are more active on the ground substance than on the fibrous component of connective tissue (59,160,235).

5. EXPERIMENTAL ARTHRITIS

Several different types of experimental arthritis can be induced in animals. Their similarity to human disease is matter of debate. However, not entirely unsuccessful attempts have been made to devise animal models of the various rheumatoid diseases. *Adjuvant-induced arthritis in rat* is probably the best and most widely used of these "models," employed in screening programs for antiinflammatory drugs (73,82,139,152,163,164,183,184,195,198,200,202, 209,232,254,280,281,285,286,287).

It has been suggested that adjuvant-induced arthritis in rat constitutes a delayed hypersensitivity response to mycobacterial antigens, probably represented by the wax D fraction of mycobacteria. Evidence in favor of this hypothesis includes the following: transmission of the disease to normal animals by sensitized lymphocytes from afflicted animals, prevention of disease by excision of lymph nodes draining the site of adjuvant injection, immunity in animals exposed to tolerogenic doses of adjuvant early in life (198,200,280,281). It has been also suggested that adjuvant arthritis is an autoimmune disease, the altered collagen or a combination of the wax D fraction with a tissue constituent being the responsible antigen (165,201,223,250). The hypothesis that adjuvant disease is the result of latent PPLO or other infection did not find much support since antibiotics proved ineffective and it is possible to induce the disease in germ-free animals (139,144,145,211) (Table 18).

Killed mycobacteria (M. butyricum, M. tubercolosis, M. phlei), suspended or emulsified in mineral or paraffin oil (0.2-1.0 mg of mycobacteria in 0.1 ml), are injected intradermally into rat tail or hind paw. According to some authors (204,312), the tail is the preferred site of injection. The time course of the disease has been described (196,198). When the hind paw is injected, it shows a pronounced swelling shortly afterward which then persists for several weeks. This is usually considered a primary reaction. A few days after the injection (from 7 to 15 days, depending on the strain of animal used), the contralateral paw as well as the front paws

TABLE 18. Adjuvant arthritis

Mineral Oil + Killed M. Butyricum

Primary reaction	— At site of injection
	— Few hours after injection
	— Severe edema, granulation (necrosis)
	— Very long lasting
Secondary reaction	— At distal sites (small joints)
	— 10-15 days after injection
	— Edema, lymphocyte infiltration
	— Fibroblast proliferation, synovitis, pannus, very long lasting
Delayed hypersensitivity reaction	— Latency period
	— Disease transferred by thoracic duct lymphocytes
	— Suppressive effect of draining-lymph-node excision and whole-body irradiation
"Active" Drugs	— Steroids
	— Aspirin like compounds
	— Gold salts
	— Immunosuppressants

swell, and "arthritic" nodules appear on the ears and tail. This is, strictly speaking, the syndrome termed "adjuvant arthritis," i.e., the delayed systemic response. The reaction that occurs at the injection site does not have the same significance as the disseminated arthritis. Remissions and exacerbations of the disease have been reported (203). Hematological (286), biochemical (3,93,95) and histopathological changes (35,110,139,198,200) have been recorded. Various strains of rats differ in their response to the injection of an arthritogenic adjuvant (95,216,223,326), the most sensitive being inbred Lewis rats. Young and old animals are relatively resistant to the disease, probably because they seem to be immunologically compromised (49,96,304).

The most objective measurement for assessing the course of the disease and the effects of antiinflammatory drugs is the determination of the magnitude of swelling of the hind paws (321). If the adjuvant has been injected into the plantar tissue of one hind paw, then the edema of that paw may be used to evaluate the in-

TABLE 19. Parameters for assessing course of adjuvant
arthritis and/or drug interaction

Parameter	References
Arthritic lesions	286, 250, 47
Joint "score" or other scoring methods	104, 31, 216, 198
Hind-paw size	320, 183, 312, 228, 6
Grip strength	207
Paw temperature	284
Joint histopathology	209
Erythrocyte sedimentation rate	209
Albumin/globulin ratio	95, 209
Plasma fibrinogen	209, 95
Heat-coagulable protein (inflammation units)	95, 11
Lysosomal enzyme activity	208

flammatory response to the injection of the adjuvant and the increase in the size of the other paw to estimate the delayed, immunologically mediated component of the disease. The degree of joint involvement (138,211,286), the subjective scoring of the incidence and severity of the lesions on the paws, ears and tail (31, 104,147,216), and the grip of the animals (207,284) have also been used to assess the severity of the disorder. Some other parameters have been employed to describe its course and/or the effect of drugs on the syndrome. These are summarized in Table 19.

As previously mentioned, the development of adjuvant arthritis depends on the presence and functional integrity of lymphocytes. The arthritic syndrome can be alleviated or prevented by: lymphocytotoxic drugs and antilymphocyte globulin (47), removal of lymphocytes by cannulation of the thoracic duct (303), neonatal thymectomy (223), and extirpation of the lymph nodes draining the site of adjuvant injection (95,184,222). Furthermore, pharmacological doses of estrogens (264,284), thyroidectomy (251) and alloxan diabetes (146) alleviate the disease. The latter may also be inhibited through immunosuppression by antigenic competition (89,108,130, 201, 203) (Table 20).

The severity of the disorder may be modified by steroidal and non-steroidal antiinflammatory drugs (104,167,183,199,209,228,239, 286,320). Agents able to interfere with immunological reactions will be discussed in Chapters 17, 18 and 19.

The effect of drugs on the established disease (104,167,228,

TABLE 20. ED_{50} and relative potency of several antiinflammatory agents as measured by therapeutic test in arthritic rats

Drug	$ED_{50} \pm$ S.E. mg/Kg	Relative Potency (95% confidence limits)
Phenylbutazone	13.27 ± 2.68	1
Aspirin	279.00 ± 24.60	0.04 (0.03-0.07)
Aminopyrine	129.95 ± 25.28	0.13 (0.08-0.23)
Mefenamic acid	20.10 ± 5.77	0.88 (0.47-1.66)
Hydrocortisone	12.42 ± 3.03	1.02 (0.56-1.87)
Prednisolone	3.49 ± 0.96	3.61 (1.92-6.77)
Indomethacin	0.22 ± 0.05	57.4 (33.7- 102)

312) has been determined since this may be more relevant to the clinical situation. Other investigators have chosen "prophylactic" treatment (104,204,219,285) which can serve to detect both antiinflammatory and immunosuppressive substances. Cyclophosphamide, however, has proved active both as a prophylatic and therapeutic agent (6,11), suggesting, together with other findings, that this compound is endowed with true antiinflammatory properties. Valid comparative bioassays for non-steroidal antiinflammatory drugs have been performed both after prophylactic or therapeutic administration (104,312,320). The amount of either steroidal or non-steroidal antiinflammatory substances needed to produce a significant effect on adjuvant-induced arthritis seems to correlate with the doses clinically active in humans (286,312). Indomethacin is, perhaps, overestimated in the above assay, but it is known that the rat is peculiarly sensitive to the therapeutic and toxic effects of this drug (286,320).

Whether gold preparations are efficacious in adjuvant arthritis is a matter of debate. Both positive (88,138) and negative (6,183, 285) findings have been reported. The results obtained with chloroquine are more consistent and indicate that this compound is rather inactive (104,183,207,286).

Infective, chemical, endocrine, immunological and physical means have been employed to experimentally induce arthritis in animals (57,86,136,197,248,290,318). Very few of these methods, however, have been used to evaluate new antirheumatic compounds. However, examples of the above procedures that will be mentioned here are 6-sulfanylamidoindazole (6-SAI)-induced arthritis in rats and antigen-induced arthritis in rabbits.

Several oral or subcutaneous administrations of 6-SAI to adult rats regularly resulted in acute, self-limiting arthritis and peri-arthritis confined primarily to the hind paws (174,177). The onset of the disease becomes apparent 5-9 days after the beginning of 6-SAI treatment; the maximum inflammatory response occurs about the 11th-13th day; the inflammatory reaction subsides by about the 25th days (174,177,231). The incidence of this arthritis is related to the dose of 6-SAI and the age of the animals. Monkeys and mice are reported not to develop the disease (174). Histologically, the lesions are not suppurative and proliferative. Lymphocytes are present in all stages of inflammation, preceding the appearance of fibroblasts which are the more consistent and striking cellular components (177). The "arthritogenic" effect of 6-SAI is independent of: crystal formation in the periarticular tissues, provocation of latent mycoplasma infections, kinin production through activation of the Hageman factor, immediate or delayed hypersensitivity response, and induction of an anaphylactoid reaction (38,177,331). Steroidal and non-steroidal antiinflammatory drugs prevent paw swelling in rats given 6-SAI. Chloroquine, gold preparations and certain immunosuppressives (with the exception of cycloleucine) are ineffective in this case (217,231) (Table 21).

Animal models in which inflammatory arthritis is produced by immunological mechanisms constitute particularly attractive tools for investigating the pathophysiology of the rheumatoid process and the possible effects of therapeutic agents on this disease.

Because the cellular infiltrate in adjuvant arthritis is qualitatively different from that of rheumatoid synovitis, interest was aroused in *antigen-induced arthritis in rabbits*. This model has certain important features that suggest it may be a satisfactory research tool. It is immunologically induced, the resulting synovitis is associated with a pronounced local response in which lymphocytes and plasma cells predominate, and becomes a chronic condition, often lasting several months (65,97,98,136). Heterologous fibrin (65), egg albumin (39,299), bovine-serum albumin (40), autologous and homologous IgG derivatives (99) have been used to induce chronic synovitis. Mediators of cellular immunity are produced by cells accumulating in the chronically inflamed synovial tissue, which supports the view that a local immune response to retained antigen plays an important role in maintaining the chronic inflammatory process (136). Furthermore, in the case of IgG-induced arthritis it was shown that only in those animals which demonstrated cellular immunity by skin hypersensitivity and inhibition of macrophage migration was it possible to cause significant synovitis (99). Very

TABLE 21. Effect of antiinflammatory agents on 6-SAI*-induced periarthritis in rats

Drug	Dose	Mean Dorsoplantar Hind-paw Diameter on Day 12
	mg/kg p.o.	mm ± S.E.
No treatment		3.7 ± 0.03
6-SAI (Control)	125	0.1 ± 0.43
6-SAI + phenylbutazone	25	3.8 ± 0.04
	10	3.8 ± 0.10
6-SAI + oxyphenbutazone	50	3.8 ± 0.06
	25	3.9 ± 0.08
6-SAI + sulfinpyrazone	25	3.9 ± 0.08
6-SAI + indomethacin	0.5	3.9 ± 0.05
6-SAI + acetylsalicylic acid	200	4.4 ± 0.2
6-SAI + paramethasone	0.25	3.6 ± 0.04
6-SAI + hydrocortisone	5	3.8 ± 0.05
6-SAI + 6-mercaptopurine	3	7.6 ± 0.58
6-SAI + methotrexate	0.5	5.9 ± 1.34
6-SAI + chloroquine	10	7.2 ± 0.77

*6-SAI = 6-sulfanylamidoindazole
6-SAI was given at a daily dose of 125 mg/kg p.o. for 12 days. The test agents were administered daily at the doses indicated, commencing 1 day prior to the beginning of 6-SAI treatment.

little information concerning the effect of drugs on the above syndrome is available at present (99,299). However, cortisone, phenylbutazone, antilymphocyte serum, but not cyclophosphamide and chloroquine, are active in this test.

6. IN VITRO METHODS OF ASSAY

Many of the assay methods discussed below have been developed after the discovery of some special property of a given class of known antiinflammatory drugs, which could be exploited for screening compounds of the same type. Therefore, these methods seem of particular value for the rapid evaluation of a series of compounds whose prototype has been demonstrated to be antiinflammatory by other means.

A screening method for non-steroidal antiinflammatory drugs, based on the *inhibition of protein denaturation*, has been proposed

(178,179,180). Phenylbutazone and salicylate in concentrations comparable to those which can be attained in sera of rheumatoid patients were effective inhibitors of protein denaturation (181). Antimalarial antirheumatics, antihistamines, immunosuppressives and steroids failed to inhibit denaturation (105,181). It may be assumed that the effects on denaturation are a consequence of drug-binding to a specific site of the albumin molecule (302). It has also been found that the results of this test correlate with those obtained in ultraviolet erythema (181) and urate-crystal-induced synovitis but not with drug activity in carrageenin edema (106).

An inhibitory effect of non-steroidal antiinflammatory drugs on *erythrocyte lysis* has been described. The action of these compounds has been evaluated on heat-induced hemolysis of canine red blood cells (27,28) and on hypotonic lysis of human red blood cells (129). It is likely that the erythrocyte-stabilizing assay represents another form of the protein-stabilizing test previously mentioned. Its specificity is doubtful, however, since phenothiazines, barbiturates and serotonin antagonists, such as LSD-25, have a similar activity (27, 28). Furthermore, this assay does not distinguish between analogs of indomethacin that have very different in vivo effects and, in general, it seems to have little predictive value (94).

In view of the numerous reports on the role of released lysosomal materials as mediators of inflammation, evaluation of drug *effects on lysosomes* has been suggested as a possible in vitro assay. Early studies had illustrated that certain glucocorticoids and chloroquine inhibit, in vitro, the release of acid hydrolases from isolated rat and rabbit liver lysosome fractions (294,295,297,298). More recently, several non-steroidal antiinflammatory drugs were demonstrated to stabilize, in vitro, lysosomes of rat and rabbit liver and of polymorphonuclear leukocytes (124,125,126,128,176,261). Other reports, however, revealed some inconsistencies in these findings (30,159). The conditions of the assay appear to be of particular importance (123), especially, the use of the "heavy" lysosomal fraction (3500 g), employment of a buffer during lysosome isolation and maintaining a relatively low sucrose concentration during enzyme release (124,298). Moreover, it has been found that the "stabilizing" effect of both steroidal and non-steroidal antiinflammatory drugs on lysosomes from human polymorphonuclear leukocytes is more marked when the cells are previously incubated with serum-treated zymosan particles (127) (Table 22).

Platelet aggregation induced in vitro by thrombin, collagen, connective tissue particles, antigen-antibody complexes or IgG-

TABLE 22. Effect of antiinflammatory drugs on the stability of human neutrophil lysosomes in vitro

	% Inhibition of β-Glucuronidase Release	
Drug	Untreated Neutrophils 10^{-6}M	Zymosan-treated Neutrophils 10^{-6}M
Methylprednisolone sodium succinate	14 ± 1.1	53 ± 4.9
Hydrocortisone sodium succinate	12 ± 0.8	32 ± 3.4
Paramethasone acetate	7 ± 0.9	33 ± 3.0
Phenylbutazone	16 ± 1.4	30 ± 2.8
Indomethacin	11 ± 1.0	32 ± 3.4
Acetylsalicylic Acid	9 ± 0.9	29 ± 2.4
Chloroquine phosphate	5 ± 0.4	3 ± 1.3
Gold sodium thiomalate	1 ± 0.2	3 ± 0.8
Paracetamol (Acetaminophen)	5 ± 0.8	4 ± 0.8

coated polystyrene particles is inhibited by aspirin (66,293,328), phenylbutazone (74,189,190), indomethacin and fenamic acids (188,328). To determine the effects of antiinflammatory drugs, aliquots of platelet-rich plasma are incubated with the test compound for various periods of time. Aggregation is then induced by the addition of appropriate substances (328). When ADP is used for this purpose, secondary but not primary aggregation is inhibited by antiinflammatory drugs (327). Consequently, the protocol of the experiment must be changed.

The in vitro measurement of the *inhibition of prostaglandin biosynthesis* as an assay for non-steroidal antiinflammatory compounds has acquired great popularity after it was observed that these drugs inhibit prostaglandin release from human platelets (238) and perfused dog spleen (69), and suppress prostaglandin

TABLE 23. Inhibition of prostaglandin synthesis in homogenates or subcellular fractions I_{50} concentrations of some aspirin-like drugs*

Enzyme Preparation	Prostaglandin	Meclofenamic acid	Niflumic acid	Indomethacin	Mefenamic acid	Flufenamic acid	Naproxen	Phenylbutazona	Acetylsalicylic acid	Ibuprofen
Cell-free guinea-pig lung homogenate	$F_{2\alpha}$			0.75					35.0	
Dog-spleen microsomes	$F_{2\alpha}$	0.1	0.11	0.3	0.71			7.25	37.0	
	E_2			0.17						
Rabbit-brain homogenates	E_2			3.6					61.0	
	E_2			7.0			100		15000	
Bovine seminal-vesicle enzymes	Total PGs			2.0	15.0	48.0	220	420	820	1200
	E_2	13.0		38.0			370	1400	9000	2000
	$F_{2\alpha}$	17.0		30.0			480	1200	10000	2300
Sheep seminal-vesicle enzymes	E_2		1.21	0.45	2.1	2.5	6.1	12.6	83.0	1.5
	Total PGs								9000	

*I_{50} concentrations are expresses as μM.

formation in cell-free homogenates of guinea-pig lung (273). Almost all the non-steroidal antiinflammatory agents tested so far are potent inhibitors of prostaglandin synthetase. While the original experiments were performed with cell-free homogenates of guinea-pig lung (273), these drugs proved effective against virtually every synthetase preparation investigated to date, even though their relative potencies vary (177). "Microsomal" preparations of tissue homogenates have been widely used, mainly from sheep seminal vesicles, since this fraction is rich in synthetizing enzymes and practically devoid of inactivating ones. A variety of techniques for measuring prostaglandins formed from the added precursor, arachidonic acid, have been used: radiometry (78,265,321,324), spectrophotometry (78,260), immunochemistry (34,158), gas-liquid chromatography—mass spectrometry (118,119). The basic findings are substantially similar, regardless of the type of assay, and indicate that the potency of non-steroidal antiinflammatory drugs decreases in the following orders: melclofenamic acid > niflumic acid, indomethacin > mefenamic acid > flufenamic acid > phenylbutazone > ibuprofen > acetylsalicylic acid. That inhibition of prostaglandin synthetase is a property peculiar to non-steroidal antiinflammatory drugs is suggested by the fact that many other pharmacologically active compounds are ineffective against this enzyme at concentrations of 1.0-5.0 mM (111). The in vitro activities of the antiinflammatory agents generally rank in the same order as those in vivo (carrageenin edema), and the concentrations required are within the range of plasma levels found after therapeutic dosages in man, even when plasma binding is taken into consideration (79). Especially impressive is the in vitro distinction between two pairs of enantiomers, which corresponds to their in vivo efficacy (260),265,321). So far little effort has been made to differentiate between the effects on E- and F-type prostaglandin production. This may be pertinent in view of the often antagonistic effects of the two different classes of prostaglandins (Table 23).

Additional in vitro methods of assay include: uncoupling of oxidative phosphorylation (301,302), fibrinolytic activity (112,221) and acid urate displacement (21).

7. MODELS OF ACUTE GOUT

Once it became apparent that microcrystalline sodium urate was responsible for initiating an attack of gout, this knowledge was employed in the development of animal models of this disorder.

Suspensions of monosodium urate were injected into the suplantar region of the hind paw of rats to obtain a swelling, or into their interscapular region—to produce granuloma (266). The urate-induced paw swelling has been used to explore the pharmacological effects of colchicine and of several of its analogs (50,266,329). The urate-induced paw swelling in mice has also been employed as a model of acute gout (72).

A bird model of pseudo-gout, based on intra-articular injection of microcrystalline sodium urate has been developed (75,76). The length of time during which the bird stood on one leg was taken as a measure of the extent of inflammatory reaction: colchicine is effective here in the same range of doses found to be active in mice (72) and rats (266,329). Tests with vinblastine and vincristine were negative.

Intra-articular injections of sodium urate in dogs have been used to produce another model of gout (67,169). The inflammatory reaction characterized by a typical three-legged gait is suppressed by indomethacin and phenylbutazone (218). Colchicine was not tested.

Animal models for evaluating potential uricosuric activity of drugs in man have not been particularly successful (114). The reasons for this are the basic differences in the renal mechanisms for handling urate in various species and the presence of uricase in many species other than man.

The chimpanzee is quite similar to man in the renal handling of urate (68). Probenecid, sulfinpyrazone, zoxazolamine and salicylate are active in this species (68).

The ability of uricosuric agents to delay renal clearance of phenol red in rat has found application in an assay for uricosuric activity (151). The obvious advantage in employing rats is offset by the need to use huge doses of drugs in order to demonstrate some pharmacological activity.

REFERENCES

1. Adams, S. S., Hebborn P., and Nicholson, J. S.: J. Pharm. Pharmacol. *20*: 305, 1968.
2. Adams, S. S., McCullough, K. F., and Nicholson, J. S.: Arch. Int. Pharmacodyn. Ther. *178*:115, 1969.
3. Anderson, A. J.: Ann. Rheum. Dis. *29*:307, 1970.
4. Ankier, S. I., and Whiteside, M. L.: Biochem. Pharmacol. *18*:2197, 1969.
5. Arrigoni-Martelli, E.: Pharm. Pharmacol. *19*:617, 1967.
6. Arrigoni-Martelli, E., and Bramm, E.: Agents Actions *5*:264, 1975.

7. Arrigoni-Martelli, E., Bramm, E., and Binderup, L.: Pharmacology, *14*: 405, 1976.
8. Arrigoni-Martelli, E., and Conti, I.: Farmaco (Prat.) *19*:134, 1964.
9. Arrigoni-Martelli, E., and Kramer, M.: Boll. Soc. Ital. Biol. Sper. *34*:1130, 1958.
10. Arrigoni-Martelli, E., and Restelli, A.: Eur. J. Pharmacol. *19*:191, 1972.
11. Arrigoni-Martelli, E., Schiatti, P., and Selva, D.: Pharmacol. Res. Commun. *3*:239, 1971.
12. Arrigoni-Martelli, E., Schiatti, P. F., and Selva, D.: Pharmacology *5*:212, 1971.
13. Arrigoni-Martelli, E., Selva,D., and Schiatti, P. F.: J. Int. Med. Res. *1*: 120, 1973.
14. Atkinson, D. C., and Hicks, R.: Br. J. Pharmacol. *41*:480, 1971.
15. Bailey, K. R., and Sheffner, A. L.: Biochem. Pharmacol. *16*:1175, 1967.
16. Barcelo, R., Riopel, P., and Legresley, L. P.: Can. Med. Assoc. J. *88*:562, 1963.
17. Bartos, F.: Experientia *22*:716, 1966.
18. Benitz, K. F., and Hall, L. M.: Arch. Int. Pharmacodyn. Ther. *144*:185, 1963.
19. Benzer, H., Blümel, G., and Piza, F.: Wien, Klin. Wochenschr. *75*:881, 1963.
20. Benzi G., and Frigo, G. M.: Farmaco (Prat.) *19*:327, 1964.
21. Bluestone, R., Kippen, I., Klinenberg, J. R., and Whitehouse, M. E.: J. Lab. Clin. Med. *76*:88, 1970.
22. Bobalik, G. R., and Bastian, J. W.: Arch. Int. Pharmacodyn. Ther. *166*: 466, 1967.
23. Bogden, A. E., Glenn, E. M., Koslowske, T., and Rigiero, C. S.: Life Sci. *6*:965, 1967.
24. Bonta, J. L., De Vos, C. J., and Bolding, W. H.: Acta Physiol. Pharmacol. Neerl. *14*:48, 1966.
25. Boris, A., and Stevenson, R. H.: Arch. Int. Pharmacodyn. Ther. *153*:205, 1965.
26. Bourne, G. H.: Br. J. Exp. Pathol. *32*:377, 1951.
27. Brown, J. H., and Mackey, H. K.: Proc. Soc. Exp. Biol. Med. *128*:504, 1968.
28. Brown, J. H., Mackey, H. K., and Riggilo, D. A.: Proc. Soc. Exp. Biol. Med. *125*:837, 1967.
29. Brown, D. M., and Robson, R. D.: Nature *202*:812, 1964.
30. Brown, J. H., and Schwartz, N. L.: Proc. Soc. Exp. Biol. Med. *131*:614, 1969.
31. Brown, J. H., Schwartz, N. L., Mackey, H. K., and Murray, H. L.: Arch. Int. Pharmacodyn. Ther. *183*:1, 1970.
32. Brownlee, G.: Lancet *1*:157, 1950.
33. Burford, R. G., and Gowdey, C. W.: Arch. Int. Pharmacodyn. Ther. *173*: 56, 1968.
34. Burke, G.: Prostaglandins *2*:413, 1972.
35. Burstein, N. A., and Waksman, B. H.: Yale J. Biol. Med. *37*:177, 1964.
36. Bush, I. E., and Alexander, R. W.: Acta Endocrinol (Kbh.) *35*:268, 1960.
37. Clark, S.: J. Pathol. *99*:93, 1969.
38. Cole, B. C., Miller, M. L., and Ward, J. R.: Proc. Soc. Exp. Biol. Med. *130*: 994, 1969.

39. Consden, R., Doble, A., Glynn, L. E., and Nind, A. P. P.: Ann. Rheum. Dis. *30*:307, 1971.
40. Cooke, T. D., and Jasin, H. E.: Arthritis Rheum. *15*:327, 1972.
41. Cotran, R. S.: Exp. Mol. Pathol. *6*:143, 1967.
42. Cotran, R. S., and Majno, G.: Ann. N. Y. Sci. *116*:750, 1964.
43. Coulon, R., Charlier, R., and Vandersmissen, V.: Arch. Int. Pharmacodyn. Ther. *99*:474, 1954.
44. Courvoisier, S., and Ducrot, R.: Arch. Int. Pharmacodyn. Ther. *102*:33, 1955.
45. Crunkhorn, P., and Willis, A. L.: Br. J. Pharmacol. *41*:49, 1971.
46. Curran, R. C., Lovell, D., and Clark, A. E.: J. Pathol. *91*:429, 1966.
47. Currey, H. L. F., and Ziff, M.: J. Exp. Med. *127*:185, 1968.
48. Cygielman, S., and Robson, J. M.: J. Pharm. Pharmacol. *15*:794, 1963.
49. Dalmasso, A. P., Martinez, C., Sjødin, K., and Good, R. A.: J. Exp. Med. *118*:1089, 1963.
50. Denko, C. W., and Whitehouse, M. W.: Pharmacology *3*:229, 1970.
51. Di Pasquale, G., and Meli, A.: J. Pharmacol. *17*:379, 1965.
52. Di Pasquale, G., Rassaert, C. L., and McDougall, E.: J. Pharm. Sci. *59*:267, 1970.
53. Di Rosa, M., Giroud, J. P., and Willoughby, D. A.: J. Pathol. *104*:15, 1971.
54. Di Rosa, M., Papadimitriou, J. M., and Willoughby, D. A.: J. Pathol. *105*:239, 1971.
55. Di Rosa, M., and Sorrentino, L.: Eur. J. Pharmacol. *4*:340, 1968.
56. Di Rosa, M., and Willoughby, D. A.: J. Pharm. Pharmacol. *23*:297, 1971.
57. Doebel, K. J., Graeme, M. L., Gruenfeld, N., Ignarro, L. J., Piliero, S. J., and Wasley, J. W. F.: Ann. Rep. Med. Chem. p. 225, 1970.
58. Domenjoz, R.: Ann. N. Y. Acad. Sci. *86*:263, 1960.
59. Domenjoz, R.: Med. Pharmacol. Exp. *14*:321, 1966.
60. Domenjoz, R., and Morsdorf, K.: In "Non-Steroidal Antiinflammatory Drugs," S. Garattini and M. N. G. Dukes, eds. Excerpta medica, Amsterdam, 1965, p. 162.
61. Domenjoz, R., Theobald, W., and Mörsdorf, K.: Arzneim. Forsch. *5*:488, 1955.
62. Donner, F. R.: "Animal Experiments in Pharmacological Analysis," Charles Thomas, Springfield, Illinois, 1971.
63. Dorfman, R. I., and Dorfman, A. S.: Proc. Soc. Exp. Biol. Med. *119*:859, 1965.
64. Ducrot, R., Julou, L., Marai, R., Bardone, M. C., Guyonnet, J. C., and Loiseau, G.: In "Non-Steroidal Antiinflammatory Drugs," S. Garattini, and M. N. G. Duke, eds. Exerpta Medica, Amsterdam, 1965, p. 259.
65. Dumonde, D. C., and Glynn, L. E.: Br. J. Exp. Pathol. *43*:373, 1962.
66. Evans, G., Packham, M. A., Nishizawa, E. E., Mustard, J. F., and Murphy, E. A.: J. Exp. Med. *128*:877, 1968.
67. Faires, J. S., and McCarty, D. J., Jr.: Lancet *2*:282, 1962.
68. Fanelli, G. M., Bohn, D. L., and Reilly, S. S.: J. Pharmacol. Exp. Ther. *177*:591, 1971.
69. Ferreira, S. H., Moncada, S., and Vane, J. R.: Nature (New Biol.) *231*:237, 1971.
70. Finney, R. S. H., and Somers, G. F.: J. Pharm. Pharmacol. *10*:613, 1958.
71. Fisher, J. W.: J. Pharmacol. Exp. Ther. *132*:232, 1961.
72. Fitzgerald, T. J., Williams, B., and Nyecki, E. M.: Proc. Soc. Exp. Biol.

Med. *136*:115, 1971.
73. Flax, M. M., and Waksman, B. H.: Int. Arch. Allergy *23*:331, 1963.
74. Fleming, J. S., Bierwagen, M. E., Losada, M., Campbell, J. A. L., King, S. P., and Pindell, M. H.: Arch. Int. Pharmacodyn. Ther. *186*:120, 1970.
75. Floersheim, G. L., Brune, K., and Seiler, K.: Agents Actions *3*:20, 1973.
76. Floersheim, G. L., Brune, K., and Seiler, K.: Agents Action *3*:24, 1973.
77. Flower, R. J.: Pharmacol. Rev. *26*:33, 1974.
78. Flower, R. J., Cheung, H. S., and Cushman, D. W.: Prostaglandins *4*: 325, 1973.
79. Flower, R. J., Gryglewski, R., Herbaczynska-Cedro, K., and Vane, J. R.: Nature (New Biol.) *238*:104, 1972.
80. Flower, R. J., and Vane, J. R.: Nature *240*:410, 1972.
81. Formanek, K., Förster, O., and Stoklaska, E.: Arzneim. Forsch. *18*:943, 1968.
82. Formanek, K., Rosak, M., and Steffen, C.: Int. Arch. Allergy. *24*:39, 1964.
83. Fukuhara, M., and Tsurufuji, S.: Biochem. Pharmacol. *18*:475, 1969.
84. Fukuhara, M., and Tsurufuji, S.: Biochem. Pharmacol. *18*:2409, 1969.
85. Garattini, S., Jori, A., Bernardi, D., Carrara, C., Paglialunga, S., and Segre, D.: "Non-Steroidal Antiinflammatory Drugs," S. Garattini, and M. N. G. Dukes, eds. Excerpta Medica, Amsterdam, 1965, p. 151.
86. Gardner, D. L.: Ann. Rheum. Dis. *19*:297, 1960.
87. Gardner, D. L.: Ann. Rheum. Dis. *19*:369, 1960.
88. Gerber, R. C., Whitehouse, M. W., and Orr, K. J.: Proc. Soc. Exp. Biol. Med. *140*:1379, 1972.
89. Gery, I., and Waksman, B. H.: Int. Arch. Allergy Appl. Immunol. *31*:57, 1967.
90. Giordano, M., and Junge-Hulsing, G.: Z. Rheumaforsch. *22*:99, 1963.
91. Giordano, M., and Scapaginini, N.: Med. Pharmacol. Exp. *17*:445, 1967.
92. Giri, S. N., Joshi, B., and Peoples, S. A.: Clin. Exp. Pharmacol. Physiol. *2*:193, 1975.
93. Glenn, E. M., Bowman, B. J., Kooyers, W., Koslowske, T., and Myers, M. L.: J. Pharmacol. Exp. Ther. *155*:157, 1967.
94. Glenn, E. M., Bowman, B. J., Lyster, S. C., and Rohloff, N. A.: Proc. Soc. Exp. Biol. Med. *138*:235, 1971.
95. Glenn, E. M., Gray, J., and Kooyers, W.: Am. J. Vet. Res. *26*:1195, 1965.
96. Glenn, E. M., Miller, W. L., and Schlagel, C. A.: Recent Prog. Horm. Res. *19*:107, 1963.
97. Glynn, L. E.: Ann. Rheum. Dis. *27*:105, 1968.
98. Glynn, L. E.: Ann. Rheum. Dis. *28* (Suppl. 6) : 1969.
99. Goldberg, V. M., Lance, E. M., and Davis, P.: Arthritis Rheum. *17*:993, 1974.
100. Goldstein, S., and Schnak, M.: Arch. Int. Pharmacodyn. Ther. *144*:269, 1963.
101. Görög, P., and Szporny, L.: Med. Pharmacol. Exp. *16*:635, 1964.
102. Göszy, B., and Kátó, L.: Nature *178*:1352, 1956.
103. Göszy, B., and Kátó, L.: Rev. Can. Biol. *19*:425, 1960.
104. Graeme, M. L., Fabry, E., and Sigg, E. B.: J. Pharmacol. Exp. Ther. *153*: 373, 1966.
105. Grant, N. H., Alburn, H. E., and Kryzanauskas, C.: Biochem. Pharmacol. *19*:715, 1970.

106. Grant, N. H., Alburn, H. E., and Singer, A. C.: Biochem. Pharmacol. *20*: 2137, 1971.
107. Green, A. Y., Murray, P. A., and Wilson, A. B.: Br. J. Pharmacol. *41*: 132, 1971.
108. Greenwood, B. M., Voller, A., and Hervick, E. M.: Ann. Rheum. Dis. *29*: 321, 1970.
109. Gross, F.: Arch. Exp. Pathol. Pharmakol. *211*:421, 1950.
110. Gryfe, A., Sanders, P. M., and Gardner, D. L.: Ann. Rheum. Dis. *30*:24, 1971.
111. Gryglewski, R., Flower, R. J., Herbaczynska-Cedro, K., and Vane, J. R.: In Proceedings, 5th International Congress of Pharmacology, 1972, p. 90.
112. Gryglewski, R. J., and Gryglewska, T. A.: Biochem. Pharmacol. *15*:1171, 1966.
113. Gupta, N., and Levy, L.: Fed. Proc. *29*:419 Abs 1970.
114. Gutman, A. B.: Adv. Pharmacol. *4*:91, 1966.
115. Haining, C. G.: Br. J. Pharmacol. Chemother. *21*:104, 1963.
116. Halpern, B. N., Liacopoulos, P., and Liacopoulos Briot, M.: Arch. Int. Pharmacodyn. Ther. *119*:56, 1959.
117. Ham, E. A., Cirillo, K. J., Zanetti, M., Shen, T. Y., and Kuehl, F. A.: In "Prostaglandins in Cellular Biology," P. W. Ramwell, and B. B. Phariss, eds. Plenum Press, New York, 1972, p. 345.
118. Hamberg, M.: Biochem. Biophys. Res. Commun. *49*:720, 1972.
119. Hamberg, M., and Samuelsson, B.: J. Biol. Chem. *247*:3495, 1972.
120. Hartmann, F., and Walpurger, G.: Z. Rheumaforsch. *26*:12, 1967.
121. Hertting, G., and Stoklaska, E.: Arch. Exp. Pathol. Pharmakol. *231*:562, 1957.
122. Hurley, J. C., and Spector, W. G.: J. Pathol. *89*:245, 1965.
123. Hyttel, J., and Jørgensen, A.: Eur. J. Pharmacol. *11*:383, 1970.
124. Ignarro, L. J.: Biochem. Pharmacol. *20*:2847, 1971.
125. Ignarro, L. J.: Biochem. Pharmacol. *20*:2861, 1971.
126. Ignarro, L. J.: Biochem. Pharmacol. *22*:1296, 1973.
127. Ignarro, L. J.: Agents Actions *4*:241, 1974.
128. Ignarro, L. J., and Colombo, C.: Nature (New Biol.) *239*:155, 1972.
129. Inglot, A. D., and Wolna, E.: Biochem. Pharmacol. *17*:269, 1968.
130. Isakovic, K., and Waksman, B. H.: Proc. Soc. Biol. Med. *119*:676, 1965.
131. Isikowa, H., Mori, Y., and Tsufuruji, S.: Eur. J. Pharmacol. *7*:201, 1969.
132. Ishioka, T., Honda, Y., Sagara, A., and Shimamoto, T.: Acta Endocrinol. *60*:177, 1969.
133. Jahn, U., and Adrian, R. W.: Arzneim. Forsch. *19*:36, 1969.
134. Jancsó-Gábor, A., Szolcsányi, J., and Jancsó, M.: J. Pharm. Pharmacol. *19*:486, 1967.
135. Jaquet, H.: Arch. Int. Pharmacodyn. Ther. *144*:161, 1963.
136. Jasin, H. E., Cooke, T. D., Hurd, E. R., Smiley, J. D., and Ziff, M.: Fed. Proc. *32*:147, 1973.
137. Jasmin, G.: In "Rheumatology Annual Review," Vol. 1. Karger, Basel, 1967, p. 107.
138. Jessop, J. D., and Currey, H. L. F.: Ann. Rheum. Dis. *27*:577, 1968.
139. Jones, R. S., and Ward, J. R.: Arthritis Rheum. *6*:23, 1963.
140. Jori, A., Bentivoglio, A., and Garattini, S.: J. Pharm. Pharmacol. *13*:617, 1961.

141. Jori, A., and Bernardi, D.: Med. Pharmacol. Exp. *14*:500, 1966.
142. Judah, J. D., and Willoughby, D. A.: J. Pathol. *83*:657, 1962.
143. Julou, L., Guyonnet, J. C., Ducrot, R., Garret, C., Bardone, M. C., Maignan, C., and Pasquet, J.: J. Pharmacol. *2*:259, 1971.
144. Kapusta, M. A., and Mendelson, J.: Proc. Exp. Biol. Med. *126*:496, 1967.
145. Kapusta, M. A., and Mendelson, J.: Arthritis Rheum. *12*:463, 1969.
146. Kellet, D. N.: J. Pharm. Pharmacol. *17*:184, 1965.
147. Klamer, B., Kimura, E. T., and Makstenieks, M.: Pharmacology *1*:283, 1968.
148. Klein, L., and Weiss, P. H.: Proc. Natl. Acad. Sci. USA *56*:277, 1966.
149. Kobayashi, S., and Takagi, H.: Arzneim. Forsch. *18*:1352, 1968.
150. Kramer, M.: Arch. Exp. Pathol. Pharmakol. *228*:340, 1956.
151. Kreppel, E.: Med. Exp. *1*:285, 1959.
152. Kulka, D. P., Houssay, R. H., and Clausen, J. L.: Arthritis Rheum. *8*:452, 1965.
153. Kuzell, W. C.: Ann. Rev. Pharmacol. *8*:357, 1968.
154. La Belle, A., and Tislow, R.: J. Pharmacol. Exp. Ther. *99*:19, 1950.
155. Lancaster, M. G., and Vegad, J. L.: Nature *213*:840, 1967.
156. Léger, J., Masson, G., and Prado, L. J.: Proc. Soc. Exp. Biol. Med. *64*:366, 1947.
157. Lerner, J. L., Turkheimer, A. R., Bianchi, A., Singer, F. M., and Borman, A.: Proc. Soc. Exp. Biol. Med. *116*:385, 1964.
158. Levy, B., and Lindner, H. R.: Br. J. Pharmacol. *43*:236, 1971.
159. Lewis, D. A., Capstick, R. B., and Ancill, R. J.: J. Pharm. Pharmacol. *23*:931. 1971.
160. Likar, L. J., Mason, M. M., and Rosenkrantz, H.: Endocrinology *72*:393, 1963.
161. Logan, G., and Wilhelm, D. A.: Br. J. Exp. Pathol. *47*:286, 1966.
162. Logan, G., and Wilhelm, D. A.: Br. J. Exp. Pathol. *47*:300, 1966.
163. Lowe, J. S.: Biochem. Pharmacol. *13*:633, 1964.
164. Lucherini, T., Cecchi, E., Porzio, F., and D'Amore, A.: Minerva. Med. *55*:4059, 1964.
165. Mackay, I. R., and Burnet, F. M.: In "Autoimmune Disease." Charles Thomas, Springfield, Illinois, 1963, p. 149.
166. Maros, T., Száva, J., Rettegi, K., Lázár, L., and Seres-Sturm, F. M.: Z. Orthop. *98*:106, 1964.
167. Martell, R. R., Klicius, J., and Herv, F.: Can. J. Physiol. *52*:791, 1974.
168. McCandless, E. L.: Fed. Proc. *21*:166, 1962.
169. McCarty, D. J., Jr., Phelps, P., and Pyenson, J.: J. Exp. Med. *124*:99, 1966.
170. McQueen, A., and Hurley, J. V.: Pathology *3*:191, 1971.
171. Meier, R., Schuler, W., and Desaulles, P.: Experientia *6*:469, 1950.
172. Meyer, R. K., Stucki, J. C., and Auslebrook, K. A.: Proc. Soc. Exp. Biol. Med. *84*:624, 1953.
173. Mielens, Z. E., Drobeck, H. P., Rozitis, J., Jr., and Sansone, V. J.: Toxicol. Appl. Pharmacol. *14*:293, 1969.
174. Mielens, Z. E., and Rozitis, J., Jr.: Proc. Soc. Exp. Biol. Med. *117*:751, 1964.
175. Miles, A. A., and Miles, E. M.: J. Physiol. (Lond.) *118*:228, 1952.
176. Miller, W. S., and Smith, J. G.: Proc. Soc. Exp. Biol. Med. *122*:634, 1966.

177. Miller, M. L., Ward, J. R., Cole, B. C., and Swinyard, E. A.: Arthritis Rheum. *13*:222, 1970.
178. Mizushima, Y.: Arch. Int. Pharmacodyn. Ther. *149*:1, 1964.
179. Mizushima, Y.: Lancet *1*:169, 1965.
180. Mizushima, Y.: Lancet *2*:443, 1966.
181. Mizushima, Y., and Suzuki, H.: Arch. Int. Pharmacodwyn. Ther. *157*:115, 1965.
182. Mueller, M. N., and Kappas, A.: Proc. Soc. Exp. Biol. Med. *117*:845, 1964.
183. Newbould, B. B.: Br. J. Pharmacol. *21*:127, 1963
184. Newbould, B. B.: Ann. Rheum. Dis. *23*:392, 1964.
185. Niemegeers, C. J. E., Verbruggen, F. J., and Janssen, P. A. J.: J. Pharm. Pharmacol. *16*:810, 1964.
186. Northover, B. J.: J. Pathol. Bacteriol. *87*:395, 1964.
187. Northover, B. J., and Subramanian, G.: Br. J. Pharmacol. *16*:163, 1961.
188. O'Brien, J. R.: Lancet *1*:894, 1968.
189. Packham, M. A., and Mustard, J. F.: Proc. Soc. Exp. Biol. Med. *130*:72, 1969.
190. Packham, M. A., Warrior, E. S., Glynn, M. F., Senyi, A. S., and Mustard, J. F.: J. Exp. Med. *126*:171, 1967.
191. Papadimitrious, J. M., Shilkin, K. B., Archer, J. M., and Walters, M. N. J.: Exp. Mol. Pathol. *6*:347, 1967.
192. Parrat, J. R., and West, G. B.: J. Physiol. (Lond.) *139*:27, 1957.
193. Parrat, J. R., and West, G. B.: Br. J. Pharmacol. *13*:65, 1958.
194. Paulus, H. E., and Whitehouse, M. W.: In "Search for New Drugs," A. A. Rubin, ed. Dekker, New York, 1972, p. 1.
195. Pearson, C. M.: Proc. Soc. Exp. Biol. Med. *91*:95, 1956.
196. Pearson, C. M.: Arthritis Rheum. *7*:80, 1964.
197. Pearson, C. M.: In "Arthritis," J. L. Hollander, ed. Lea and Febiger, Philadelphia, 1966, p. 119.
198. Pearson, C. M., Waksman, B. H., and Sharp, J. T.: J. Exp. Med. *113*:485, 1961.
199. Pearson, C. M., and Wood, F. D.: Arthritis Rheum. *2*:440, 1959.
200. Pearson, C. M., and Wood, F. D.: Am. J. Pathol. *42*:73, 1963.
201. Pearson, C. M., and Wood, F. D.: Immunology *16*:157, 1969.
202. Pearson, C. M., Wood, F. D., McDaniel, E. G., and Daft, S. F.: Proc. Soc. Exp. Biol. Med. *112*:91, 1963.
203. Pearson, C. M., Wood, F. D., and Vande-Sande, B.: Arthritis Rheum. *8*:460, 1965.
204. Perper, R. J., Alvarez, B., Colombo, C., and Schroder, H.: Proc. Soc. Exp. Biol. Med. *137*:506, 1971.
205. Perper, R. J., Sanda, M., Chinea, G., and Oronsky, A. L.: J. Lab. Clin. Med. *84*:378, 1974.
206. Perper, R. J., Sanda M., Chinea, G., and Oronsky, A. L.: J. Lab. Clin. Med. *84*:394, 1974.
207. Perrine, J. W., and Takesue, E. J.: Arch. Int. Pharmacodyn. Ther. *174*:192, 1968.
208. Piliero, S. J., and Colombo, C.: J. Pharmacol. Exp. Ther. *165*:294, 1969.
209. Piliero, S. J., Graeme, M. L., Sigg, E. B., Chinea, G., and Colombo, C.: Life Sci. *5*:1057, 1966.
210. Prodi, G., and Romeo, G.: Br. J. Exp. Pathol. *48*:40, 1967.

211. Quagliata, F., Sanders, P. M., and Gardner, D. L.: Ann. Rheum. Dis. *28*: 163, 1969.
212. Randall, L. O., and Selitto, J. J.: Arch. Int. Pharmacodyn, Ther. *111*:409, 1957.
213. Rebuck, J. W., and Crowley, J. H.: Ann. N. Y. Acad. Sci. *59*:757, 1965.
214. Robert A., and Nezamis, J. E.: Acta Endocrinol. (Kbh.) *25*:105, 1957.
215. Rosenkilde, H.: In "Pharmacological Techniques in Drug Evaluation," J. H. Nodine, and P. E. Siegler, eds. Yearbook Publishers, Chicago, 1964, p. 492.
216. Rosenthale, M. E.: Arch. Int. Pharmacodyn. Ther. *188*:14, 1970.
217. Rosenthale, M. E., and Gluckman, M. J.: Experientia *24*:1229, 1968.
218. Rosenthale, M. E., Kassarich, J., and Schneider, F., Jr.: Proc. Soc. Exp. Biol. Med. *122*:693, 1966.
219. Rosenthale, M. E., and Nagra, C. L.: Proc. Soc. Exp. Biol. Med. *125*:149, 1967.
220. Roskowski, A. P., Rooks, V. H., Tomolonis, A. J., and Miller, L. M.: J. Pharmacol. Exp. Ther. *179*:114, 1971.
221. Roubal, Z., and Nemecek, O.: Nature *212*:861, 1966.
222. Ryzewska, A. G.: Ann. Rheum. Dis. *26*:506, 1967.
223. Ryzewska, A. G., Ryzewski, J., and Dabrowski, M.: In "Inflammation Biochemistry and Drug Interactions," A. Bertelli, and J. C. Houck, eds. Excerpta Medica, Amsterdam, 1969, p. 275.
224. Sancilio, L. F.: J. Pharmacol. Exp. Ther. *168*:199, 1969.
225. Sancilio, L. F., and Rodriguez, R.: Proc. Soc. Exp. Biol. Med. *123*:707, 1966.
226. Saxena, P. N.: Arch. Int. Pharmacodyn. Ther. *126*:228, 1960.
227. Schiatti, P. F., Selva, D., and Arrigoni-Martelli, E.: Boll. Chim. Farm. *109*:33, 1970.
228. Schiatti, P., Selva, D., Arrigoni-Martelli, E., Lerner, L. J., Sardi, A., Diena, A., and Maffii, G.: Arzneim. Forsch. *24*:2003, 1974.
229. Schlamowitz, S. T., De Graff, A. C., and Schubert, M.: Circulation *1*:833, 1950.
230. Selye, M.: Proc. Soc. Exp. Biol. Med. *82*:328, 1953.
231. Sigg, E. B., Graeme, M. L., and John, M.: J. Pharmacol. Exp. Ther. *157*: 214, 1967.
232. Silverstein, E., and Sokoloff, L.: Arthritis Rheum. *3*:485, 1960.
233. Silvestrini, B.: In "Non-Steroidal Antiinflammatory Drugs," S. Garattini, and M. N. G. Dukes, eds. Excerpta Medica, Amsterdam, 1965, p. 180.
234. Sim, M. F.: In "Non-Steroidal Antiinflammatory Drugs," S. Garattini, and M. N. G. Dukes, eds. Excerpta Medica, Amsterdam, 1965, p. 207.
235. Smith, Q. T.: J. Invest. Dermatol. *42*:353, 1964.
236. Smith, W. L., and Lands, W. E.: J. Biol. Chem. *21*:6700, 1971.
237. Smith, D. B., O'Neill, A. N., and Perlin, A. S.: Can. J. Chem. *33*:1352, 1955.
238. Smith, J. B., and Willis, A. L.: Nature (New Biol.) *231*:235, 1971.
239. Sofia, R. D., Knobloch, L. C., and Vassar, H. B.: J. Pharmacol. Exp. Ther. *193*:918, 1975.
240. Sokoloff, L.: J. Natl. Cancer Inst. *20*:965, 1958.
241. Sokoloff, L.: Lab. Invest. *8*:1209, 1959.
242. Sokoloff, L.: Adv. Vet. Sci. *6*:193, 1960.

243. Spector, W. G.: J. Pathol. Bacteriol. *72*:367, 1956.
244. Spector, W. G., and Willoughby, D. A.: Nature *181*:708, 1958.
245. Spector, W. G., and Willoughby, D. A.: J. Pathol. *77*:1, 1959.
246. Spector, W. G., and Willoughby, D. A.: Bacteriol. Rev. *27*:117, 1963.
247. Spector, W. G., and Willoughby, D. A.: In "Evaluation of Drug Activities: Pharmacometrics," D. R. Laurence, and A. L. Bacharach, eds. Academic Press, New York, 1964, p. 815.
248. Stastny, P., and Ziff, M.: Rheumatology *1*:189, 1967.
249. Steele, R. H., and Wilhelm, D. L.: Br. J. Exp. Pathol. *48*:592, 1967.
250. Steffen, C., and Wick, G.: Z. Immunitaetsforsch. *141*:169, 1967.
251. Steinetz, B., Giannina, T., Butler, M., and Popick, F.: Proc. Soc. Exp. Biol. Med. *133*:401, 1970.
252. Stern, P.: Arzneim. Forsch. *15*:819, 1965.
253. Stevens, J. E., and Willoughby, D. A.: J. Pathol. *97*:367, 1969.
254. Stoerk, H. C., Bielinski, T., and Budzilovich, T.: Arch. Pathol. *30*:616, 1954.
255. Studer, A., and Reber, K.: "Rheumatismus als Problem der experimentellen Medizin." Steinkopft, Darmstad, 1959.
256. Swingle, K. F., Harrington, J. K., Hamilton, R. R., and Kvam, D. C.: Arch. Int. Pharmacodyn. Ther. *192*:16, 1971.
257. Swingle, K. F., Jaques, L. W., and Kvam, D. C.: Proc. Soc. Exp. Biol. Med. *132*:608, 1969.
258. Swingle, K. F., and Shidemann, F. E.: Pharmacologist *9*:243, 1967.
259. Sykes, J-A. C., and Maddox, I. S.: Nature (New Biol.) *237*:59, 1972.
260. Takeguchi, C., and Sih, C. J.: Prostaglandins *2*:169, 1972.
261. Tanaka, K., and Iizyka, Y.: Biochem. Pharmacol. *17*:2023, 1968.
262. Theobald, W.: Arch. Int. Pharmacodyn. Ther. *103*:17, 1955.
263. Theobald, W., and Domenjoz, R.: Arzneim. Forsch. *8*:18, 1958.
264. Toivanen, P., Siikala, H., Laiho, P., and Paavilainen, T.: Experientia *23*:560, 1967.
265. Tomlinson, R. V., Ringold, H. J., Qureshi, M. C., and Forchielli, E.: Biochem. Biophys. Res. Commun. *46*:552, 1972.
266. Trnavsky, K., and Kopecky, S.: Med. Exp. *15*:322, 1966.
267. Trnavsky, K., and Lapárorá, V.: Med. Pharmacol. Exp. *16*:171, 1967.
268. Turk, J. L., Willoughby, D. A., and Stevens, J. E.: Immunology *14*:683, 1968.
269. Valtonen, E. J.: Acta Derm. Venereol. (Stockh.) *46*:292, 1966.
270. Van Arman, C. G., Begany, A. J., Miller, L. M., and Pless, H. H.: J. Pharmacol. Exp. Ther. *150*:328, 1965.
271. Van Arman, C. G., Risley, E. A., and Kling, P. J.: Pharmacologist *13*:284, 1971.
272. Van Cauwenberge, H., and Franchimont, P.: Arch. Int. Pharmacodyn. Ther. *170*:74, 1967.
273. Vane, J. R.: Nature (New Biol.) *231*:232, 1971.
274. Varsa-Handler, E. E., Handler, E. S., and Gordon, A. S.: Proc. Soc. Exp. Biol. Med. *124*:562, 1967.
275. Vinegar, R., Macklin, A. W., Truax, J. F., and Selph, J. L.: Pharmacologist *13*:284, 1971.
276. Vinegar, R., Schreiber, W., and Hugo, R.: J. Pharmacol. Exp. Ther. *166*:96, 1969.

277. Vogel, G., and Marek, M. L.: Arzneim Forsch. *11*:1051, 1961.
278. Volkman, A., and Gowans, J. L.: Br. J. Exp. Pathol. *46*:50, 1965.
279. Wagner-Jauregg, T., and Jahn, N.: Helv. Physiol. Pharmacol. Acta *21*: 65, 1963.
280. Waksman, B. H., Pearson, C. M., and Sharp, J. T.: J. Immunol. *85*:403, 1960.
281. Waksman, B. H., and Wennerstein, C.: Int. Arch. Allergy *23*:129, 1963.
282. Walters, M. N. I., and Willoughby, D. A.: J. Pathol. Bacteriol. *90*:641, 1965.
283. Walz, D. T., and Berkoff, C. E.: Proc. Soc. Exp. Biol. Med. *135*:760, 1970.
284. Walz, D. T., Di Martino, M. J., Kurch, I. M., and Zuccarello, W.: Proc. Soc. Exp. Med. *136*:907, 1971.
285. Walz, D. T., Di Martino, M. J., and Misher, A.: J. Pharmacol. Exp. Ther. *178*:223, 1971.
286. Ward, J. R., and Cloud, S. R.: J. Pharmacol. Exp. Ther. *152*:116, 1966.
287. Ward, J. R., and Jones, R. S.: Arthritis Rheum. *5*:557, 1962.
288. Wasserman, K., Loeb, L., and Mayerson, H. S.: Circ. Res. *3*:594, 1955.
289. Watnick, A. S., Taber, R. I., and Tabachnick, I. I. A.: Arch. Int. Pharmacodyn. Ther. *190*:78, 1971.
290. Weiner, M., and Piliero, S. J.: Ann. Rev. Pharmacol. *10*:171, 1970.
291. Weis, J.: Med. Exp. *8*:1, 1963.
292. Weisbach, J. A., Burns, C., Macko, E., and Douglas, B.: J. Med. Chem. *6*:91, 1963.
293. Weiss, H. J., Aledorf, L. M., and Kochwa, S.: J. Clin. Invest. *47*:2169, 1968.
294. Weissmann, G.: Fed. Proc. *23*:1038, 1964.
295. Weissmann, G., and Dingle, J. T.: Exp. Cell Res. *25*:207, 1961.
296. Weissmann, G., Hirschhorn, R., Pras, M., Sessa, G., and Bevons, V. A. H.: Biochem. Pharmacol. *16*:1957, 1967.
297. Weissmann, G., and Thomas, L.: J. Exp. Med. *116*:433, 1962.
298. Weissmann, G., and Thomas, L.: Recent Prog. Horm. Res. *20*:215, 1964.
299. Wepsic, H. T., and Hollingsworth, J. W.: Yale, J. Biol. Med. *41*:273, 1968.
300. Whitehouse, M. W.: Fortschr. Arzneim. Forsch. *8*:321, 1965.
301. Whitehouse, M. W.: Biochem. Pharmacol. *16*:753, 1967.
302. Whitehouse, M. W., and Skidmore, I. F.: J. Pharm. Pharmacol. *17*:668, 1965.
303. Whitehouse, M. W., and Whitehouse, D. J.: Arthritis Rheum. *11*:519, 1968.
304. Wigzell, H., and Stjernsward, J.: J. Natl. Cancer Inst. *37*:513, 1966.
305. Wilhelmi, G.: Schweiz. Med. Wochenschr. *79*:577, 1949.
306. Wilhelmi, G.: Schweiz. Med. Wochenschr. *80*:936, 1950.
307. Wilhelmi, G.: Schweiz. Med. Wochenschr. *88*:185, 1958.
308. Wilhelmi, G.: Arch. Exp. Pathol. Pharmakol. *246*:51, 1963.
309. Wilhelmi, G.: In "Non-Steroidal Antiinflammatory Drugs," S. Garattini, and M. N. G. Dukes, eds. Excerpta Medica, Amsterdam, 1965, p. 174.
310. Wilhelm, G., and Domenjoz, R.: Arzneim Forsch. *1*:151, 1951.
311. Willoughby, D. A., Dunn, C. J., Yamamoto, S., Capasso, F., Deporter, D. A., and Giroud, J. P.: Agents Actions *5*:35, 1975.
312. Winder, C. V., Lembke, L. A., and Stephens, M. D.: Arthritis Rheum. *12*: 472, 1969.
313. Winder, C. V., Wax, J., Burr, V., Been, M., and Rosiere, C. E.: Arch. Int. Pharmacodyn. Ther. *116*:261, 1958.

314. Winder, C. V., Wax, J., Scotti, L., Scherrer, R. A., Jones, E. M., and Short, F. W.: J. Pharmacol. Exp. Ther. *138*:405, 1962.
315. Winder, C. V., Wax, J., Serrano, B., Jones, E. M., and McPhee, M. L.: Arthritis Rheum. *6*:36, 1963.
316. Winder, C. V., Wax, J., and Welford, M.: J. Pharmacol. Exp. Ther. *148*: 422, 1965.
317. Winter, C. A.: In "Non-Steroidal Antiinflammatory Drugs," S. Garattini, and M. N. G. Dukes, eds. Excerpta Medica, Amsterdam, 1965, p. 190.
318. Winter, C. A.: Ann. Rev. Pharmacol. *6*:157, 1966.
319. Winter, C. A.: Fortschr. Arzneim. Forsch. *10*:139, 1966.
320. Winter, C. A., and Nuss, G. W.: Arthritis Rheum. *9*:394, 1966.
321. Winter, C. A., Risley, E. A., and Nuss, G. W.: Proc. Soc. Exp. Biol. Med. *111*:544, 1962.
322. Winter, C. A., Risley, E. A., and Nuss, G. W.: J. Pharmacol. Exp. Ther. *141*:369, 1963.
323. Witte, S., Schricker, K. T., and Schmid, E.: Arzneim. Forsch. *11*:619, 1961.
324. Yoshimoto, A., Ito, H., and Tomita, K.: J. Biochem. *68*:487, 1970.
325. Young, D. A. B.: Proc. Soc. Exp. Biol. Med. *116*:220, 1964.
326. Zidek, Z., and Perlik, F.: J. Pharm. Pharmacol. *23*:289, 1971.
327. Zucker, M. B., and Peterson, J.: Proc. Soc. Exp. Biol. Med. *127*:547, 1968.
328. Zucker, M. B., and Peterson, J.: J. Lab. Clin. Med. *76*:66, 1970.
329. Zweig, M. H., Maling, H. M., and Webster, M. E.: J. Pharmacol. Exp. Ther. *182*:344, 1972.

Chapter 12

Experimental Evaluation of Compounds Interfering with Immunopathological Events

Pathways leading to tissue damage in different immunological diseases can be divided into two main components:

1. An afferent system which includes the processing of the antigen and its interaction with the precursors of immunologically competent cells. The antigen-sensitive cells are of two types: T (thymus-derived) lymphocytes and B (bone-marrow-derived) lymphocytes. T and B cells differ in their developmental origin, their surface immunoglobulin content, and the functional and immunological characteristics of their progeny. B cells give rise to antibody-secreting cells and small lymphocytes which carry B cell immunologic memory, whereas T cells give rise to lymphocytes which are effector cells in cellular immunity, carry T cell memory and probably interfere with some of the B cell functions (Table 24).

2. An efferent system where antibodies and sensitized cells interact with soluble or cellular antigens to produce immunological in-

TABLE 24. Principal characteristics of B and T lymphocytes

Characteristics	B Lymphocytes (BL)	T Lymphocytes (TL)
Origin	Bone marrow	Bone marrow
Duration of life	Days-Weeks	Months-Years
Recirculation	Slight	Intensive
Principal localization:		
Spleen	Red pulp	White pulp Surrounding arterioles
Lymph node	Zone below medullary capsule, Germinal centers Follicular centers	Deep cortical Perifollicular Perifollicular
Response in LTT:*		
to PHA**	−	++
to various antigens (Ag)	−	++
Response in LMIT†	−	++
Immunity functions:		
cellular immunity	−	++
humoral immunity induction	++	++ (Recognition and transport of some Ag to B lymphocyte)
Antibody synthesis	++	−
Memory	+?	++
Sensitivity to antilymphocyte serum	+	+++

*LTT   = Lymphocyte transformation test
**PHA   = Phytohemagglutinin
†LMIT = Leucocyte migration inhibition test

flammation, as exemplified by cytotoxic or cytolytic reactions, anaphylactic responses caused by the release of pharmacologically active mediators, immune-complex disease resulting in migration of polymorphonuclear leukocytes and subsequent discharge of lysosomal enzymes, and a cellular hypersensitivity re-

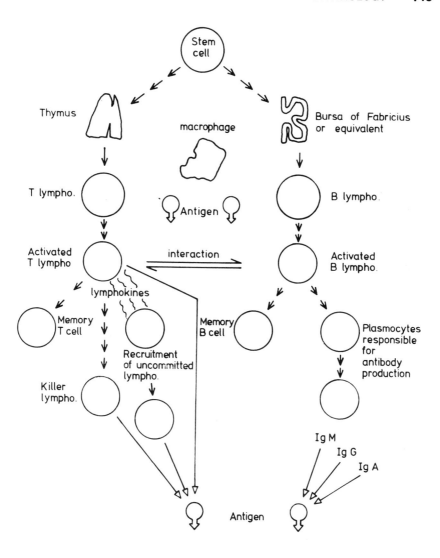

FIG. 14. Schematic representation of humoral and cellular immune response

action during which several soluble lymphocyte products (lymphokines) are released (Fig. 14).

Compounds which can interfere with these immunopathological events may act at different levels and through different mechanisms (12,46,61), and their antiinflammatory activity is not necessarily just the consequence of their capacity to suppress the immune response (1,21,39,47,144,154).

1. HUMORAL HYPERSENSITIVITY

Effects of agents on humoral hypersensitivity can be evaluated both in vivo and in vitro. The in vivo method is more commonly used and involves *systemic anaphylaxis*—an immediate allergic manifestation resulting from the union of antigen with specific antibody. The latter is the first in a series of reactions leading to the release of various pharmacologically active mediators. Experimentally, anaphylaxis occurs when an animal is injected systematically with antigen on two occasions, or once with serum from a sensitized animal and then with antigen. When antigen is administered the first time, it is known as the "sensitizing dose" and stimulates antibody production; the second injection is the "challenging dose" and causes anaphylactic shock. Systemic anaphylaxis provides a tool for evaluating how a drug influences not only the antigen-antibody interaction but also the effects of allergic mediators. Because of interspecies differences in respect to both of these parameters (16), the above test should be performed for each drug in at least rat and guinea pig. An example of species-dependent variations in drug sensitivity is provided by cyclophosphamide and 6-mercaptopurine which are both active in rat (132) but only the former is effective in guinea pig (99,100). Similarly, cycloleucine produces a response in rat but not in guinea pig (132). In addition to the antimetabolites (70,99,100), glucocorticoids (73,91) also prevent anaphylactic shock, suppressing the selection and the proliferation of immunocompetent cells. Salicylates, antihistamines and kinin inhibitors (36, 45,124,169) probably act through a blockade of humoral receptor sites in the organs involved in the development of anaphylactic shock.

There are several mechanisms by which anaphylactic shock can be prevented in animals: 1. suppression of immunocompetent cells; 2. inhibition of antigen-antibody reaction; 3. prevention of release of various mediators; 4. blockade of humoral receptor sites. Other reactions concerned with an immediate type of hypersensitivity are those generally elicited in the skin. They include active local and passive cutaneous anaphylaxis.

An example of the first type is the *Arthus reaction*. It can be induced with different procedures. The active Arthus reaction is elicited by intracutaneous injection of specific antigen into an animal with a high level of circulating antibody. The passive reaction is brought about by injecting antibody intravenously and then challenging the animal with intracutaneous antigen. The reverse passive reaction occurs when the antigen is injected intravenously and the antibody intracutaneously. No matter how it is produced, the Arthus reaction begins typically with erythema and edema but may progress to necrosis if the level of circulating antibody is sufficiently high. It is a truly inflammatory response where the accumulation of polymorphs and release of lysosomal enzymes play a major role; it also represents the simplest form of immune-complex-induced disease, characterized by a localized acute necrotizing vasculitis due to the precipitation of antigen-antibody-complement complex in the vessel walls, with consequent immigration of polymorphonuclear leukocytes (28,34,35). Due to its pathogenesis, the Arthus reaction can be prevented by cytotoxic agents (77), decomplementation (15, 34,165) and antilymphocytic serum (152,159). Immunosuppressive agents, such as 6-mercaptopurine, block the reaction without depressing circulating anitbodies, thus suggesting a peripheral antiinflammatory effect (22).

Passive cutaneous anaphylaxis (PCA) is based on the liberation of vasoactive substances upon interaction of intravenous antigen and subcutaneous antibody in the skin (6,25,111,112). The inhibition by peripheral antagonists of the vascular effects of mediators of allergy, such as antihistamine and antiserotonin drugs, can be demonstrated in this test. Cortisone, antilymphocyte serum, oxyphenbutazone and cyclophosphamide are inactive here (76,111, 159). The validity of the PCA reaction as a test for detecting agents able to block the immune response is the discovery of the unique effect of disodium cromoglycate (37). This agent selectively suppresses in vivo the specific immunological mediators. The use of PCA for identifying and characterizing disodium cromoglycate is based on the capacity of rats to produce homocytotropic reaginic antibody, essentially as in the Prausnitz-Kustner test in allergic humans (64,84,110) (Table 25).

The cellular production of immunoglobulins is widely used for the in vitro evaluation of agents expected to interfere with immediate hypersensitivity reactions. Three tests have been described.

The *antibody-forming cell plaque test* (49,78,79,81) involves localized hemolysis, with single antibody-forming cells suspended in a semisolid medium containing erythrocytes and complement. The antibody-forming cells (generally spleen, but also lymph nodes or

TABLE 25. Some features of Arthus reaction and of passive
cutaneous anaphylaxis

	Arthus Reaction	Passive Cutaneous Anaphylaxis
Animal species	Rabbit	Guinea pig Rat
Presence of antigen-antibody complexes	Needed	Not needed
Accumulation of PMN	Needed	Not needed
Antihistamine and antiserotonin	Not active	Active
Non-steroidal anti-inflammatory drugs	Active(?)	Not active
Complement depletion	Active	Not active
Cyclophosphamide	?	Not active
Disodium cromoglycate	Not active	Active

thymus cells) are obtained from animals sensitized 4-5 days previously with heterologous erythrocytes. The cells are then incorporated in agar containing the erythrocytes and complement. An halo of hemolysis forms around the lymphoid cells and, therefore, the number of antibody-forming cells can be counted. The substances under study can be administered in vivo or used to treat the lymphoid cells in vitro. In either case the test measures the inhibition of the proliferation of antibody-producing cells rather than the decrease in antibody formation by individual cells (155). Inhibitors of respiration and protein synthesis reduce plaque formation (136, 143). Actinomycin D (79,128), cycloleucine (134), 6-mercaptopurine (13,128), cyclophosphamide (70,155), cytosine arabinoside (67,128) and L-asparaginase (59,72) are also effective in this respect. An increase in the number of antibody-forming cells has been shown after incubation with dibutyryl cAMP (167).

The more recently developed *rosette inhibition* test depends on an in vitro interaction between lymphocytes from spleen or blood of immunized animals and erythrocytes. The erythrocytes adhere to the lymphocytes, forming rosettes around them that can be counted. This process is complement-independent and involves cells producing either IgM or IgG antibodies (173,175). Several immunosuppressive agents and antilymphocyte serum have been found active in the rosette test (7,8,105).

Probably, the most commonly used system for evaluating the antiimmune activity of drugs is the *passive hemoagglutination* technique which involves coating pretreated erythrocytes with antigen and measuring their agglutination by specific antibodies (14, 28,40,55,141,147). A number of different types of agents have been tested, including steroids (50,55), protein synthesis inhibitors (58, 60,106) and immunosuppressants (44,50,70). With this method, it is possible to demonstrate either a drug-induced immunological tolerance or enhancement (33,38,63,140) and an effect on a particular type of immunoglobulin by the inactivation of IgM antibody with mercaptoethanol (55,58,70).

2. CELLULAR HYPERSENSITIVITY

Tests for cellular (delayed-type) hypersensitivity include those involving stimulation of delayed response in whole animals and others based on the measurement of some function in immunologically competent lymphocytes. It should be kept in mind that humoral antibody response can occur concomitantly and either enhance or inhibit the cell-mediated reaction.

A. In vivo tests for cellular hypersensitivity

These can be subdivided into three groups:
1. Contact dermatitis induced by different procedures.
2. Homograft responses, including homologous disease.
3. Experimental autoimmune diseases.

Contact dermatitis, induced with various sensitizing chemicals or drugs, represents a cellular or delayed-type hypersensitivity reaction (109,153). Basically, the test consists of sensitizing the skin of an animal with an agent that is also capable of sensitizing human skin. An increase in the proportion of large pyroninophylic cells occurs in the cortex of draining lymph modes, reaching a peak 3-4 days after sensitization. Subsequently, the proportion of these cells diminishes and a relative accumulation of small lymphocytes takes place 4-6 days after sensitization. If at that time the animals are challenged with a small non-irritating dose of the sensitizing agent, an inflammatory response takes place that attains a maximum within 24-48 hours after the challenge. This reaction appears to mimic the cellular proliferative effects and is sensitive to the same drugs as other forms of delayed hypersensitivity (98,99,100, 107,132). Using contact dermatitis in the guinea pig, it has been shown that if cyclophosphamide is administered before sensitization, the reaction is enhanced (98,151) whereas it is inhibited when this drug is given early after sensitization (148). These and other observations (150) suggested that the B lymphocytes, the target for cyclophosphamide, modulate the T-lymphocyte reaction occurring in the contact-sensitivity response (150). It has also been shown that the tolerance which can be induced to contact sensitization (122, 123) is reversible with appropriate cyclophosphamide treatment.

Homograft rejection is mediated by blood-borne, immunologically activated lymphoid cells. Experimental transplantation of vascularized tissue could, therefore, represent a useful method for evaluating agents that retard the rejection of grafted organs, such as, for example, the kidney. However, investigations assessing drug activity and toxicity in a dose-response relationship are scarce, and controlled studies differ considerably in their findings (11,27,68, 176). In addition, technical difficulties and the time-consuming and costly procedures required, especially when animals other than rodents are used, have hampered the application of the homograft response as a method for testing immunosuppressants.

The graft versus host reaction has found a wider application. This phenomenon occurs when lymphocytes or lymphoid tissue from immunologically mature donors are injected into allogeneic recipients whose antigens are sufficiently distinct from those of the donor cells to elicit a response. The injected cells produce a local and/or systemic attack against the antigens of the lymphoid system of the recipient who is unable to eliminate these foreign cells. The severity of the response is measured in various ways, such as lymphoid poliferation, splenomegaly and stimulation of macrophage activity (9,10,24,56,62,96,113,137,139,142). This reaction is a useful model of delayed immune mechanisms and it has been employed to test a variety of immunosuppressants, such as cyclophosphamide (10,20, 62,96,113,137), methotrexate (10,20,24,96,113,137,139,142) and 6-mercaptopurine (9,113,139,168). Among the drugs tested, only cyclophosphamide has been found active when the disease is clinically evident (113). Since cytotoxic agents can induce hypoplasia

TABLE 26. Graft versus host reaction

Drug	Administered to	Species	References
Cyclophosphamide	Recipient	Mouse	62, 113
	Recipient	Rat	10, 20, 137
	Recipient or donor	Guinea pig	24
Methotrexate	Recipient	Rat	10, 20, 137
	Recipient or donor	Guinea pig	24
	Recipient	Mouse	113, 139
	Recipient	Dog	142
6-Mercaptopurine	Recipient	Mouse	9, 113, 139
Asparaginase	Donor	Mouse	169
	Recipient	Rat	20
Methchloretamine	Recipient	Mouse	113
	Recipient	Rat	10

of the lymphoid system, they should be used at doses below those that can depress spleen weight (9). Furthermore, it should be taken into account that the antiimune potency of a drug may vary, depending on the strain of host and donors utilized (135) (Table 26).

Experimental *autoimmune* diseases involve various autoallergic reactions readily produced in laboratory animals and satisfy most of the criteria accepted for characterizing the human syndrome. They offer several advantages in evaluating compounds expected to interfere with immunopathological events. These disorders can be produced by tissue-specific immunization, have a prolonged and remittent course, exhibit signs of delayed hypersensitivity—although circulating antibodies may be present—and can usually be transferred only through lymphocytes. In addition to examining the effects of drugs on the clinical signs and symptoms peculiar to the particular animal model, other aspects of the disease can also be studied, including hematological, biochemical, histopathological and immunological parameters. Since the disease condition in these experimental models is generally subacute, different treatment schedules can be used in investigating the test compounds, thus, allowing a more thorough determination of their effects.

Among the experimental autoimmune diseases, *adjuvant-in-duced arthritis* is the more widely utilized model. It has been extensively discussed in the previous chapter. The considerable body of data, gathered from many laboratories, indicates that this type of arthritis represents both a reproducible and quantifiable method for drug evaluation and is a suitable model for investigating immunosuppressive agents. Using the different stages of this experimental disease, it is possible to differentiate immunosuppressants from steroidal non-steroidal antiinflammatory drugs (5,90,108,118, 130,133,160,161,171). Recent observations show that adjuvant-induced arthritis can also be employed to detect immunostimulant activities (2,3). D-Penicillamine and levamisole have been found to enhance the intensity of the secondary reaction of adjuvant arthritis, i.e., the response which is accepted to be an expression of delayed hypersensitivity (2,3) (see also below and Chapter 17).

Experimental allergic encephalomyelitis is an autoimmune disease of probably cellular type. It can be induced in a variety of animal species by injecting homologous, heterologous or isologous nervous tissue incorporated in complete or incomplete Freund adjuvant. Upon intradermal inoculation with emulsified nervous tissue, a local inflammatory response takes place which develops into a granulomatous reaction extending along the draining lymphatics. Lymphocyte-bound antibodies appear. Clinical symptoms of the disease are seen 11-15 days after inoculation and consist of ataxia or paresis, followed by flaccid paralysis that causes a dragging of hindquarters. Death occurs in more severely affected animals but there may also be a remission of neurological signs, especially in rats. The disease can be transferred to recipients by lymphocytes from animals with allergic encephalomyelitis. This experimental autoimmune reaction is a useful model for studying the pathophysiology of demyelinating disease and the pharmacology of agents effective in immunoinflammatory disorders (114,115,131,138,157,158). Immunosuppressants, steroids and antilymphocyte serum have been found active when administered to animals at various clinical stages of the disease (95). It must be taken into account, however, that lesions of the central nervous system may be histologically apparent in the absence of clinical signs (116). It should also be noted that, in contrast to adjuvant arthritis, experimental allergic encephalomyelitis is not affected by non-steroidal antiinflammatory drugs.

A variety of experimental models of delayed hypersensitivity has been described. These employ a number of different types of antigens in rats, mice and guinea pigs, and several parameters for assessing the response. Among the more widely used antigens are sheep red blood cells which induce a delayed hypersensitivity reaction in mice; the response is determined either by measuring the swelling of the food pad or by counting the number of spleen cells producing antibody (87,92,93,94,102,127). Recently, the delayed hypersensitivity reaction elicited either in rat paw (4) or pleural cavity (48) has been proposed as a model for evaluating compounds that interfere with immunological (cell-mediated) reactions. Rats are sensitized with Bordetella pertussis mixed with Freund incomplete adjuvant. The sensitizing injection is administered into the plantar surface of one hind paw and one fore paw. After 7-13 days, the rats are challenged either intrapleurally or in the other hind paw and the intensity of the reaction is assessed by measuring the volume and cellularity of the pleural exudate or the swelling of the challenged hind paw, respectively. An important feature of this model is that D-penicillamine and levamisole enhance the response while indomethacin suppresses it. These models seem, therefore, useful for distinguishing the effects of antiinflammatory drugs from those of such substances as D-penicillamine, which have a specific activity in rheumatoid arthritis.

B. In vitro tests for cellular hypersensitivity

As previously mentioned, the terms "cellular hypersensitivity" or "cell-mediated immunity" denote those biological and clinical phenomena that seem to result from interaction between sensitized lymphocytes and specific antigen (149), and in which classical humoral antibodies need not be involved. These sensitized lymphocytes are thymus-derived (32); their various activities may be expressed or indirectly amplified by soluble non-antibody mediators appearing as a result of antigen-lymphocyte interaction. In fact, simple biochemical fractionation reveals that some of these activities are concentrated in the chromatographic and electrophoretic fractions different from those containing the classical immunoglobulins (52, 53,54,121,125,126). Since they were first observed (19,42,51), it has become evident that soluble non-antibody products of lymphocyte activation in vitro possess a number of biological activities that influence the in vitro and in vivo expression of cellular immune response (17,43,52). Some of the soluble factors described and their relevant biological features are reported in Table 27 (see also Chapter 10). The term "lymphokines" was coined to indicate these soluble factors (54) and to suggest the existence of autopharmacolog-

TABLE 27. Outline of non-antibody lymphocyte activation products

Lymphokine	Biological Activity
Lymphocyte mitogenic factor	Enhancement of lymphocyte DNA synthesis
Inflammatory factor	Inflammatory response (increased vascular permeability) to intradermal injection
Cytotoxic factor	Cytotoxicity to fibroblast monolayer
Chemotactic factor	Increased passage of mononuclears through millipore membranes
Migration-inhibition factor	Inhibition of polymorpho- and mononuclears migration from capillary tubes
Macrophage activation factor	Enhancement of metabolic phagocytic activity of macrophages
Interferon-like factor	Interference with virus pathogenicity in cultured cells

ical non-antibody mediators of T-cell response to antigen. Similar biological activities are generated during lymphocyte activation by certain lectins (97,120,121). This is obviously of potential interest for in vitro testing of compounds which may affect cellular hypersensitivity. It has yet to be shown, however, that lymphokines are present in vivo at the site of active reaction of cell-mediated immunity and that agents which would specifically block lymphokine action would also suppress the in vivo induction or expression of cellular immune response (18) (Table 27).

Other major shortcomings of in vitro drug testing must be considered: inability to detect compounds that need to be metabolized to exert their effects, toxicity to cells, drug binding to culture medium.

Methodologies for determining lymphocyte response to activators and for measuring lymphokines have been recently described in great detail (104,156) (see also Chapter 10).

Cellular activation, including the measurement of the proportion of cells undergoing morphological transformation, number of cells undergoing mitosis, uptake of labeled amino-acids, purine or pyrimidine bases (52,54,57,65,84,174) has been used to evaluate the

TABLE 28. Drug effects on various in vitro models of cellular
hypersensitivity - bibliographic references

	Lymphocyte Activation in Vitro	Migration inhibition (Macrophage)	Polymorpho-nuclear Leukocyte Migration	Lymphocyte Cytotoxicity
6-Mercaptopurine	84	82	164	
Methotrexate	29			
Actinomycin D	75	41	30	26, 75
Puromycin	75	41	163	75, 66
Cycloheximide				26, 66, 101
Cytosine-arabinoside	84	82		
Steroids	69, 171	31	162, 164	75, 101, 129
L-Asparaginase	72, 103, 169			
Azathioprine			164	173
Non-steroidal A.I.	171		119, 164	
Chloroquine (and analogs)	84		164	

effect of several compounds (69,72,74,75,103,168,170).

Inhibition of macrophage migration from cell explants in capillary tubes (19,42,51,145,146) and of chemotactic factors for polymorphonuclear leukocytes (23,85,166) has been used for assaying immunosuppressants (30,41,82,83,130,163), and steroidal and non-steroidal drugs (86,119,162).

Among the various methods available for measuring different reactions (117) *lymphocyte cytotoxicity* (54,88,89,117) has also been used as a tool for evaluating immunosuppressive agents (26, 66,71,75,101,129,172) (Table 28).

REFERENCES

1. Arinoviche, R., and Loewi, C.: Ann. Rheum. Dis. *29*:32, 1970.
2. Arrigoni-Martelli, E., and Bramm, E.: Rheumat. Rehabil. *15*:207, 1976.
3. Arrigoni-Martelli, E., and Bramm, E.: Agents Actions *5*:264, 1975.
4. Arrigoni-Martelli, E., Bramm, E., Huskisson, E. C., Willoughby, D. A., and Dieppe, P. A.: Agents Actions, *6*:613, 1976.
5. Arrigoni-Martelli, E., Schiatti, P. F., and Selva, D.: Pharmacol. Res. Commun. *3*:239, 1971.
6. Austen, K. F.: In "The Inflammatory Process," B. W. Zweifact, L. M. Grant, and R. T. McClusky, eds. Academic Press, New York, 1965, p. 589.
7. Bach, J. F., and Dormont, J.: Transplantation *11*:96, 1971.

8. Bach, J. F., Gigli, L., Dardenne, M., and Dormont, J.: Immunology *22*: 625, 1972.
9. Barnes, B. A., Schad, P. B., and Pinn, V. W.: Transplantation *4*:154, 1966.
10. Beck, F. J., Levy, L., and Whitehouse, M. W.: Br. J. Pharmacol. *49*:293, 1973.
11. Berenbaum, M. C.: Br. Med. Bull. *21*:140, 1965.
12. Berenbaum, M. C.: Pharm. J. *203*:671, 1969.
13. Berenbaum, M. C.: Clin. Exp. Immunol. *8*:1, 1971.
14. Berenbaum, M. C., and Brown, I. M.: Immunology *7*:65, 1964.
15. Bice, D., Schwartz, H. J., Lake, W. W., and Salvaggio, J.: Int. Arch. Allergy Appl. Immunol. *41*:628, 1971.
16. Bloch, K. J.: Prog. Allergy *10*:84, 1967.
17. Bloom, B. R.: Adv. Immunol. *13*:101, 1971.
18. Bloom, B. R.: Adv. Immunol. *14*:340, 1971.
19. Bloom, B. R., and Bennett, B.: Science *153*:80, 1966.
20. Bonney, W. W., Feldbush, T. L., and Newfeld, S. E.: J. Pharmacol. Exp. Ther. *190*:576, 1974.
21. Borel, Y., Fauconnet, M., and Miescher, P. A.: Int. Arch. Allergy Appl. Immunol. *33*:583, 1968.
22. Borel, Y., and Schwartz, R. S.: J. Immunol. *92*:754, 1964.
23. Boyden, S.: J. Exp. Med. *115*:453, 1962.
24. Brent, L., and Medawar, P.: Proc. R. Soc. (Lond. [B]) *165*:281, 1966.
25. Broklehurst, W. E.: In "Handbook of Experimental Immunology," D. M. Weir, ed. Davis, Philadelphia, 1967, p. 745.
26. Brumer, K. T., Mauel, J., Cerottini, J. C., and Chapuisfi B.: Immunology *14*:181, 1968.
27. Calne, R. Y., Alexandre, C. P. J., and Murray, J. E.: Ann. N. Y. Acad. Sci. *99*:743, 1962.
28. Campbell, D. H., Garvey, J. S., Cremer, N. E., and Sussdorf, D. H.: "Methods in Immunology," Benjamin, New York, 1963, p. 215.
29. Caron, G. A.: In "Proceedings, 3rd Annual Leucocyte Culture Conference," W. O. Rieke, ed. Appleton, New York, 1969, p. 287.
30. Carruthers, B. M.: Can. J. Physiol. Pharmacol. *45*:269, 1967.
31. Casey, W. J., and McCall, C. E.: Immunology *21*:225, 1971.
32. Cerottini, J. C., and Dumonde, D. D.: In "Progress in Immunology," B. Amos, ed. Academic Press, New York, 1971, p. 1459.
33. Chaumougan, D., and Schwartz, R. S.: J. Exp. Med. *124*:363, 1966.
34. Cochrane, C. G.: In "The Inflammatory Process," B. W. Zweifach, L. H. Grant, and R. T. McClusky, eds. Academic Press, New York, 1968, p. 613.
35. Cochrane, C. G., and Dixon, F. J.: In "Textbook of Immunopathology," Vol. 1, P. A. Miescher, and H. J. Müller-Eberhard, eds. Grune and Stratton, New York, 1968, p. 94.
36. Collier, H. O. J., and James, G. W. L.: Br. J. Pharmacol. *30*:283, 1967.
37. Cox, J. S. G., Beach, J. E., Blair, A. M. J. M., Clarke, A. J., King, L., Lee, T. B., Loveday, D. E. E., Moss, G. F., Orr, T. S. C., Ritchie, T., and Sheard, P.: Adv. Drug Res. *5*:115, 1970.
38. Cruchaud, A.: J. Immunol. *96*:832, 1966.
39. Currey, H. L. F.: Clin. Exp. Immunol. *9*:879, 1971.
40. Daniel, T. M., Weygand, J. G. M., Jr., and Stavitsky, A. B.: J. Immunol. *90*:741, 1963.

41. David, J. R.: J. Exp. Med. *122*:1125, 1965.
42. David, J. R.: Proc. Natl. Acad. Sci. USA *56*:72, 1966.
43. David, J. R.: Fed. Proc. *30*:1730, 1971.
44. Davies, G. E.: Immunology *14*:393, 1968.
45. Dawson, W., Starr, M. S., and West G. B.: Br. J. Pharmacol. *27*:249, 1966.
46. Denman, E. J.: Clin. Exp. Immunol. *5*:217, 1969.
47. Denman, E. J., Denman, A. M., Greenwood, B. M., Gall, D., and Health, R. B.: Ann. Rheum. Dis. *29*:220, 1970.
48. Dieppe, P. A., Willoughby, D. A., Huskisson, E. C., and Arrigoni-Martelli, E.: Agents Actions, *6*:618, 1976.
49. Dresser, D. W., and Wortis, H. H.: In "Handbook of Experimental Immunology," D. M. Weir, ed. Davis, Philadelphia, 1967, p. 1054.
50. Dukor, P., and Dietrich, F. M.: Int. Arch. Allergy Appl. Immunol. *34*:32, 1968.
51. Dumonde, D. C.: Br. Med. Bull. *23*:9, 1967.
52. Dumonde, D. C., Howson, W. T., and Wolstencroft, R. A.: In "Immunopathology: 5th International Symposium," P. A. Miescher, and B. Grabar, eds. Schwabe, Basel, 1968, p. 263.
53. Dumonde, D. C., Page, D. A., Matthew, M., and Wolstencroft, R. A.: Clin. Exp. Immunol. *10*:25, 1972.
54. Dumonde, D. C., Wolstencroft, R. A., Panavi, G. S., Matthew, M., Morley, J., and Howson, W. T.: Nature *224*:38, 1969.
55. Durkin, H. G., and Thorbecke, G. J.: J. Immunol. *106*:1079, 1971.
56. Elkins, W. L.: Prog. Allergy *15*:78, 1971.
57. Farrow, M. C., and Van Dyke, K.: Chemotherapy *16*:76, 1971.
58. Fisher, D. S., Cassidy, E. P., and Welch, A. D.: Biochem. Pharmacol. *15*:1013, 1966.
59. Friedman, H., and Chakrabarty, A. K.: Immunology *21*:989, 1971.
60. Frisch, A. W., and Davies, G. H.: J. Immunol. *88*:269, 1962.
61. Gerebetzoff, A., Lambert, P. H., and Miescher, P. A.: Ann. Rev. Pharmacol. *12*:287, 1972.
62. Glucksberg, H., and Fefer, A.: Transplantation *13*:300, 1972.
63. Goh, K. O., Miller, D. G., and Diamond, H. D.: J. Immunol. *86*:606, 1961.
64. Goose, J., and Blair, A. M. J. N.: Immunology *16*:749, 1969.
65. Gordon, B. L., and Ford, D. K.: In "Essentials of Immunology," Davis, Philadelphia, 1971, p. 17.
66. Granger, G. A.: Am. J. Pathol. *60*:469, 1970.
67. Gray, O. D., Mickelson, M. M., and Crim, J. A.: Transplantation *6*:805, 1968.
68. Halasz, N. A., Orloff, J., and Hirose, F.: Transplantation *2*:453, 1964.
69. Halpern, B., Ky, N. T., and Amache, N.: J. Allergy *40*:168, 1967.
70. Harrison, E. F., and Fuguay, M. E.: Proc. Soc. Exp. Biol. Med. *139*:957, 1972.
71. Henney, C. S., and Lichtenstein, L. M.: J. Immunol. *107*:610, 1971.
72. Hersch, E. M.: Transplantation *12*:368, 1971.
73. Hicks, R.: J. Pharm. Pharmacol. *21*:202, 1969.
74. Hirschhorn, R., Grossman, J., Troll, W., and Weissmann, G.: J. Clin. Invest. *50*:1206, 1971.
75. Holm, G.: Exp. Cell Res. *48*:334, 1967.

76. von Horsch, A., and Rapp, W. Arzneim Forsch. *21*:769, 1971.

77. Humphrey, J. M.: Br. J. Exp. Pathol. *36*:268, 1955.

78. Ingraham, J. S., and Bussard, A. J. Exp. Med. *119*:667, 1964.

79. Jerne, N. K., Nordin, A. A., and Henry, C.: In "Cell-Bound Antibodies," S. Amos, and H. Kaprowski, eds. Wistar Institute Press, Philadelphia, 1963, p. 109.

80. Kabat, E. A.: "Structural Concepts in Immunology and Immunochemistry," Holt, New York, 1968, p. 248.

81. Kaliss, N.: Transplantation *12*:146, 1971.

82. Kaplan, S., and Calabresi, P.: Clin. Res. *13*:543, 1965.

83. Kaplan, S., and Calabresi, P.: Clin. Res. *14*:333, 1966.

84. Kasakura, S.: J. Immunol. *105*:1162, 1970.

85. Keller, H. U., Borel, J. F., Wilkinson, P. C., Hess, M. W., and Cottier, H.: J. Immunol. Meth. *1*:165, 1972.

86. Keller, H. U., and Sorkin, E.: In "Non-Steroidal Antiinflammatory Drugs," S. Garattini, and M. N. G. Dukes, eds. Excerpta Medica, Amsterdam, 1965, p. 134.

87. Kerckhaert, J. A. M., Van den Berg, G. J., and Willers, J. M. N.: Ann. Immunol. *125C*:415, 1974.

88. Kolb, W. P., and Granger, G. A.: Proc. Natl. Acad. Sci. USA *61*:1250, 1968.

89. Kolb, W. P., and Granger, G. A.: Cell Immunol. *1*:122, 1970.

90. Komarek, A., and Dietrich, F. M.: Arch. Int. Pharmacodyn. Ther. *193*: 349, 1971.

91. Laddu, A. R., and Sanyal, R. K.: Int. Arch. Allergy Appl. Immunol. *33*: 593, 1968.

92. Lagrange, P. H., Mackaness, G. B., and Miller, T. E.: J. Exp. Med. *139*: 528, 1974.

93. Lagrange, P. H., Mackaness, G. B., and Miller, T. E.: J. Exp. Med. *139*: 1529, 1974.

94. Lagrange, P. H., Mackaness, G. B., Miller, T. E., and Ishibashi, T.: J. Exp. Med. *139*:543, 1974.

95. Levine, S., Sowinski, R., and Kies, M. W.: Clin. Exp. Immunol. *6*:503, 1970.

96. Levy, L.: Arch. Int. Pharmacodyn. Ther. *211*:8, 1974.

97. Mackler, B. F., Wolstencroft, R. A., and Dumonde, D. C.: Nature (New Biol.) *239*:139, 1972.

98. Maguire, H. C., and von Ettore, L.: J. Invest. Dermatol. *48*:39, 1967.

99. Maguire, H. C., and Maibach, H. J.: J. Allergy *32*:406, 1961.

100. Maibach, H. J., and Maguire, H. C.: Int. Arch. Allergy Appl. Immunol. *29*:209, 1966.

101. Manuel, J., Rudolf, H., Chapuis, B., and Brunner, K. T.: Immunology *18*: 517, 1970.

102. Measel, J. W., Jr.: Infect. Immun. *11*:350, 1975.

103. Mersh, E. M., and Brown, B. W.: Cancer Res. *31*:834, 1971.

104. Morley, J., Wolstencraft, R. A., and Dumond, D. C.: In "Cellular Immunology,"Vol. 2, D. M. Weir, ed. Blackwell, Oxford, 1973, p. 28.1.

105. Munro, A., Bewick, M., Manuel, L., Cameron, J. S., Ellis, F. G., Boulton-Jones, M., and Ogg, C. S.: Br. Med. J. *3*:271, 1971.

106. Nathan, H. C., Bieber, S., Elion, G. B., and Hitchings, C. H.: Proc. Soc.

Exp. Biol. Med. *107*:796, 1961.
107. Nehlsen, S. L.: Clin. Exp. Immunol. *9*:63, 1971.
108. Newbould, B. B.: Br. J. Pharmacol. *24*:632, 1965.
109. Oort, J., and Turk, J. L.: Br. J. Exp. Pathol. *46*:147, 1965.
110. Orr, T. S. C., Pollard, M. C., Gwilliam, J., and Cox, J. S. G.: Clin. Exp. Immunol. *7*:745, 1970.
111. Ovary, Z.: Prog. Allergy *5*:459, 1958.
112. Ovary, Z.: In "Immunological Methods," J. F. Ackroyed, ed. Blackwell, Oxford, 1964, p. 239.
113. Owens, A. H., and Santos, G. E.: Transplantation *2*:378, 1971.
114. Paterson, P. Y.: Adv. Immunol. *5*:131, 1966.
115. Paterson, P. Y.: In "Textbook of Immunology," P. A. Miesched, and H. J. Müller-Eberhard, eds. Grune and Stratton, New York, 1968, p. 132.
116. Paterson, P. Y., Hanson, M. A., and Gerner, E. W.: Proc. Soc. Exp. Biol. Med. *124*:928, 1967.
117. Perlmann, P., and Holm, G.: Adv. Immunol. *11*:117, 1969.
118. Perper, R. J., Alvarez, B., Colombo, C., and Schroder, H.: Proc. Soc. Exp. Biol. Med. *137*:506, 1971.
119. Phelps, P., and McCarty, D. J., Jr.: J. Pharmacol. Exp. Ther. *158*:546, 1967.
120. Pick, E., Brostoff, J., Krejci, J., and Turk, J. L.: Cell. Immunol. *1*:92, 1970.
121. Pick, E., Krejci, J., and Turk, J. L.: Nature *225*:236, 1970.
122. Polak, L., Geleick, H., and Turk, J. L.: Immunology *28*:939, 1975.
123. Polak, L., and Turk, J. L.: Nature *249*:654, 1974.
124. Raab, W.: Experientia *24*:250, 1968.
125. Remold, H. G., and David, J. R.: J. Immunol. *107*:1090, 1970.
126. Remold H. G., Katz, A. B., Haber, E., and David, J. R.: Cell. Immunol. *1*:133, 1970.
127. Renoux, G., and Renoux, M.: J. Immunol. *133*:779, 1974.
128. Rose, N. R., Haber, J. A., and Calabresi, P.: Proc. Soc. Exp. Biol. Med. *128*:1121, 1968.
129. Rosenau, W., and Moon, H. D.: J. Immunol. *89*:422, 1962.
130. Rosenthale, M. E., Datko, L. J., Kassarich, J., and Rosanoff, E.: J. Pharmacol. Exp. Ther. *180*:501, 1972.
131. Rosenthale, M. E., Datko, L. J., Kassarich, J., and Schneider, E.: Arch. Int. Pharmacodyn, Ther. *179*:251, 1969.
132. Rosenthale, M. E., and Gluekman, M. J.: Experientia *24*:1229, 1968.
133. Rosenthale, M. E., and Margules, D. L.: Proc. Soc. Exp. Biol. Med. *130*:339, 1969.
134. Rubin, B. A., and Tint, H.: Transplant. Proc. *3*:819, 1971.
135. Russell, P. S.: Ann. N. Y. Acad. Sci. *87*:445, 1960.
136. Sabet, T. Y., and Friedman, H.: Int. Arch. Allergy Appl. Immunol. *42*:161, 1972.
137. Santos, G. W., and Owens, A. H.: Nature *210*:139, 1966.
138. Scheinberg, L. C., Kies, M. W., and Alvord, E. C.: Ann. N. Y. Acad. Sci. *122*:1-570, 1965.
139. Schwarz, R. S., and Beldoth, L.: Transplantation *3*:79, 1965.
140. Schwartz, R. S., and Dameshek, W.: J. Clin. Invest. *38*:1394, 1959.
141. Stavitsky, A. N.: J. Immunol. *72*:360, 1954.

142. Storb, R., Epstein, R. B., Graham, T. C., and Thomas, G. D.: Transplantation *9*:240, 1970.
143. Strander, H.: Immunology *10*:45, 1966.
144. Swanson, M. A., and Schwartz, R. S.: N. Engl. J. Med. *277*:163, 1967.
145. Søborg, M.: Acta Med. Scand. *185*:221, 1969.
146. Søborg, M., and Bendixen, G.: Acta Med. Scand. *181*:247, 1967.
147. Takatsky, G., Furesz, J., and Farkas, E.: Acta. Physiol. Scand. *5*:241, 1954.
148. Turk, J. L.: Int. Arch. Allergy *24*:191, 1964.
149. Turk, J. L.: Br. Med. Bull. *23* (1) : 1967.
150. Turk, J. L., and Parker, D.: Immunology *24*:751, 1973.
151. Turk, J. L., Parker, D., and Poulter, C. W.: Immunology *23*:493, 1972.
152. Turk, J. L., and Polak, L.: Lancet *1*:130, 1969.
153. Turk, J. L., and Stone, S. H.: In "Cell-Bound Antibodies," S. Amos, and H. Kaprowski, eds. Wistar Institute Press, Philadelphia, 1963, p. 51.
154. Turk, J. L., and Willoughby, D. A.: Lancet *1*:249, 1967.
155. Ueki, E. M., and Long, J.: J. Pharmacol. Exp. Ther. *158*:365, 1967.
156. Waithe, W. I., and Hirschhorn, K.: In "Cellular Immunology," Vol. 2, D. M. Weir, ed. Blackwell, Oxford, 1973, p. 25.1.
157. Waksman, B. H.: Int. Arch. Allergy Appl. Immunol. *14* (Suppl.) : 1, 1959.
158. Waksman, B. H., and Adams, R. D.: Am. J. Pathol. *41*:135, 1962.
159. Waksman, B. H., Arbouys, S., and Arnason, B. G.: J. Exp. Med. *114*:997, 1961.
160. Walz, D. T., and Berkoff, C. E.: Proc. Soc. Exp. Biol. Med. *135*:760, 1970.
161. Walz, D. T., Di Martino, M. J., and Misher, A.: J.Pharmacol. Exp. Ther. *178*:223, 1971.
162. Ward, P. A.: J. Exp. Med. *124*:209, 1966.
163. Ward, P. A.: Biochem. Pharmacol. *17* (Suppl.) : 99, 1968.
164. Ward, P. A.: Am. J. Pathol. *64*:521, 1971.
165. Ward, P. A., and Cochrane, G. G.: J. Exp. Med. *121*:215, 1965.
166. Ward, P. A., Offen, C. D., and Montgomery, F. R.: Fed. Proc. *30*:1721, 1971.
167. Watts, H. G.: Transplantation *12*:229, 1971.
168. Weksler, M. E., and Weksler, B. B.: Immunology *21*:137, 1971.
169. West, G. B.: Clin. Pharmacol. Ther. *4*:749, 1963.
170. Whitehouse, M. W.: J. Pharm. Pharmacol. *19*:590, 1967.
171. Whittington, H.: Br. J. Pharmacol. *40*:167P, 1970.
172. Wilson, D. B.: J. Exp. Med. *122*:167, 1965.
173. Wilson, J. D.: Immunology *21*:233, 1971.
174. Wolstencroft, R. A., and Dumonde, D. C.: Immunology *18*:599, 1970.
175. Zaalberg, O. B., Van der Meul, V. A., and Van Twisk, M. J.: J. Immunol. *100*:451, 1968.
176. Zukoski, C. F., Callaway, J. M., and Rhea, W. G.: Transplantation *1*:293, 1963.

Chapter 13

Evaluation of Clinical Efficacy

The generally recognized difficulty of proving the effectiveness of antiinflammatory drugs in patients with arthritis is partly due to the fact that our methods for assessing inflammation clinically are not sufficiently refined. The selection of relevant diagnostic indices and a sound experimental design constitute the essential prerequisites for a meaningful trial. A further basic premise is that the study should identify and evaluate the reversible features of the disease (29). No allegations are, in fact, made that classical antiinflammatory agents cure the underlying disease, or even completely prevent tissue injury or progressive loss of function. Long-term investigations are not needed to demonstrate the beneficial effects of the many non-steroidal agents currently available but, on the other hand, the results of short-term trials (2-4 weeks) can hardly be considered meaningful in the treatment of patients with a disease such as rheumatoid arthritis. If yet another drug of this type were to be introduced, the only rationale for doing so would be a lack of toxicity and continued efficacy. In such a case, a long-term study would be justified and emphasis should be placed on a careful evaluation of undesirable side effects.

1. EXPERIMENTAL DESIGN

There are several reasons why experimental design is of primary importance. The most obvious is the inherent biological variability of patients with rheumatoid arthritis. A second problem arises because drugs commonly used to treat this disease have a less than dramatic effect on its course. Finally, the methods commonly employed for assessing rheumatoid arthritis are relatively insensitive and the difficulty of evaluating inflammatory activity in clinical practice (28) has been generally acknowledged.

The best protocol is one which is developed jointly by the pharmacologist, clinical investigator and statistician. A double-blind design is mandatory; pairing of patients for a number of variables, such as age, sex, duration and severity of the disease, is highly desirable but is not often practical. Consequently, the standard protocol for short-term evaluation of an antiinflammatory agent is the double-blind cross-over study in which treatment periods are randomly allocated, usually by Latin square design (9,45). The patient acts as his own control and it is assumed that the unavoidable spontaneous changes in disease activity will be equally distributed between the various treatment periods. One major disadvantage of the cross-over clinical trial is the problem of carry-over effects; however, these can be minimized by inserting a wash-out period in between the treatments. It has already been mentioned that there is great variability among patients with rheumatoid arthritis. Since, for the purpose of drug evaluation, patient homogeneity is important, it is most helpful to define the patient group to be studied according to the classification of the American Rheumatism Association (48).

Every new compound should be tested against a placebo at an early stage in its evaluation. Moreover, the use of a placebo for comparing a known active drug with a new compound will increase the sensitivity of a double-blind study and will give some indication of the patient's capacity to respond. It should be taken into account that the placebo response in patients with a chronic disease, such as rheumatoid arthritis, is in the order of 30% It is a common practice to study a new antiinflammatory drug in a fixed dose. However, one basic prerequisite for managing any chronic disease is that the dosage of the drug selected be tailored to the individual patient. In addition, it has been shown that similarly conducted trials with the same compound but at different dose levels may produce divergent results (34). Therefore, it is of greatest importance to conduct dose-response studies and to employ at least two different dose levels at some stage of the evaluation. With certain notable exceptions (40, 41, 43), the emphasis in rheumatological drug evaluation has been on short-term studies. However, as mentioned before, only long-term investigations can provide meaningful information on treating this disease in a real life situation. There are several problems associated with long-term studies which could be at least partially solved with multicenter clinical trials (40,41,43).

2. METHODS OF ASSESSMENT

Almost all the indices currently used for assessing rheumatoid arthritis are based upon the cardinal signs of inflammation: redness, heat, swelling, pain and loss of function. In addition, muscle weakness, morning stiffness, fatigue and several laboratory determinations of, e.g., erythrocyte sedimentation rate; concentrations of rheumatoid factor and serum protein; and radioisotope parameters may also be employed. There is not a single "ideal" measurement which reflects total disease activity in rheumatoid arthritis and, therefore, we depend on the selection of a number of perhaps less satisfactory criteria. Several composite indices have been suggested (27,33) and shown to be useful in determining the efficacy of new compounds, even if none of them have proven superior to a simple demonstration of pain relief (7,11,34).

In these composite indices, both subjective and objective evaluations are included.

The subjective assessment should be quantifiable, and both inter- and intra-observer errors must be measured and taken into account when reporting the final results (4,18). When information on the subjective indices is being collected, the queries should be arranged in such order that no "leading" question is posed. Questions should always be asked in the same sequence and a separate data sheet should be used on each occasion (23).

Pain is generally the main complaint of the patient suffering from rheumatoid arthritis. Its intensity or its relief can be only evaluated through a statement from the sufferer. Numerous studies attest to the validity of employing the patient's own assessment in measuring the efficacy of new drugs, compared to placebo or to established analgesic preparations (17,21,25,26,31,32). Various methods for recording pain have been employed. A percentage system, with all patients beginning at 100% and moving up or down the scale according to progress, has been suggested (7). This method, however, has no descriptive limits and different patients with the same severity of pain may assign it a varying position on the scale (15). A nominal scale overcomes the problems of descriptive limits to some extent but in calculating the response, it is assumed that the divisions on such a scale are all of equal length. It has been pointed out that not all the steps may, in fact, be of equal value and a decrease in pain from severe to moderate is of greater importance to the patient than a change from slight to none (20,30). The assignment of a numerical scale to each category of pain intensity or its relief probably makes little difference. It seems more relevant to extend the scale from four to nine points in order to differentiate between minor effects of drugs (15,22). Indirect methods for measuring pain, such as the algometer, dolorimeter (35), or catecholamine excretion rates (15) are unlikely to find wide acceptance in clinical practice.

Although numerous methods have been proposed for quantitating *joint tenderness* in rheumatoid arthritis (6,19,27,33,46,49), no entirely satisfactory system has even evolved so far. The problem arises from the fact that joint tenderness depends on a number of variables, such as the severity of the inflammatory process, the pain threshold of the patient, the amount of pressure applied, the patient's reaction to pain, and his attitude toward disease and physician. Moreover, inherent in the method are variations due to differences among investigators in the manner of applying pressure, and the frequently asymmetrical distribution of the inflammatory process around and within a joint.

The articular index of joint tenderness of Ritchie et al. (46) is based on a summation of a number of quantitative indicators of pain when the joint is subjected to firm digital pressure at the articular margin. There is a close correlation between this index and that employed by the cooperative clinics of the American Rheumatism Association (6). The latter index determines the clinical activity by the presence of tenderness on pressure, pain on passive movement, or soft-tissue swelling.

Reduction of hand *grip strength* is extremely common in rheumatoid arthritis. It is measured by using a folded standard sphygmomanometer cuff inflated to 30 mmHg and attached to an ordinary mercury columnar sphygmomanometer registering at least

300 mmHg. The measurement of grip strength is not a simple assessment of muscle strength since various factors, such as deformities—particularly of the metacarpo-phalangeal and proximal interphalangeal joints—pain, stiffness, effusion into tendon sheaths and arthritic involvement of the more proximal joints, may considerably influence the results. It is considered to be a single, reliable and reproducible test (8,28).

The measurement of *digital joint size* provides a useful index of antiinflammatory drug activity in rheumatoid arthritis. Since first suggested (14), it has been widely employed, with minor technical modifications (use of Geigy gauge instead of standard jeweller'rings), in a number of clinical trials (2,3,5,11,12,24). The reduction in digital joint circumference was shown to have occurred in joints with soft-tissue swelling and this is one factor limiting the value of the above test as a routine index of joint inflammation in clinical trials.

Assessment of the duration and severity of *morning stiffness* has been widely employed as an index of the rheumatoid condition (28). Although morning stiffness is an almost invariable feature of active rheumatoid arthritis, and both severity and duration decrease with reduction in disease activity, its quantitation is hindered by the same difficulties as exist in estimating pain. Methods for objective measurement of morning stiffness have been described (1,55).

Time to walk 50 feet is another functional test which has been employed. Like the measurement of grip strength, it can be influenced by a number of factors, such as the presence of joint deformities and, possibly, diurnal variations.

Attempts have been made to employ *aspirin or paracetamol consumption* throughout a clinical trial of a new compound as a measure of its efficacy (28,34). The potential usefulness of this parameter is a matter of debate. It should be mentioned that, during a multicenter clinical trial of indomethacin, the use of salicylates, when needed, was allowed (6). The results of this study indicated no difference between indomethacin and placebo. It was then shown (57,58) that the salicylate impairs indomethacin absorption. A subsequent clinical trial (56) performed according to the criteria of the American Rheumatism Association and where aspirin consumption was measured showed a significantly higher activity of indomethacin vs. placebo.

A raised *erythrocyte sedimentation rate* is an invariable feature of active rheumatoid arthritis. However, its usefulness as an indicator of drug activity in short-term clinical trials is questionable since, frequently, continued elevated values have been observed in patients whose clinical conditions, by other criteria, have shown considerable improvement (28). A number of other *laboratory tests* also indicates changes in the activity of rheumatoid arthritis and includes determinations of hemoglobin, serum iron, albumin, globulin, C-reactive protein (38,42) and rheumatoid factor. The more popular assays for rheumatoid factor, such as the Waaler-Rose or latex test, are positive in more than 60% of rheumatoid patients. These tests revals the presence of anti-IgG antibodies in 100% of positive subjects (51). More refined techniques as, for example, immunoabsorption, show the presence of anti-IgG antibodies even in subjects rheumatoid factor negative (47). A review of biochemical and hematological data in rheumatoid arthritis and drug interactions has been published recently (54).

Radioisotope studies have found wide application in rheumatology during the past few years. Radioisotopes may be administered either intravenously or intra-articularly but, in both instances, clear-cut differences between normal and inflamed joints are apparent (5,10,37,36,44). Numerous radioisotopes have been used to investigate joints but, currently, radioactive technetium (^{99m}Tc) is most commonly employed for this purpose (10,11,16,36). It is safe because it does not emit primary β radiation and has a short half-life of only 6 hours. The local accumulation of intravenously administered ^{99m}Tc has been shown to reflect not only vascularity but also tissue volume and, in some instances, that of synovial fluid (13,37,53). Results of joint scanning have been found to correlate well with other clinical parameters of the respective inflammation (10,11,13,36,44). The radioactivity in a joint may be recorded by scintillation scanning (52,53) or by continuous external directional counting above it and measuring the peak isotope uptake (5,10). With this method it is possible to detect changes following effective antiinflammatory therapy (5).

3. DIAGNOSTIC CRITERIA OF RHEUMATOID ARTHRITIS (48)

A. Classical rheumatoid arthritis

This diagnosis must meet seven of the following criteria. In criteria 1 through 5, listed below, the joint signs or symptoms must be continuous for at least 6 weeks. (Any one of the features listed under "Exclusions" will eliminate a patient from this and all other categories.)

1. Morning stiffness.
2. Pain on motion or tenderness in at least one joint (observed by physician).
3. Swelling (soft-tissue thickening or fluid, not bony overgrowth alone) in at least one joint (observed by physician).
4. Swelling (observed by physician) of at least one other joint (any interval free of joint symptoms between the two joint involvements may not exceed 3 months).
5. Symmetrical joint swelling (observed by physician), with simultaneous involvement of the same joint on both sides of the body (bilateral involvement of proximal interphalangeal, metacarpophalangeal, or metatarsophalangeal joints is acceptable without absolute symmetry). Terminal phalangeal joint involvement will not satisfy this criterion.
6. Subcutaneous nodules (observed by physician) over bony prominences, on extensor surfaces or in juxta-articular regions.
7. Radiological changes typical of rheumatoid arthritis (which must include at least bony decalcification localized in the involved joints or most pronounced adjacent to them and not just degenerative changes). Degenerative changes do not exclude patients from any group classified as rheumatoid arthritis.
8. Positive agglutination test—demonstration of the "rheumatoid factor" by any method which, in two laboratories, has been positive in not over 5% of normal controls—or positive streptococcal agglutination test (the latter is now obsolete).
9. Poor mucin precipitate from synovial fluid (with shreds and cloudy solution).
10. Characteristic histological changes in synovium, with three or more of the following: marked villous hypertrophy; proliferation of superficial synovial cells, often with palisading; marked infiltration of chronic inflammatory cells (lymphocytes or plasma cells predominating), with tendency to form "lymphoid nodules"; deposition of compact fibrin either on surface or interstitially; foci of necrosis.
11. Characteristic histological changes in nodules showing granulomatous foci with central zones of cell necrosis, surrounded by a palisade of proliferated macrophages, and peripheral fibrosis and chronic inflammatory cell infiltration, predominantly perivascular.

B. Definite rheumatoid arthritis

This diagnosis requires five of the above criteria. In criteria 1 through 5, the joint signs or symptoms must be continuous for at least 6 weeks.

C. Probable rheumatoid arthritis

This diagnosis must satisfy three of the above criteria. In at least one of the criteria 1 through 5, the joint signs or symptoms must be continuous for at least six weeks.

D. Possible rheumatoid arthritis

This diagnosis must meet two of the following conditions, and the total duration of joint symptoms must be at least 3 weeks.
1. Morning stiffness.
2. Tenderness or pain on motion (observed by physician), with history of recurrence or persistence for 3 weeks.
3. History or observation of joint swelling.
4. Subcutaneous nodules (observed by physician).
5. Elevated sedimentation rate or C-reactive protein.
6. Iritis (of dubious value as a criterion, except in the case of juvenile rheumatoid arthritis).

E. Exclusions

1. Typical rash of systemic lupus erythematosus (with butterfly distribution, follicle plugging and areas of atrophy).
2. High concentration of lupus erythematosus cells (four or more in two smears prepared from heparinized blood incubated not over 2 hours) (or other clear-cut evidence of systemic lupus erythematosus).
3. Histological evidence of periarteritis nodosa with segmental necrosis of arteries, associated with nodular leukocytic infiltration extending perivascularly and tending to include many eosinophils.
4. Weakness of neck, trunk and pharyngeal muscles, or persistent muscle swelling, or dermatomyositis.
5. Definite scleroderma (not limited to the fingers). (The latter is an arguable point.)
6. Clinical picture characteristic of rheumatic fever, with migratory joint involvement and evidence of endocarditis, especially if accompanied by subcutaneous nodules, or erythema margi-

natum, or chorea. (An elevated antistreptolysin titer will not rule out the diagnosis of rheumatoid arthritis).

7. Clinical picture characteristic of gouty arthritis, with acute attacks of swelling, redness, and pain in one or more joints, especially if relieved by colchicine.
8. Tophi.
9. Clinical picture characteristic of acute infectious arthritis of bacterial or viral origin with: an acute focus of infection or in close association with a disease of known infectious origin; chills; fever; and an acute joint involvement, usually migratory at the beginning (especially if there are organisms in the joint fluid or the patient responses to antibiotic therapy).
10. Tubercle bacilli in the joints or histological evidence of joint tuberculosis.
11. Clinical picture characteristic of Reiter's syndrome, with urethritis and conjunctivitis associated with acute joint involvement, usually migratory at first.
12. Clinical picture characteristic of the shoulder-hand syndrome, with unilateral involvement of shoulder and hand, with diffuse swelling of hand, followed by atrophy and contractures.
13. Clinical picture characteristic of hypertrophic osteoarthropathy, with clubbing of fingers and/or hypertrophic periostitis along the shafts of the long bones, especially if an intrapulmonary lesion (or another appropriate underlying disorder) is present.
14. Clinical picture characteristic of neuroarthropathy, with condensation and destruction of bones of involved joints and with associated neurological findings.
15. Homogentisic acid in urine, detectable grossly with alkalinization.
16. Histological evidence of sarcoid or positive Kveim test.
17. Multiple myeloma as evidenced by marked increase in plasma cells in the bone marrow, or Bence-Jones protein in urine.
18. Characteristic skin lesions of erythema nodosum.
19. Leukemia or lymphoma, with characteristic cells in peripheral blood, bone marrow or tissues.
20. Agammaglobulinemia.

4. CRITERIA FOR CLINICAL ASSESSMENT OF ANTIINFLAMMATORY ACTIVITY (39)

Patients should have active adult rheumatoid arthritis in order to qualify for trials of new drugs. They either should never have received antirheumatic agents or, if they have, these drugs should be withdrawn for a sufficiently long period to dissipate their effects and permit an acute rebound of the disease prior to the patient's inclusion in the study. Concomitant therapy for the disorder should be limited to salicylates.

A. Phase 1

Patients should, in general, be hospitalized, but this requirement will depend on any previous experience with the drug.

Patients should be closely followed for evidence of adverse effects by clinical observation and appropriate laboratory "safety" tests, including simple examination of all stools for occult blood. For efficacy, twice-weekly evaluations are recommended in accordance with the indications given below under point 5.A.1 (Efficacy assessment).

In order to obtain the desired information, treatment should last up to 4 weeks; the drug doses should be administered on an open basis, and be varied from patient to patient within the probable dose range and according to the safety findings obtained in trials with normal volunteers. Some patients should receive the highest doses tolerated in the latter trials.

B. Phases 2 and 3

Early Phase 2: These investigations may be performed on outpatients. They may begin as relatively short-term (i.e., 2 weeks), open-label (non-placebo controlled) trials, followed by double-blind studies with low, medium, and high doses, where the efficacy of the test drug is compared at different dose levels to a placebo. If necessary for the patient's comfort, a non-antiinflammatory analgesic may be added (e.g., codeine) but the reasons for doing so must be specified and only one particular analgesic should be used for the patients in a given study; furthermore, no analgesic drug combinations should be employed.

Additional early studies, lasting about 6-8 weeks, may include a comparison of the investigational drug with an adequate antiinflammatory dose (usually more than 3.6 g/day) of aspirin or other established antiinflammatory agents.

Greater efficacy than aspirin should not be required since antiinflammatory drugs with less frequent or serious side effects than aspirin are what is needed clinically.

Some other studies which might be considered for this phase are those that may show additional benefits of the test drug, compared to maintenance treatment alone.

Patients should be monitored at close intervals for adverse effects, through both clinical observation and laboratory safety tests (including stool examinations for occult blood). Efficacy assessments, may be made weekly or at least every 2 weeks, with signal joints evaluated every week. When studies last only 2 weeks, efficacy assessment should be made weekly.

Late Phase 2 and Phase 3: The next or expanded phases of clinical investigation continue to be directed toward safety and efficacy evaluation in the long-term management (pain and inflammation) of rheumatoid arthritis, and consist of open-label or controlled studies.

These controlled studies, should extend over several months to a year, be double-blind and involve comparison with a placebo. Because of the duration of these investigations and the practicalities of obtaining a patient population large enough to undergo meaningful clinical trials, most subjects will be on some concomitant therapy. Such therapy should be maintained at constant dosage levels. The conditions of this type of study should be truly double-blind.

Patients should be randomized, so that those who are on various concomitant drugs are distributed proportionately between the groups given placebo or the test compound. If patients are on concomitant therapy, placebo studies can continue for up to one year.

Although it would be desirable to perform investigations where each would be limited to patients with similar degrees of disease severity, it is recognized that this cannot be done, except in cooperative clinical trials.

Since patients in late Phase 2 and Phase 3 will usually be on concomitant therapy, it is important to note on the chart whether the baseline Activity Index was obtained while on such therapy or if and when the latter was discontinued.

Three examples of studies designed to permit the assessment of drug efficacy and safety are outlined below:

1. Parallel comparison of drug and placebo added to background (i.e., concomitant) therapy.
   a. Subjects: outpatients with active adult rheumatoid arthritis.
   b. Number of subjects: to be determined after reviewing earlier studies.
   c. Duration of treatment: 24 weeks or longer.

    d. Dosing: random, blind assignment to drug or placebo, with the same background treatment continued throughout the study.

    e. Assessment: safety—hematocrit, WBC and differential, urinalysis, BUN, alkaline phosphatase, SGOT, and any other indicated, at appropriate intervals. Efficacy—every 4 weeks.

2. Comparison of drug to aspirin or other active agent.

    a. Subjects: disease and activity as in point 1 above, except that the patient must not have received any of the long-acting types of antirheumatic agents in the recent past.

    b. Number of subjects: to be determined after reviewing earlier studies and the literature pertaining to other active agents.

    c. Duration of treatment: 12 to 16 weeks.

    d. Dosing: random blind assignment to test drug or identically appearing aspirin (or other active agent) in a daily specified adequate, antiinflammatory dose.
Assessment: safety—as in point 1 above. Efficacy—every 4 weeks, and chronic disease evaluation at the beginning and end of trial.

3. Studies of an open dosing nature but closely monitored provide descriptive data on efficacy and, especially, safety. Some of these studies may result in double-blind assessments of the steroid-sparing action of the new drug.

    a. Subjects: disease and activity as in point 1 above.

    b. Number of subjects: as necessary to gain enough experience with respect to safety or to assess special effects.

    c. Duration for each subject: 6 to 12 months.

    d. Dosing: flexible but defined doses administered on an open or double-blind basis.
Assessment: safety: see point 1 above. Efficacy—every 4 weeks, and chronic disease assessment at beginning and end of trial.

Patients in drug-evaluation studies should be seen by the investigator at approximately the same time of the day on each visit. Baseline data should be obtained which is appropriate for the study design. A sufficient number of such data should be collected to provide a basis for clinical assessment of disease activity and, in controlled studies, a statistical evaluation of variability of the recorded measurements.

Change in Functional Class should be registered in all studies. The data obtained on each visit from the Efficacy Assessment should always be recorded so that the effect of the investigational drug on every measurement and observation may be reviewed for all studies.

5. EFFICACY ASSESSMENT

A. All studies

Items 1 and 2 should be assessed in all studies; other items are appropriate for drug trials.

1. Number of painful joints: 68 joints are assessed. To be included are: temporomandibular (2), sternoclavicular (2), and acromioclavicular (2), radiocarpal, carpal, and carpometacarpal are collectively designated as wrist (2). Ankle (2) is the mortise. Tarsus (2) includes as a single unit subtarsal, transverse tarsal, and tarsometatarsal joints. The eight IP joints (proximal and distal) of the four lateral toes are counted as four units.
   Press on joint and move through a full range of motions.
   Pain upon either maneuver represents a positive result.
   Record which joints are positive.

2. Number of swollen joints: 66 joints are assessed. The hips are omitted from the above list. Synovial fluid and/or soft-tissue swelling but not bony overgrowth represent a positive result. Record which joints are positive.

3. Duration of morning stiffness: ask the patient to think of recent mornings. When did he awake? When did the sensation of stiffness begin to wear off?

4. Grip strength: it is best to use a sphygmomanometer cuff which has been sewn into a cloth bag that fits it snugly after the cuff has been folded twice, its dimensions thus being reduced to $\frac{1}{3}$ of the original ones. Inflate to 20 mmHg. With arm unsupported, the patient should grasp and squeeze three times, and the sustained values noted. The procedure is repeated for the other hand. The six values are averaged and the mean is recorded.

5. Time required to walk 50 feet: Specify what walking aids are required. Use a stopwatch to record the time required to walk (not run) a marked off 50-foot distance from a standing start. Record to the nearest tenth of a second.

6. Erythrocyte sedimentation rate: (only the Westergren method is recommended). Two ml of whole blood are added to 0.5ml of 3.8% sodium citrate. The mixture is drawn up to 200 mm in a 300×2.5-mm tube and allowed to stand in a precisely vertical position for one hour. The clear zone over the red cells is then measured in millimeters.

7. Principal observer's evaluation of patient's condition on day of assessment, which should be made and recorded before obtaining the patient's opinion. This evaluation should be graded descrip-

tively and with consistency (i.e., very good, good, fair, poor, very poor).

8. Patient's opinion of condition on day of assessment. This should also be graded descriptively with consistency.

B. Chronic studies

For studies of 6 months or longer, four further modes may be considered in addition to the above:

1. Record ARA (Steinbrocker) functional capacity (class)—as described by Steinbrocker et al. (49)—before, during and at end of drug trial. Although this is highly recommended for chronic studies, it may also be of value in those of less than a 6-month duration.

2. ARA anatomical stage, as described by Steinbrocker et al. (49), recorded before and at end of drug trial.

3. Of secondary importance: hand X-rays made at beginning and end of the trial, without knowledge of drugs or clinical course.

4. Of secondary importance: serum samples from beginning and end of trial may be obtained for rheumatoid factor titer values, without knowledge as to which serum is first or last, or information on drugs or clinical course.

REFERENCES

1. Bäcklund, L., and Tiselius, P.: Acta Rheum. Scand. *13*:275, 1967.
2. Beales, D. L., Burry, H. C., and Grahame, R.: Br. Med. J. *2*:483, 1972.
3. Boardman, P. L., and Hart, F. D.: Br. Med. J. *4*:264, 1967.
4. Cochrane, A. L., Chapman, P. J., and Oldham, P. D.: Lancet *1*:1007, 1951.
5. Collins, K. E., Deodhar, S., Nuki, G., Whaley, K., Buchanan, W. W., and Dick, W. C.: Ann. Rheum. Dis. *30*:401, 1971.
6. Cooperating Clinics Committee of the American Rheumatism Association: Clin. Pharmacol. Ther. *8*:11, 1967.
7. Copeman, W. S. C.: Br. Med. J. *2*:849, 1950.
8. Cousins, G. E.: Res. Q. *26*:273, 1955.
9. Cox, D. R.: "Planning of Experiments." Wiley and Son, New York, 1958.
10. Dick, W. C.: Semin. Arthritis Rheum. *1*:301, 1972.
11. Dick, W. C., Grayson, M. F., Woodburn, A., Nuki, G., and Buchanan, W. W.: Ann. Rheum. Dis. *29*:643, 1970.
12. Freemont-Smith, K., and Bayles, T. B.: J. Am. Med. Assoc. *192*:103, 1965.
13. Green, F. A., and Hays, M. T.: Ann. Rheum. Dis. *31*:278, 1965.
14. Hart, F. D., and Clark, C. J.: Lancet *1*:775, 1951.
15. Hart, F. D., and Huskisson, E. C.: Lancet *1*:28, 1972.
16. Hays, M. T., and Green, F. A.: Ann. Rheum. Dis. *31*:272, 1972.
17. Hewer, A. J. H., Keele, C. A., Keele, K D., and Nathan, P. W.: Lancet *1*: 431, 1949.

18. Hill, A. B.: Ann. Rheum. Dis. *25*:107, 1966.
19. Hollander, J. L., and Young, D. G.: Arthritis Rheum. *6*:277, 1963.
20. Houde, R. W., and Wallenstein, S. L.: Drug Addict. Narcot. Bull. Appendix C: 417, 1953.
21. Houde, R. W., Wallenstein, S. L., and Rogers, A.: Clin. Pharmacol. Ther. *1*:163, 1960.
22. Huskisson, T., Shenfield, G., Taylor, R. T., and Hart, F. D.: Rheumatol. Phys. Med. (Suppl.) : 88, 1970.
23. Jacobsen, M.: Br. J. Psychiat. *111*:545, 1965.
24. Jasani, M. K., Downie, W. W., Samuels, B. M., and Buchanan, W. W.: Ann. Rheum. Dis. *27*:457, 1968.
25. Keats, A. S., Beccher, H. K., and Mosteller, F. C.: J. Appl. Physiol. *1*:35, 1950.
26. Keele, C. A.: Lancet *2*:683, 1948.
27. Lansbury, J.: Arthritis Rheum. *1*:505, 1958.
28. Lansbury, J.: In "Arthritis and Allied Diseases," 7th edition. J. L. Hollander, ed. Lea and Febiger, Philadelphia, 1966, p. 269.
29. Lansbury, J.: Arthritis Rheum. *11*:599, 1968.
30. Lasagna, L.: Ann. N. Y. Acad. Sci. *86*:28, 1960.
31. Lasagna, L., and Beccher, H. K.: J. Am. Med. Assoc. *156*:230, 1954.
32. Lee, L. E., Jr.: J. Pharmacol. Exp. Ther. *75*:161, 1942.
33. Mainland, D.: Arthritis Rheum. *10*:71, 1967.
34. Mason, R. M., Barnado, D. E., Fox, W. R., and Weatherall, M.: Ann. Rheum. Dis. *26*:373, 1967.
35. McCarty, D. J., Gatter, R. A., and Phelps, P.: Arthritis Rheum. *8*:551, 1965.
36. McCarty, D. J., Polcyn, R. E., and Collins, P. A.: Arthritis Rheum. *13*:21, 1970.
37. McCarty, D. J., and Polcyn, R. E., Collins, P. A., Gottschalk, A.: Arthritis Rheum. *13*:11, 1970.
38. McConkey, B., Crockson, R. A., and Crockson, A. P.: Q. J. Med. *41*:115, 1972.
39. McMillen, J., Leer, J. A., Ridolfo, A., Decker, J., Paulus, H. E., Ehrlich, G., Rothermich, H., Godfrey, R., and Zvaifler, N.: Drug Res. Rep. *14*:52, 1971.
40. Medical Research Council and Nuffield Foundation: Br. Med. J. *2*:695, 1955.
41. Medical Research Council and Nuffield Foundation: Ann. Rheum. Dis. *19*: 95, 1960.
42. Mowatt, A., Hothersall, T. E., and Aitcheson, W. R. T.: Ann. Rheum. Dis. *28*:303, 1969.
43. Multicentre Trial Group: Lancet *1*:275, 1973.
44. Oka, M., Rekonen, A., and Ruotsi, A.: Acta Rheum. Scand. *16*:271, 1970.
45. Prineas, R. J.: Med. J. Aust. *2*:245, 1971.
46. Ritchie, D. M., Boyle, J. A., McInnes, J. M., Jasani, M. K., Dalakos, T. G., Grieveson, P., and Buchanan, W. W.: Q. J. Med. *37*:393, 1968.
47. Roitt, M., and Torrigiani, G.: In "Immune Complex Disease," L. Ronomo and I. L. Turk, eds. Carlo Erba Foundation, Milan, 1970, p. 73.
48. Ropes, M. W., Bennett, G. A., Cobb, S., Jacox, R., and Jesser, R. A.: Arthritis Rheum. *2*:16, 1959.
49. Steinbrocker, O.: Arch. Phys. Med. Rehabil. *30*:289, 1949.
50. Steinbrocker, O., Traeger, C. H., and Batterman, R. C.: J. Am. Med. Assoc. *140*:659, 1949.

51. Torrigiani, G., and Roitt, M.: Ann. Rheum. Dis. *26*:334, 1967.
52. Weiss, R. E., Maxfield, W. S., Murison, P. J., and Hidalgo, J. U.: Arthritis Rheum. *8*:976, 1965.
53. Whaley, K., Pack, A. I., Boyle, J. A., Dick, W. C., Downie, W. W., Buchanan, W. W., and Gillespie, F. C.: Clin. Sci. *35*:547, 1968.
54. Wilding, P., Kendall, M. J., Holder, R., Grimes, J. A., and Farr, M.: Clin. Chim. Acta *64*:185, 1975.
55. Wright, V., and Johns, R. J.: Bull. Johns Hopkins Hosp. *106*:215, 1960.
56. Wright, V., Walker, W. C., and McGuire, R. J.: Ann. Rheum. Dis. *28*:157, 1969.
57. Yesair, D. W., Callahan, M., Remington, L., and Kensler, C. J.: Biochem. Pharmacol. *19*:1579, 1970.
58. Yesair, D. W., Remington, L., Callahan, M., and Kensler, C. J.: Biochem. Pharmacol. *19*:1591, 1970.

Chapter 14

Possible Mechanisms of Action of Non-Steroidal Antiinflammatory Drugs

Since inflammation is a complex process that can be induced by a variety of means and can be mediated by a number of only partly known mechanisms with multiple manifestations, it will not be surprising if antiinflammatory agents exert their effects through a spectrum of different modes of action. Generally, the drugs in clinical use exhibit antipyretic and analgesic activity in addition to edema-inhibiting properties, and such side-effects as ulcerogenicity. Historically, the tests used for evaluating these compounds have been selected because they respond to drugs known to be useful in rheumatoid disease. The compounds active in these tests are loosely termed "antiinflammatory" and, occasionally, "antirheumatic," although it would be better to reserve this term for the drug of the future. One consequence of the imprecision of terminology has been the tendency to suggest a number of mechanisms of action that, on one hand, are frequently pharmacological curiosities produced in laboratory situations and entirely divorced from human clinical relevance and, on the other, seem more related to the disease being inadequately treated rather than to the animal models which respond considerably more dramatically to the same drug. Therefore, we are confronted with a confused picture of claims and counterclaims attesting to the inadequacy of each.

This chapter will review the suggested mechanism of action of non-steroidal antiinflammatory drugs but no attempt will be made to consider in detail the action of individual compounds, except by way of example. In fact, no drugs have so far been produced for the treatment of rheumatoid arthritis that are basically different from salicylates; furthermore, none of them seem to hold much more promise for patients than temporary relief. Completely different agents need to be developed which would accomplish much more than simply suppressing the symptoms and signs of rheumatoid arthritis.

1. EFFECTS ON PAIN

The analgesic effect of salicylates and phenylbutazone involves a peripheral component of action, probably due to an interference with the function of pain-producing substances (29). The existence of peripheral analgesic mechanisms has been suggested also by experiments on vaso-isolated but neurally intact dog spleen, using bradykinin as the pain-producing substance (110,111). In these experiments, acetylsalicylic acid and phenylbutazone were found effective at doses of 3.8 and 10.0 mg/kg, respectively. Very similar results in regard to suppression of pain and normalization of electrical activity in afferent nerve fibers have been obtained when visceral pain was elicited by the injection of KCl and acetylcholine into the femoral, coronary or internal carotid arteries (77). The excitation potentials in afferent fibers, generated by a cutaneous inflammatory focus, were suppressed by salicylates and phenylbutazone but, on the other hand, the electrical phenomena caused by stimulation of normal skin areas were not influenced by these drugs (185). In experiments on rabbit vagal fibers, differences between centrally acting analgesics and antiinflammatory agents have been described, suggesting a peripheral site of action for the latter (156).

The possibility that the analgesic effect of non-steroidal antiinflammatory agents is attributable to an interference with putative mediators of inflammation or with their receptors is also supported by the results of human experiments (112). The pain evoked by intraperitoneal bradykinin is, in fact, inhibited by acetylsalicylic acid in dose-dependent manner. It is of interest that it is possible to demonstrate similar dose-response curves for acetylsalicylic acid in rheumatoid arthritis by rather more conventional techniques (15).

Evidence is accumulating that prostaglandins sensitize pain receptors to chemical and mechanical stimulation (54,58,202), and that an increased release of prostaglandin-like material occurs in the outflow of dog isolated spleen when perfused with bradykinin (58). In these experimental conditions, aspirin-like drugs increase the pain threshold and concomitantly reduce prostaglandin outflow (58). These observations fit in with the hypothesis (54) that the analgesia produced by aspirin-like drugs can be explained by the removal of the facilitation caused by endogenously released prostaglandins, which normally lead to hyperalgesia as a result of mechanical or chemical stimulation. More recent experiments (125) further support the conclusion that aspirin-like drugs are analgesic because they inhibit prostaglandin synthesis, thereby preventing the sensitization of pain receptors. In this connection, it is of interest that these drugs can prevent the writhing response elicited by bradykinin, among other substances, but are inactive against that induced by prostaglandins (34) (Table 29).

2. EFFECTS ON CELLS

Several types of cells with multiple functions are implicated in the inflammatory process. Polymorphonuclear and mononuclear leukocytes, lymphocytes and platelets participate to a different extent and through a variety of mechanisms in the development and persistence of inflammation. Schematically, the non-steroidal antiinflammatory drugs may affect both the movement of the cells toward the site of inflammation or their functions once they have arrived there. For the purpose of the present discussion, these two aspects will be considered separately since such a distinction between movement and function can be regarded as arbitrary.

A. Cell movement

The in vivo chemotaxis involves the purposeful migration of viable leukocytes through intact vascular endothelium toward the site of inflammation. The non-steroidal antiinflammatory drugs interfere with such a migration.

Evidence has been accumulated demonstrating that these agents are mainly active on the migration of mononuclear cells.

TABLE 29. Approximate relative analgesic potency of
some non-steroidal antiinflammatory drugs

Experimental Procedure	Approximate Relative Potency		References
Phenylquinone writhing (mice)	Acetylsalicylic ac.	= 1	15
	Aminopyrine	= 2.1	
	Phenylbutazone	= 1	
Acetylcholine writhing (mice)	Acetylsalicylic ac.	= 1	14
	Flufenamic ac.	= 1.2	
	Meclofenamic ac.	= 3.2	
	Mefenamic ac.	= 2.1	
Intra-arterial bradykinin (rats)	Acetylsalicylic ac.	= 1	16
	Phenylbutazone	= 0.5	
	Aminopyrine	= 4.9	
Pressure on inflamed paw (rats)	Acetylsalicylic ac.	= 1	17
	Phenylbutazone	= 1.7	
	Indomethacin	= 2.8	
	Flufenamic ac.	= 1.5	
	Ibuprofen	= 2.9	
Intra-arterial bradykinin (dogs)	Acetylsalicylic ac.	= 1	4
	Phenylbutazone	= 1.6	

In fact, indomethacin does not prevent polymorphonuclear cell accumulation at the intradermal site prepared for a local Schwartzman reaction in rabbits although it inhibits the development of this reaction on subsequent challenge (186). Similar results have been obtained in studies of inflammation in dog knee joint (187). Previous findings were, however, at variance showing that indomethacin reduces polymorphonuclear cell migration in dogs with crystal-induced synovitis (145).

The extensive depletion of polymorphonuclear cells results in partial suppression of the late phase of carrageenin edema in rats (44,188). The residual edema and monocytic infiltration is eliminated by indomethacin, phenylbutazone, and acetylsalicylic and mefenamic acids (44). In rats depleted of histamine, serotonin and kininogen but not of polymorphonuclear cells, there is a good correlation between suppression of edema by the above antiinflammatory agents and monocyte migration (44). In addition, phenylbuta-

TABLE 30. Inhibition of swelling and leukocyte chemotaxis in vivo
(rat, carrageenin edema)

Compound	Swelling	% Inhibition of Mononuclear Chemotaxis	Polymorphonuclear
Paramethasone 1 mg/kg p.os.	57	60	62
Indomethacin 2 mg/kg p.os.	28	31	8
Phenylbutazone 100 mg/kg p.os.	34	38	0
Mefenamic ac. 200 mg/kg p.os.	27	41	7
Acetylsalicylic ac. 150 mg/kg p.os.	26	28	2

zone inhibits in vitro the migration of peritoneal macrophages from capillary tubes (44).

Dextran-induced pleurisy in rats involves migration of both polymorphonuclear and mononuclear cells but at different times (87). It has been shown that antiinflammatory drug treatment, at high doses, inhibits only mononuclear infiltration (45). In calcium pyrophosphate-induced pleurisy, the polymorphonuclear response and—to a greater extent—mononuclear immigration were reduced by indomethacin pretreatment (204).

With the technique of the adoptively transferred ^{51}Cr isologous leukocytes in rats bearing carrageenin inflammation, it has been demonstrated that methylprednisolone inhibits the in vivo chemotaxis of both mononuclear and polymorphonuclear cells, whereas phenylbutazone, indomethacin and flufenamic acid block mononuclear but not neutrophil chemotaxis (142) (Table 30).

The mechanism whereby antiinflammatory drugs interfere with mononuclear-cell chemotaxis is unclear. However, these compounds have the capacity to affect the integrity of cell membranes. The macrophage cell membrane is unique in having a heavy mucopolysaccharide exterior coat which probably correlates with the ability of this cell type to adhere to fixed surfaces (23). Indomethacin, phenylbutazone, mefenamic acid and corticosteroids all interfere with cellular synthesis of mucopolysaccharides in several tissues (47,200). With the exception of corticosteroids, these compound are uncouplers of oxidative phosphorylation (201) which is known to interfere with selective membrane permeability (162). Some other properties of these compounds, such as the inhibition of protein synthesis (64), are probably unrelated to the inhibition of mononuclear cell chemotaxis since cyclophosphamide has no effect in this regard (142).

Direct cellular toxicity cannot, however, be ruled out (44).

B. Cell function

In view of the numerous reports dealing with the escape of lysosomal enzymes from within their bounds during acute and chronic inflammation (196), the possibility that antiinflammatory agents may inhibit or reduce lysosomal membrane labilization has been carefully scrutinized.

Early studies illustrated that certain glucocorticoids and chloroquine inhibited in vitro the release of acid hydrolases from isolated rat and rabbit liver lysosome fractions (195,197,198,199). More recently, several non-steroidal antiinflammatory drugs were demonstrated to stabilize, in vitro, lysosomes of rat (88,91,122,176) and rabbit liver (89), and of polymorphonuclear leukocytes (93,141). An important common finding from these studies was that lysosomal membrane stabilization was confined for the most part to drugs possessing antiinflammatory activity. Some reports, however, were inconsistent with this general finding but this may have been largely due to differences in methodology (19,50,118). The possibility that lysosomes from different tissues have a different sensitivity to drug effects has also been demonstrated (88,89). Moreover, it has been shown that lysosomes from induced or stimulated rat (93) or human (92) neutrophils were more responsive to the membrane-stabilizing action of several antiinflammatory drugs (82,92) than were those from peripheral or untreated cells.

In vivo findings further support the hypothesis, based on previous in vitro data, that antiinflammatory agents stabilize lysosomes against disruption produced by various means. The increased lysosomal fragility in liver of rats with adjuvant arthritis is partially restored by treatment with paramethasone, indomethacin and phenylbutazone (94). In addition, studies with normal rats revealed that these drugs possess the capacity to stabilize liver lysosomes in vivo (90). Mefenamic acid, however, was inactive and indomethacin was active only at high doses. Phenylbutazone was found to reduce the lysosomal enzyme level in the supernatant of homogenates of arthritic paws of rats (149). However, in the perfusate collected from inflamed paw, the increased lysosomal enzyme content was significantly reduced by indomethacin while phenylbutazone and acetylsalicylic acid were inactive (8). Sodium salicylate was unable to affect the lysosomal content of the joint wash of avian microcrystal arthritis (21), and the lysosomal release in the exudate of carrageenin pleurisy was not reduced by indomethacin, phenylbutazone, acetylsalicylic and flufenamic acid (5).

A possible explanation of these apparently conflicting results could lie in the different susceptibility of liver compared to leukocyte lysosomes to the drugs in question, as previously observed in in vitro experiments (89).

In recent years, there has been an increasing interest in the effects of antiinflammatory drugs on platelets, because of the possible role of these cells in the development of inflammatory reactions and the assumption that a drug that controlled platelet function in vivo may also be able to prevent some forms of thrombosis. In this context, two aspects of platelet function have been investigated: the release of stored amines (histamine, serotonin) and aggregation.

Many compounds with antiinflammatory properties have been shown to inhibit the release reaction induced by collagen fibers added to human platelet-rich plasma. These drugs include phenylbutazone and sulfinpyrazone (139), acetylsalicylic acid (51,193), indomethacin, and mefenamic and flufenamic acid (209). Inhibitory effects of these agents were also observed when the release reaction was induced by thrombin (51,138), or by ADP, or epinephrine (208,209). Indomethacin is some 20 times more active than acetylsalicylic acid in terms of concentrations required to produce half-maximal effects, but the plateau levels of inhibition produced by the two drugs are identical (209).

The decreased synthesis of prostaglandins by human platelets in vitro, following administration of indomethacin or acetylsalicylic acid, will be discussed in the next paragraph. It should be mentioned here that, under the conditions used for this assay, the thrombin-induced release reaction was not inhibited, thus suggesting dissociation of these two platelet functions.

Agents which elicit the release reaction, such as ADP, epinephrine and collagen, also cause platelet aggregation. When ADP or epinephrine are used as the inducing stimulus, two waves of aggregation can be visualized, the first attributable to the direct action of exogenous stimulus, the second to that of ADP liberated in the release reaction.

Acetylsalicylic acid given orally or added in vitro completely inhibits the second wave of biphasic aggregation but has no effect on the first wave (133,194,208). Even with a single oral dose of acetylsalicylic acid as low as 150 mg, this effect may persist for several days (133). Meclofenamic acid, indomethacin, ibuprofen, ibufenac, phenylbutazone and mefenamic acid are active in vitro (134). After oral dosing, indomethacin shows marked but transient activity, the smallest effective dose being 0.035 mg/kg (135). Several workers have shown that the collagen-induced aggregation may also be inhibited by acetylsalicylic acid given orally (98,138,193) or added in vitro (51,134). Other non-steroidal antiinflammatory drugs, including those that inhibit the second wave of aggregation caused by epinephrine, are also able to prevent collagen-induced aggregation (134). Furthermore, chloroquine and hydroxychloroquine have been reported to block collagen-induced aggregation (98), with the latter inhibiting the action of ADP (98). In view of the claim that hydroxychloroquine prevents postoperative thrombosis (24), these effects should be further investigated.

Relatively little work has been done on the possible effect of non-steroidal antiinflammatory drugs on lymphocyte function despite the known role of these cells in several inflammatory processes. Acetylsalicylic acid (as well as related drugs) has been reported to inhibit both in vitro and in vivo the lymphocyte response to mitogens (20,38,136,164,178). However, the concentrations used in vitro were frequently high and in the presence of serum, which strongly bound these drugs, the inhibitory effect disappeared (64). Other in vivo studies revealed lymphocyte function to be depressed in rheumatoid patients and, in some cases, when the disease was controlled with acetylsalicylic acid, an improvement of lymphocyte response to mitogens was seen (115). In animal experiments, there is little to suggest any effects of non-steroidal antiinflammatory drugs on any lymphocyte function (10,43,60,97,192).

3. EFFECTS ON MEDIATORS

The list of endogenous substances responsible for the characteristic changes at the molecular and cellular levels in the inflamed tissue has increased logarithmically in recent years and yet there is no clear evidence that any single one of them is more than an "innocent bystander" in the inflammatory process. It has been reported by many authors that non-steroidal antiinflammatory agents can inhibit many of the effects of *histamine*: for instance, histamine-induced injury to the capillary wall and histamine shock in guinea pigs (96,107,172). Furthermore, these drugs are reported to prevent the formation of histamine (158) as well as its release following administration of antigens to sensitized guinea pigs (78, 179) or to mast cells of sensitized animals (131,132). As will be seen from the dates of the above references, histamine research lost popularity when it became clear that the histamine response which could be modified by therapy was limited to the early phase of the vascular reaction in inflammation (169). There has, however, been a resurgence of interest provoked by the recent demonstration of the existence of H_2 receptors (14), of their possible role in the autoregulation of endogenous histamine release (25,109,148), and by new therapeutic possibilities implicit in the production of antagonists to these receptors (206). The entire problem of the interrelationship between inflammation, gastric secretion, foregut polypeptide hormone and histamine receptors remains an area of active research at this time.

It is surprising that, so far, there is little evidence for the existence of the characteristic interference of non-steroidal antiinflammatory agents with the specific inflammagenic properties of the *kinins*. On the other hand, we know that bradykinin exerts quite a series of effects that are obviously in no way connected with the mechanism of inflammation, but which can be inhibited in a specific way by very low doses of these drugs.

An extensive investigation has been performed on the effects of non-steroidal antiinflammatory agents on bronchoconstriction induced by bradykinin in the guinea pig (28,33,35,36). Antagonistic effects were observed with calcium acetylsalicylate, aminopyrine, phenazone, mefenamic and flufenamic acids, while mepyramine, atropine and LSD 25 were unable to modify the bronchiolar response. On the other hand, the antiinflammatory compounds were inactive against acetylcholine-, histamine- and serotonin-induced bronchoconstriction (28,33,35,36). It is interesting that the effects of the antiinflammatory compounds on tests based on the antagonism of bradykinin-induced bronchoconstriction correlate well with those on ultraviolet erythema (33,36).

The antagonism towards the increase in capillary permeability induced by bradykinin has been investigated by several authors with somewhat divergent results. Acetylsalicylic acid, phenylbutazone, flufenamic acid have been found active in rats (6) but not in rabbits (127). Other research suggests that a partial antagonism could exist (1,113) whereas certain workers did not observe any effect (27,36).

Table 31 summarizes the antagonistic effects of some antiinflammatory agents towards the increase in capillary permeability induced in rat paw by bradykinin, histamine and serotonin. The swelling of rat paw elicited by the subcutaneous injection of bradykinin is inhibited by antiphlogistic agents (114). Thermic edema, where bradykinin release seems to play an important role, is prevented by these agents (170). This finding, however, has not been confirmed (7,151). It has been found that cyproheptadine, an antiserotonin-antihistamine agent, is fairly potent in reducing the development of thermic edema (67) but it is ineffective in preventing carrageenin- or bradykinin-induced swelling (184). On the other hand, substances which hinder the activation of the kinin system, such as hexadimethrine or the soyabean tripsin inhibitors, were found to block thermic edema (67,101,184) and, at least partially, carrageenin edema (184).

The results of investigations on the effects of some antiinflammatory agents on carrageenin edema and bradykinin release in paw perfusates (coaxial perfusion) are reported in Table 32. A significant inhibition of the edema was observed at all times while bradykinin release was significantly reduced only in the more advanced phases of the reaction.

Inhibition of kinin-forming enzymes by sodium salicylate, phenylbutazone and related antiinflammatory drugs has been reported (127) but not confirmed (82). It has also been shown in vitro that indomethacin, flufenamic acid, phenylbutazone, ibufenac and acetylsalicylic acid up to a concentration of 100 mcg/ml did not inhibit the release of kinin, whereas soyabean tripsin inhibitor was markedly active (40). Inhibition of the algogenic action of bradykinin is produced by common antiinflammatory drugs, such as acetylsalicylate, phenylbutazone, acetaminophen and aminopyrine, in experiments where potentials evoked in splenic nerves were recorded or in cross-perfusion of dog spleen (77,111). In contrast, salicylates and indomethacin did not reduce the algogenic effects of bradykinin in man either when the blister base test or the venous constriction test (157) were applied.

It seems, therefore, that only in some experimental models of

TABLE 31. Antagonism of phenylbutazone, sodium salicylate, calcium acetylsalicylate and sodium mefenamate to bradykinin-, histamine-, or 5-HT-induced increase in capillary permeability in rat paw

Antagonist	Dose mg/kg i.p.	Bradykinin	Histamine	5-HT
		(μg) needed to restore response (95% fiducial limits)*		
Phenylbutazone	50	0·11 (0·07-0·15)	—	—
—	100	0·24 (0·19-0·27)	1·23 (0·96-1·57)	0·13 (0·09-0·17)
—	200	0·29 (0·24-0·32)	2·56 (1·97-3·12)	0·20 (0·15-0·24)
Sodium salicylate	100	0·07 (0·05-0·12)	—	—
—	200	0·28 (0·20-0·36)	1·47 (1·05-2·12)	0·07 (0·04-0·90)
—	400	0·41 (0·36-0·48)	4·56 (3·72-5·24)	0·23 (0·19-0·30)
Calcium acetylsalicylate	100	0·07 (0·04-0·10)	—	—
—	200	0·24 (0·18-0·30)	1·36 (1·02-1·85)	0·09 (0·10-0·13)
—	400	0·41 (0·35-0·48)	3·95 (3·15-4·71)	0·29 (0·22-0·37)
Sodium mefenamate	50	0·10 (0·07-0·16)	1·49 (1·18-1·97)	0·08 (0·04-0·10)
—	100	0·20 (0·13-0·24)	—	—
—	200	0·21 (0·16-0·26)	0·46 (0·32-0·68)	0·02 (0·01-0·05)

*After obtaining a standard response in untreated rats (a threefold increase of azovan blue dye content relative to controls) to 0·05 μg of bradykinin or to 1·0 μg of histamine or to 0·05 μg of 5-HT, a dose of antagonist was administered and the dose of bradykinin or histamine, or 5-HT giving a response comparable to the standard was then determined. The results reported are the means of 20 determinations.

TABLE 32. Percentage inhibition of edema development and bradykinin output in carrageenin reaction*

Time after carrageenin injection		Flufenamic acid 100 mg/kg	Indomethacin 5 mg/kg	Oxyphenyl-butazone 100 mg/kg	Acetylsalicylic acid 300 mg/kg
0'-45'	Edema	65 ± 9 (14)	69 ± 7 (13)	62 ± 9 (13)	58 ± 9 (12)
	Bradykinin	3.2 ± 2.1 (14)	2.7 ± 1.1 (14)	3.6 ± 1.4 (13)	2.8 ± 1.5 (12)
45'-90'	Edema	63 ± 11 (14)	72 ± 12 (12)	59 ± 7 (13)	61 ± 9 (14)
	Bradykinin	9.1 ± 1.9 (14)	8.1 ± 1.4 (13)	9.2 ± 2.6 (12)	8.1 ± 1.6 (12)
90'-135'	Edema	70 ± 8 (12)	75 ± 9 (14)	61 ± 9 (14)	57 ± 8 (14)
	Bradykinin	8.7 ± 4.7 (12)	8.3 ± 4.6 (13)	9.1 ± 6.8 (12)	9.6 ± 3.8 (12)
135'-180'	Edema	65 ± 11 (12)	70 ± 8 (13)	62 ± 11 (14)	62 ± 10 (14)
	Bradykinin	40.7 ± 13.9 (13)	41.2 ± 12.8 (13)	22.5 ± 12.7 (14)	28.6 ± 10.9 (14)
180'-225'	Edema	62 ± 12 (14)	63 ± 11 (12)	64 ± 9 (14)	59 ± 7 (14)
	Bradykinin	39.2 ± 14.2 (14)	40.2 ± 13.9 (12)	30.6 ± 11.9 (14)	30.2 ± 12.2 (14)

*The drugs were administered i.p. 30 minutes before carrageenin injection.
The values are the mean ± S.E. In brackets — the number of determinations.

TABLE 33. Summary of systems in which prostaglandin synthesis is
inhibited by non-steroidal antiinflammatory drugs

Species	Tissue	References
Man	Platelets, semen, skin, synovium cells	114, 135, 143, 149
Bull	Thyroid cells, seminal vesicles	120, 121, 122, 210
Sheep	Seminal vesicles	123, 124
Dog	Brain, spleen, kidney, myocardium	115, 118, 119, 211, 212
Cat	Cerebrospinal fluid, spleen, kidney	139, 141, 213
Rabbit	Heart, brain, spleen, retina, gut, polymorphonuclear cells, kidney	119, 129, 134, 136, 140, 144
Guinea pig	Uterus, lungs	116, 117, 130, 215, 216
Rat	Skin, uterus, inflammatory exudate	125, 132, 137, 138
Mouse	Brain, tumor cells	117, 137, 217
Toad	Bladder	218

acute inflammation does a parallelism exist between the antiinflammatory effect of certain drugs and their capacity to antagonize some
peculiar activity of bradykinin. On the other hand, while some antiinflammatory agents currently used in therapeutics can inhibit certain effects of bradykinin, other clinically active agents are devoid
of this property.

In 1971, non-steroidal antiinflammatory drugs were shown to
inhibit *prostaglandin release* from human platelets (166) and perfused dog spleen (57), and *prostaglandin synthesis* in cell-free
homogenates of guinea pig lungs (189). Inhibition of prostaglandin
synthesis by these drugs has now been demonstrated in some 30 different systems (Table 33).

In homogenates and subcellular fractions, the ID_{50} has been
estimated for several agents (61,62,63,79,165,173,174,177,189) and
it is possible to deduce the following decreasing order of potency:
meclofenamic acid > niflumic acid, indomethacin > mefenamic acid
> flufenamic acid > naproxen > phenylbutazone > acetylsalicylic
acid, ibuprofen. Several otherwise pharmacologically active agents

have been found ineffective. Various enantiomeric pairs of antiinflammatory drugs have been tested and in each case the clinically active isomer was found to be at least the more potent (61,79,177). Chloroquine is effective at high doses (72,73) while steroids have been found to be either active (71,117) or not (62).

Also in isolated tissues have the non-steroidal antiinflammatory drugs been shown to inhibit prostaglandin synthesis, but the presence of prostaglandin-metabolizing enzyme makes the evaluation of the effects more difficult. In slices of rabbit spleen, the following decreasing order of potency has been found (75) : meclofenamic acid > indomethacin > oxyphenbutazone > acetylsalicylic acid; this corresponds to the sequence obtained for tissue homogenates. Antiinflammatory agents inhibit the release of prostaglandins from many other tissues either stimulated in various ways (146,147) or in the basal condition (55,124,191). Since cells do not store prostaglandins, in most cases, release is equivalent to de novo synthesis (147). Furthermore, acetylsalicylic acid and indomethacin inhibit synthesis in human synovium (152) and in rabbit polymorphonuclear leukocytes (121) (Table 34).

Using different experimental approaches, indomethacin and acetylsalicylic acid have been shown to block prostaglandin synthesis in rats (3,168,203), mice (173), rabbits (39,168), cats (123) and guinea pigs (80) when administered orally or parenterally. The ability of antiinflammatory drugs, given in the usual clinical doses, to inhibit prostaglandin synthesis has been also demonstrated in man (80,84,166) (Table 35).

A wide variation in drug sensitivity in different tissues has been observed (13,61,62,63). For instance, the ID_{50} of indomethacin is 0,14 μM on enzyme preparation of rabbit spleen, 1,7 μM on kidney enzyme and 26 μM on conjunctival enzyme (13). These observations support the hypothesis that prostaglandin synthetase exists in multiple molecular forms in the same organism, each having a different pharmacological profile from those found in any other tissue (190) (Table 36).

The antiinflammatory compounds are known to exert inhibitory and other effects on a variety of other enzymes and cellular systems and it is especially important that the concentrations of these drugs which inhibit prostaglandin synthetase are generally much lower than those required to block other enzymes (158,159, 163). These observations suggest that, at least, antiinflammatory agents can be considered as preferential inhibitors of prostaglandin synthetase. Moreover, the concentrations required to inactivate this

TABLE 34. Inhibition of prostaglandin synthesis in isolated tissues

Tissue	Compound	References
Rabbit, PMN	Indomethacin	136
Rat uteri, pregnant	Indomethacin Acetylsalicylic acid	132, 138
Rabbit jejunum	Indomethacin	134
Rabbit heart	Indomethacin	133
Rabbit spleen slices	Meclofenamic acid Indomethacin Oxyphenbutazone Acetylsalicylic acid	129
Guinea pig lungs, perfused	Indomethacin Mefenamic acid Acetylsalicylic acid	130, 215
Dog spleen, perfused	Indomethacin Acetylsalicylic acid	115
Cat spleen, perfused	Indomethacin	213
Human synovium cells	Indomethacin	135
Human platelets	Indomethacin Acetylsalicylic acid	114

enzyme are within the plasma levels achieved by these drugs during normal therapy even when plasma binding is taken into account (31,62,80,84) (Table 37).

There are few definite data concerning the mechanism of inhibitory action of non-steroidal antiinflammatory drugs and, perhaps, one might anticipate more than one mode of action. Among the alternatives, the more likely ones appeared to be competition at the substrate level (61,79) or at cofactor site (177). However, more detailed kinetic analysis (103,105,165) did not support this hypothesis. Furthermore, it became apparent that some agents have certain "selective" effects on one or another of the steps leading to the formation of the different prostaglandins (61,117,175). Most of these drugs probably block the initial stage of the synthetase reaction, exerting this effect by combining slowly with a site which, although not the substrate, is sufficiently close to it to reduce the catalytic activity of the enzyme in a time-dependent manner (103, 105, 165). Some compounds may affect endoperoxide breakdown but this cannot be regarded as definitely proven.

TABLE 35. Inhibition of prostaglandin synthesis in whole animals and man

Site	Compound		% Inhibition	References
Rat, hypertensive, kidney (PGE$_2$, PGA$_2$)	Indomethacin	1 mg/kg	90	139
	Acetylsalicylic acid	10 mg/kg	75	
Rat, carrageenin air bleb	Indomethacin	12.5 mg/kg	80-100	137
	Acetylsalicylic acid	100 mg/kg	75	
Dog, release from kidney by angiotensin, hemorrhage, autoregulation response	Indomethacin	2 mg/kg	100	211, 212
Guinea pig, metabolite in urine	Indomethacin	5 mg/kg	98	219
Man, metabolite in urine	Indomethacin	50 mg × 4	80-100	142
	Acetylsalicylic acid	750 mg × 4	85	
Man, serum content (PGE, PGF)	Acetylsalicylic acid	3.6 g	56	143, 149
Man, biosynthesis in platelets	Acetylsalicylic acid	600 mg	80-100	114

TABLE 36. Potency (molar IC_{50} ratios) of antiinflammatory drugs against different synthetase preparations

	Dog spleen	Bovine seminal vesicles	Rabbit kidney
Acetylsalicylic acid	1	1	1
Indomethacin	217	236	709
Phenylbutazone	5	7	180
Meclofenamic acid	370	682	1801

TABLE 37. Antiinflammatory (carrageenin edema) and prostaglandin synthetase inhibitory activity of non-steroidal antiinflammatory drugs

Compound	Synthetase I_{50} (μM)	Rat Paw Edema (I_{50} moles/kg)	Peak Plasma Conc. (μM)	Plasma Protein Binding (%)
Meclofenamic acid	0·1	0·05	6·84	99·8
Niflumic acid	0·11	0·145	300	82-98
Indomethacin	0·17	0·017	5·0	90
Flufenamic acid	0·64	0·142	53·0	90
Mefenamic acid	0·71	0·282	41	48
Phenylbutazone	7·25	0·325	230-500	98
Alclofenac	14·5	0·442	120	10
Bufexamac	18·0	0·561	23·0	5
Acetylsalicylic acid	37·0	0·833	280-300	50-80
Paracetamol	660·0	Inactive	350	25

It must be mentioned that the antiinflammatory agents may also inhibit prostaglandin inactivation, even if at concentrations higher than those required to block their synthesis (137). It is not known how these drugs inhibit prostaglandin dehydrogenase, however, the salicylates are known to block several dehydrogenases (163), probably, by a competition for the cofactor site.

Since the early observations, more recent interpretations have been developed which suggest that all the actions and side effects of the antiinflammatory drugs can be explained by prostaglandin mechanisms. Prostaglandins are found in the stomach and have a direct antisecretory effect as well as augmenting mucosal blood flow. Prostaglandins may also play a role in the kidney—indomethacin certainly reduces blood flow in dog kidney (4,116). There seems to be compelling evidence that the "prostaglandin mechanism" is a very relevant mode of action of antiinflammatory drugs. This is based particularly on the in vitro distinction between enantiomers that differ markedly in in vivo efficacy, and the fact that the in vitro effects are produced at drug levels resembling those attained during clinical use of the compounds. Other possibilities, however, cannot be disregarded, especially a possible action on cell membrane and movement. In this connection, it should be mentioned, for instance, that indomethacin inhibits leukocyte motility at the approximate concentration of 0.01 μM (144) and prostaglandin synthetase at the approximate concentration of 0.2 μM. It is possible that modifications of cell membranes are the trigger for prostaglandin synthesis and some component of the prostaglandin synthetase system is the membrane receptor that some are seeking, or that a product other than prostaglandin (intermediates or by-products) is exerting the effect we desire to inhibit. As a matter of fact, during the generation of prostaglandins from different tissues, something called rabbit aorta contracting substance (RCS), is also produced (59,75,76,140) that could be a prostaglandin precursor (74), and its formation is inhibited by non-steroidal antiinflammatory drugs (59,75,76).

4. EFFECTS ON CONNECTIVE TISSUE

One common feature of rheumatic diseases is that their target organ is connective tissue, which suffers the consequence of inflammation and often undergoes extensive degeneration. Therefore, many studies of the effect of antiinflammatory agents at a biochemical level have been concerned with the influence of such compounds on connective tissue itself. Many investigations have been aimed at describing the drug-induced changes in the fundamental components of the basic substance, particularly the acid mucopolysaccharides and the structural protein of collagen fibers.

Mucopolysaccharide biosynthesis is influenced by antiinflammatory drugs at the level of glucosamine-6-phosphate formation in normal and inflamed tissues (65,75,155). Aurothiomalate has been found particularly effective, followed in decreasing order by flufenamic acid, phenylbutazone and salicylic acid. Chloroquine proved inactive in this respect (65). The incorporation of glucosamine into the polysaccharide chain is also inhibited, at least in cultures of fibroblasts, by mefenamic acid, phenylbutazone, sodium salicylate and indomethacin (100).

Both steroidal and non-steroidal compounds markedly interfere with the final step in the biosynthesis of sulfated mucopolysaccharides—the introduction of ester sulfate groups (16,17,52,83,106). Non-steroidal drugs were found to be active both in vitro and in vivo. This effect could depend on the uncoupling activity of antiinflammatory drugs (201) since it is accompanied by a decrease of ATP content in the tissue (18,153). However, indomethacin, salicylate and chloroquine inhibit sulfate incorporation even though the tissue ATP level increases (18,153).

The effect of antiinflammatory agents on *collagen metabolism* has been studied using a great variety of experimental conditions, such as measuring the in vitro incorporation of labeled ^{14}C-proline in presence of these drugs and amino acid up-take by tissue slices obtained from animals treated in vivo with antiinflammatory compounds. The effect of parenterally administered drugs on the incorporation and excretion of labeled ^{14}C-proline injected into animals has also been studied. The greatest number of investigations has been devoted to the action of antiinflammatory corticoids (48, 102,104,129,130). A comprehensive conclusion to be drawn from these studies is that the latter certainly inhibit collagen synthesis, probably because of an intracellular effect in interfering with normal messenger ribonucleic acid activity and polyribosomal function, and a possible influence on ribosomal aggregation (70).

Little information is available on the effects of non-steroidal antiinflammatory agents on collagen metabolism. High concentrations (up to 10 mM) of acetylsalicylic acid have been found effective (37,154). Prolonged administration of this drug also produced an inhibition of ^{14}C-proline up-take (181). Similar results have been obtained with phenylbutazone (53,183). In general, non-steroidal antiinflammatory drugs do not seem to cause any major changes in the content of collagen fractions from normal connective tissue (85,182,183) and have very little effect on the collagen components of granulation tissue (66,99,180).

Even when the experimental conditions of the above-mentioned

TABLE 38. Effects of non-steroidal antiinflammatory drugs on connective tissue metabolism

Effect	In Vitro	In Vivo
Inhibition of sulfated mucopolysaccharide biosynthesis	Sodium salicylate Phenylbutazone Indomethacin	Sodium salicylate Phenylbutazone
Inhibition of collagen biosynthesis	Acetylsalicylic acid Sodium salicylate Indomethacin	Phenylbutazone Chloroquine (toxic!) Cyclophosphamide
Acceleration of collagen biosynthesis, metabolism, maturation and degradation	Indomethacin	Sodium salicylate Chloroquine

studies are taken into proper account one must admit that any intervention of the antiinflammatory agents in the overall metabolism of connective tissue cannot satisfactorily explain their mechanism of action and beneficial therapeutic effects (Table 38).

5. OTHER EFFECTS

Several enzymes are inhibited by non-steroidal antiinflammatory compounds almost exclusively by virtue of displacement by the drug of the substrate or essential cofactor. This applies in case of histidine decarboxylase (160), dopa decarboxylase (159), aminotransferase (69) and dehydrogenase (41). Of greater interest is the inhibition of proteolytic enzymes, some of which are active at physiological pH and are involved in the pathogenesis of the inflammatory process (107). In a variety of experimental conditions, sodium salicylate, phenylbutazone, mefenamic acid, flufenamic acid, ibufenac, and indomethacin inhibited proteolytic enzymes (11,126, 161). On the other hand, protease inhibitors have been repeatedly demonstrated to block inflammatory processes (12,46,210). In contradiction to these findings, a loss of normally insoluble rat collagen has been demonstrated following antiinflammatory drug therapy (86,86,68). This effect could be prevented by prior treatment with cycloheximide and has been ascribed to proteolytic enzyme induction.

The displacement of substrates by non-steroidal antiinflammatory drugs—also suggested as a possible explanation of prostaglandin-synthetase inhibition—may be relevant to the phenomena of membrane and protein stabilization. In this connection, it should be mentioned that these drugs are able to competitively displace small biologically active molecules, such as tryptophan, from both circulating and tissue proteins (119,120).

6. COMMENTS

Many of the activities exerted by antiinflammatory compounds in in vitro experiments result from the presence on proteins of binding sites capable of interacting with acidic molecules bearing a hydrophobic moiety. This class of molecules includes the acidic antiinflammatory agents, but they are not the only ones in this category. The above property may be essential for one or more modes of action of these drugs but it cannot be exclusively responsible for their pharmacological activity.

Changes in cellular membranes surely occur during the development of the inflammatory process and they are probably the trigger of the process itself. The mediator release in several cell types is initiated by phenomena occurring at cellular surfaces, as exemplified by the immunological reactions that, in turn, produce a sequence of events modulated by the cyclic nucleotides. It is interesting that some evidence of an interference of non-steroidal antiinflammatory drugs with the cyclic nucleotide system is beginning to appear (26,128,143,167).

There are reasons to believe that the functions of polymorphonuclear and mononuclear cells are affected by antiinflammatory agents. One example of this, among others, is the inhibition of mononuclear migration at the inflamed site. This is an area in which the release and action of chemotactic factors are of current interest but where the prostaglandins have no great importance.

Inhibition of prostaglandin synthesis seems to be an (at least) additional essential feature of the mode of action of antiinflammatory drugs. This effect is certainly real and highly relevant even if some essential questions still remain unanswered and the exact role of different prostaglandins, their precursors and by-products in the inflammatory process needs further clarification.

The number and variety of processes thought to be involved in the initiation and maintenance of inflammatory responses which are affected by aspirin-like compounds show that these drugs are polycompetent, i.e., able to modulate more than one molecular or cellular event. It may be that they have no specific mode of action and that their overall antiinflammatory activities are due to multiple interactions with several components of various acute and chronic inflammatory reactions. The involvement of prostaglandin synthetase may be one of the points of interaction as may membrane labilization. It might well be that these processes represent primary modes of action of non-steroidal antiinflammatory drugs, although they do not necessarily constitute an adequate treatment for rheumatoid arthritis.

REFERENCES

1. Aarsen, P. N.: Br. J. Pharmacol. *27*:196, 1966.
2. Aiken, J. W., and Vane, J. R.:Pharmacologist *13*:15, 1971.
3. Aiken, J. W.: Nature *240*:21, 1972.
4. Aiken, J. W., and Vane, J. R.: J. Pharmacol. Exp. Ther. *184*:678, 1973.
5. Amendola, G., Di Rosa, M., and Sorrentino, L.: Agents Actions *5*:250, 1975.
6. Arrigoni-Martelli, E.: J. Pharm. Pharmacol. *19*:617, 1967.
7. Arrigoni-Martelli, E., Corsico, N., and Fogagnolo, E.: In "Inflammation Biochemistry and Drug Interaction," A. Bertelli and J. C. Houck, eds. Excerpta Medica Foundation, Amsterdam, 1969, p. 185.
8. Arrigoni-Martelli, E., and Restelli, A.: Eur. J. Pharmacol. *19*:191, 1972.
9. Arrigoni-Martelli, E.: Unpublished results.
10. Arrigoni-Martelli, E., Bramm, E., Huskisson, E. C., Willoughby, D. A., and Dieppe, P. A.: Agents Actions, *6*:613, 1976.
11. Bertelli, A., Donati, L., and Marck, J.: "Inflammation Biochemistry and Drug Interaction," A. Bertelli and J. C. Houck, eds. Excerpta Medica Foundation, Amsterdam, 1969, p. 66.
12. Bertelli, A., Donati, L., and Rossano, M. A.: In "Non-Steroidal Antiinflammatory Drugs," S. Garattini and M. N. G. Dukes, eds. Excerpta Medica Foundation, Amsterdam, 1965, p. 98.
13. Bhattacherjee, P., and Eakines, K.: Pharmacologist *15*:209, 1973.
14. Black, J. W., Duncan, W. A., Durant, C. J., Ganellin, C. R., and Parsons, E. M.: Nature *236*:385, 1972.
15. Boardman, P., and Hart, F. D.: Br. Med. J. *4*:264, 1967.
16. Boström, H., Moretti, A., and Whitehouse, M. W.: Biochim. Biophys. Acta *74*:213, 1963.
17. Boström, H., Berntsen, K., and Whitehouse, M. W.: Biochem. Pharmacol. *13*:413, 1964.
18. Bröhr, H. J., and Kalbhen, D. A.: Arch. Int. Pharmacodyn. Ther. *176*:380, 1968.
19. Brown, J. H., and Schwartz, N. L.: Proc. Soc. Exp. Biol. Med. *131*:614, 1969.
20. Brown, J. H., Taylor, J. L., and Biundo, J.: J. Clin. Pharmacol. *15*:553, 1975.

21. Brune, K., and Glatt, M.: Agents Actions *4*:101, 1974.
22. Burke, G.: Prostaglandins *2*:413, 1972.
23. Carr, I.: Int. Rev. Cytol. *27*:283, 1970.
24. Carter, A. E., Eban, R., and Perrett, R. D.: Br. Med. J. *1*:312, 1971.
25. Chakrin, L. W., Krell, R. D., Mengel, J., Young, D., Zaher, C., and Wardell, J. R., Jr.: Agents Actions *4*:297, 1974.
26. Ciosek, C. P., Jr., Ortel, R. W., Thanssi, N. M., and Newcombe, D. S.: Nature *251*:148, 1974.
27. Collier, H. O. J.: Actual. Pharmacol. *14*:51, 1961.
28. Collier, H. O. J.: Ann. N. Y. Acad. Sci. *104*:290, 1963.
29. Collier, H. O. J.: Nature *223*:35, 1969.
30. Collier, H. O. J., Dinneen, C. C., Johnson, C. A., and Schneider, D.: Br. J. Pharmacol. *32*:295, 1968.
31. Collier, J. G., and Flower, R. J.: Lancet *2*:852, 1971.
32. Collier, J. G., Herman, A. G., and Vane, J. R.: J. Physiol. (Lond.) *230*: 19, 1973.
33. Collier, H. O. J., and James, G. W. L.: Br. J. Pharmacol. *30*:283, 1967.
34. Collier, H. O. J., and Schneider, C.: Nature (New Biol.) *236*:141, 1972.
35. Collier, H. O. J., and Shorley, P. G.: Br. J. Pharmacol. *15*:601, 1960.
36. Collier, H. O. J., and Shorley, P. G.: Br. J. Pharmacol. *20*:345, 1963.
37. Cooper, C. W., Roty, S. B., and Talmage, R. V.: Proc. Soc. Exp. Biol. Med. *117*:881, 1964.
38. Crout, J. E., Hepburn, B., and Ritts, E. R.: N. Engl. J. Med. *292*:221, 1975.
39. Davis, H.: In "Supplementum to Advances in the Biosciences," Vol. 9, International Conference on Prostaglandins, Vienna, S. Berström and S. Bernhart, eds. Pergamon Press Vieweg, Braunschweigh, 1973. p. 55.
40. Davies, G. E., Holman, G., Johnston, T. P., and Lowe, J. S.: Br. J. Pharmacol. *28*:212, 1966.
41. Dawkins, P. D., Gould, B. J., Sturman, J. A., and Smith, M. J. M.: J. Pharm. Pharmacol. *19*:355, 1967.
42. Deffenu, G., Pegrassi, L., and Lumachi, B.: J. Pharm. Pharmacol. *18*:135, 1966.
43. Dieppe, P. A., Willoughby, D. A., Huskisson, E. C., and Arrigoni-Martelli, E.: Agents Actions *6*:618, 1976.
44. Di Rosa, M., Papadimitriou, M., and Willoughby, D. A.: J. Pathol. *105*: 239, 1971.
45. Di Rosa, M., Sorrentino, L., and Parente, L.: J. Pharm. Pharmacol. *24*: 575, 1972.
46. Domenjoz, R., and Mörsdorf, K.: In "Non-Steroidal Antiinflammatory Drugs," S. Garattini, and M. N. G. Dukes, eds. Excerpta Medica Foundation, Amsterdam, 1965, p. 162.
47. Du Poistesselin, R., and Porcile, E.: Thérapie *18*:177, 1963.
48. Ebert, P. S., and Prockop, D. J.: Biochim. Biophys. Acta *78*:390, 1963.
49. Emele, J. F., and Shanaman, J.: Proc. Soc. Exp. Biol. Med. *114*:680, 1963.
50. Ennis, R. S., Granda, J. L., and Posner, A. S.: Arthritis Rheum. *11*:756, 1968.
51. Evans, G., Packham, M. A., Nishizawa, E. E., Mustard, J. F., and Murphy, E. A.: J. Exp. Med. *128*:877, 1968.
52. Exer, B.: Acta Rheumatol. Scand. *8* (Suppl.) : 52, 1964.

53. Fegeler, K., and Gerlach, H.: Z. Rheumaforsch. *29*:107, 1970.
54. Ferreira, S. H.: Nature (New Biol.) *240*:200, 1972.
55. Ferreira, S. H., Herman, A., and Vane, J. R.: Br. J. Pharmacol. *44*:3, 1972.
56. Ferreira, S. H., and Moncada, S.: Br. J. Pharmacol. *43*:419, 1971.
57. Ferreira, S. H., Moncada, S., and Vane, J. R.: Nature (New Biol.) *231*: 237, 1971.
58. Ferreira, S. H., Moncada, S., and Vane, J. R.: Br. J. Pharmacol. *49*:86, 1973.
59. Fjalland, B.: J. Pharm. Pharmacol. *26*:448, 1974.
60. Floersheim, G. L.: Helv. Physiol. Pharmacol. Acta *22*:92, 1964.
61. Flower, R. J., Cheung, H. S., and Cushman, D. W.: Prostaglandins *4*:325, 1973.
62. Flower, R. J., Gryglewski, R., Herbaczynska-Cedro, K., and Vane, J. R.: Nature (New Biol.) *238*:104, 1972.
63. Flower, R. J., and Vane, J. R.: Nature *240*:410, 1972.
64. Forbes, I. J., and Smith, J. L.: Lancet *2*:334, 1967.
65. Fujihira, E., Tsubota, N., and Nakazowa, M.: Chem. Pharm. Bull. (Tokyo) *19*:190, 1971.
66. Fukuhara, M., and Tsufuraji, S.: Biochem. Pharmacol. *18*:475, 1969.
67. Garcia Leme, J., Hamamura, L., and Rocha e Silva, M.: Br. J. Pharmacol. *40*:294, 1970.
68. Gladner, J. A., and Houck, J. C.: In "Inflammation Biochemistry and Drug Interaction," A. Bertelli and J. C. Houck, eds. Excerpta Medica Foundation, Amsterdam, 1969, p. 133.
69. Gould, B. J., Dawkins, P. D., Smith, M. J. H., and Lawrence, A. J.: Mol. Pharmacol. *2*:526, 1966.
70. Gould, B. S., and Manner, G.: Biochem. Biophys. Acta *138*:189, 1967.
71. Greaves, M. W., and McDonald-Gibson, W. J.: Br. Med. J. *2*:83, 1972.
72. Greaves, M. W., and McDonald-Gibson, W. J.: Br. Med. J. *3*:527, 1972.
73. Gryglewski, R., Flower, R. J., Herbaczynska-Cedro, K., and Vane, J. R.: In "Proceedings of the 5th International Congress of Pharmacology," San Francisco, 1972, p. 90.
74. Gryglewski, R., and Vane, J. R.: Br. J. Pharmacol *43*:420 P, 1971.
75. Gryglewski, R., and Vane, J. R.: Br. J. Pharmacol. *45*:37, 1972.
76. Gryglewski, R., and Vane, J. R.: Br. J. Pharmacol. *46*:449, 1972.
77. Guzman, F., Braun, C., Lim, R. K. S., Potter, G. D., and Rodgers, D. W.: Arch. Int. Pharmacodyn. Ther. *149*:571, 1964.
78. Haining, C. G.: Br. J. Pharmacol. *11*:357, 1956.
79. Ham, E. A., Cirillo, K. J., Zanetti, M., Shen, T. Y., and Kuehl, F. A.: In "Prostaglandins in Cellular Biology," P. W. Ramwell and B. B. Pharriss, eds. Plenum Press, New York, 1972, pp.345-352.
80. Hamberg, M.: Biochem. Biophys. Res. Commun. *49*:720, 1972.
81. Hamberg, M., and Samuelsson, B.: J. Biol. Chem. *247*:3195, 1972.
82. Hebborn, P., and Shaw, B.: Br. J. Pharmacol. *20*:254, 1963.
83. Hersheberger, L. G., Hansen, L., and Ranney, R. E.: Proc. Soc. Exp. Biol. Med. *101*:328, 1959.
84. Horton, E. W., Jones, R. L., and Marr, G. G.: J. Reprod. Fertil. *33*:385, 1973.
85. Houck, J. C., Patel, Y. M., and Gladner, J.: Biochem. Pharmacol. *16*:1099, 1967.

86. Houck, J. C., and Sharma, V. K.: In "Inflammation Biochemistry and Drug Interaction," A. Bertelli and J. C. Houck, eds. Excerpta Medica Foundation, Amsterdam, 1969, p. 85.
87. Hurley, J. V., Ryan, C. B., and Friedman, A.: J. Pathol. *91*:575, 1966.
88. Ignarro, L. J.: Biochem. Pharmacol. *20*:2847, 1971.
89. Ignarro, L. J.: Biochem. Pharmacol. *20*:2861, 1971.
90. Ignarro, L. J.: J. Pharm. Exp. Ther. *182*:179, 1972.
91. Ignarro, L. J.: Biochem. Pharmacol. *22*:1269, 1973.
92. Ignarro, L. J.: Agents Actions *4*:241, 1974.
93. Ignarro, L. J., and Colombo, C.: Nature (New Biol.) *239*:155, 1972.
94. Ignarro, L. J., and Slywka, J.: Biochem. Pharmacol. *21*:875, 1972.
95. Jacobsen, B., and Boström, H.: Biochim. Biophys. Acta *83*:152, 1964.
96. Jacques, R., and Domenjoz, R.: Arch. Exp. Pathol. Pharmacol. *212*:124, 1950.
97. Jasani, M. K., Lewis, G. P., and Tweed, M. F.: Br. J. Pharmacol. *50*:475 P, 1974.
98. Jobin, F., and Trembolay, F.: Thromb. Diath. Haemorrh. *22*:466, 1969.
99. Jørgensen, O.: Acta Pharmacol. Toxicol. (Kbh.) *19*:251, 1962.
100. Kalbhen, D. A., Karzel, K., and Domenjoz, R.: Med. Pharmacol. Exp. *16*: 185, 1967.
101. Kaller, H., Hoffmeister, F., and Kroneberg, G.: Arch. Int. Pharmacodyn. Ther. *161*:389, 1966.
102. Kivivikko, K. J., Laitinen, O., Aer, J., and Halme, J.: Biochem. Pharmacol. *14*:1445, 1965.
103. Ku, E. C., and Wasvary, J. M.: Fed. Proc. *32*:3302, 1973.
104. Kühn, K., Iwangoff, P., Hammerstein, F., Stecher, K., Durruti, M., Holzmann, H., and Korting, G. W.: Hoppe-Seyler's Z. Physiol. Chem. *337*:249, 1964.
105. Lands, W. E. M., LeTellier, P. R., Rome, L. H., and Vanderhoek, J. Y.: In "Advances in the Biosciences," Vol. 9, International Conference on Prostaglandins, Vienna, S. Bergström and S. Bernhart, eds. Pergamon Press Vieweg, Braunschweig, 1973, pp. 15-28.
106. Lash, J. W., and Whitehouse, M. W.: Lab. Invest. *10*:388, 1961.
107. Lazarus, G. S., Daniels, J. R., Brown, R. S., Bladen, H. A., and Fullmer, H. M.: J. Clin. Invest. *47*:2622, 1968.
108. Levine, L.: Biophys. Res. Commun. *47*:88, 1972.
109. Lichtenstein, L. M., and Gillespie, E.: Nature *244*:287, 1973.
110. Lim, R. K. S.: Ann. N. Y. Acad. Sci. *104*:256, 1953.
111. Lim, R. K. S., Guzman, F., Rodgers, D. W., Goto, K., Braun, C., Dickerson, G. D., and Engle, R. J.: Arch. Int. Pharmacodyn. Ther. *152*:25, 1964.
112. Lim, R. K. S., Miller, D. G., Guzman, F., Rodgers, D. W., Rogers, R. W., Wnag, S. K., Chao, P. Y., and Shih, T. Y.: Clin. Pharmacol. Ther. *8*:521, 1967.
113. Lish, P. M., and McKinney, G. R.: J. Lab. Clin. Med. *61*:1015, 1963.
114. Lisin, N., and Leclercq, R.: C. R. Soc. Biol. *157*:1536, 1963.
115. Lockshin, M. D., Crout, J. E., Hepburn, B., and Ritts, E. R.: N. Engl. J. Med. *292*:809, 1975.
116. Lonigro, A. J., Iskovitz, H. D., Crowshaw, K., and McGiff, J. C.: Circ. Res. *32*:712, 1973.
117. Maddox, J. S.: Biochim. Biophys. Acta *306*:74, 1973.
118. Malbica, J. O.: Biochem. Biophys. Res. Comm. *44*:1457, 1971.

119. McArthur, J. N., and Dawkins, P. D.: J. Pharm. Pharmacol. *21*:744, 1969.
120. McArthur, J. N., Dawkins, P. D., and Smith, M. J. H.: J. Pharm. Pharmacol. *23*:393, 1971.
121. McCall, E., and Youlten, L. J. F.: J. Physiol. (Lond.) *234*:98, 1973.
122. Miller, W. S., and Smith, J. G.: Proc. Soc. Exp. Biol. Med. *122*:634, 1966.
123. Milton, A. S.: In "Supplementum to Advances in the Biosciences," Vol. 9, International Conference on Prostaglandins, Vienna, S. Bergström and S. Bernhart, Pergamon Press Vieweg, Braunschweig, 1973, p. 79.
124. Minkes, M. S., Douglas, J. R., and Needleman, P.: Prostaglandins *3*:439, 1973.
125. Moncada, S., Ferreira, S. H., and Vane, J. R.: Eur. J. Pharmacol. *31*:250, 1975.
126. Mörsdorf, K.: In "Inflammation Biochemistry and Drug Interaction," A. Bertelli and J. C. Houck, eds. Excerpta Medica Foundation, Amsterdam, 1969, p. 255.
127. Movat, H. Z., Poon, M. C., and Takeuchi Y.: Int. Arch. Allergy Appl. Immunol. *40*:89, 1971.
128. Newcombe, D. S., Thanassi, N. M., and Ciosek, C. P., Jr.: Life Sci. *14*: 505, 1974.
129. Nimni, M. E., and Bavetta, L. A.: Proc. Soc. Exp. Biol. Med. *117*:618, 1964.
130. Nocenti, M. R., Lederman, G. E., Furey, C. A., and Lopano, A. J.: Proc. Soc. Exp. Biol. Med. *117*:215, 1964.
131. Norn, S.: Acta Pharmacol. Toxicol. (Kbh.) *22*:369, 1965.
132. Norm, S.: Acta Pharmacol. Toxicol. (Kbh.) *25*:281, 1967.
133. O'Brien, J. R.: Lancet *1*:779, 1968.
134. O'Brien, J. R.: Lancet *1*:894, 1968.
135. O'Brien, J. R., Finch, W., and Clark, E.: J. Clin. Pathol. *23*:522, 1970.
136. Opelz, G., Terasaki, P. I., and Hirata, A. A.: Lancet *2*:478, 1973.
137. Pace Asciak, M.: Experientia *30*:590, 1974.
138. Packham, M. A., and Mustard, J. F.: Proc. Soc. Exp. Biol. Med. *130*:72, 1969.
139. Packham, M. A., Warrior, E. S., Glynn, M. F., Senyi, A. S., and Mustard, J. F.: J. Exp. Med. *126*:171, 1967.
140. Palmer, M. A., Piper, P. J., and Vane, J. R.: Br. J. Pharmacol. *49*:226, 1973.
141. Perper, R. J., and Oronski, A. L.: Arthritis Rheum. *17*:47, 1974.
142. Perper, R. J., Sanda, M., Chinea, G., and Oronski, A. L.: J. Lab. Clin. Med. *84*:394, 1974.
143. Peters, H. D., Dimmendahl, V., and Schönhöfer, P. S.: Arch Pharmacol. *282*:R74, 1974.
144. Phelps, P.: Arthritis Rheum. *12*:189, 1969.
145. Phelps, P., and McCarty, D. J., Jr.: J. Pharmacol. Exp. Ther. *158*:546, 1967.
146. Piper, P. J., and Vane, J. R.: Nature *233*:29, 1969.
147. Piper, P. S., and Vane, J. R.: Ann. N. Y. Acad. Sci. *180*:363, 1971.
148. Plaut, M., Lichtenstein, L. M., and Henney, C. S.: J. Clin. Invest. *55*:856, 1975.
149. Pollock, S. H., and Brown, J. H.: J. Pharmacol. Exp. Ther. *178*:609, 1971.
150. Poyser, N. L.: J. Endocrinol. *54*:147, 1972.

151. Rinderknecht, H., Haverback, B. J., and Aladiem, F.: Nature *213*:1130, 1967.
152. Robinson, D. R., Smith, H., and Levine, L.: In "Proceedings of the 18th Interim Scientific Session of the American Rheumatism Association Section of the Arthritis Foundation, December 1972, p. 21.
153. Roger, J., and Kalbhen, D. A.: Arzneim. Forsch. *18*:1512, 1968.
154. Rokosová-Cmuchalová, B., and Bentley, J. P.: Biochem. Pharmacol. 17 (Suppl.) : 315, 1968.
155. Schönhöfer, P.: Med. Pharmacol. Exp. *15*:491, 1966.
156. Schorderet, M.: J. Exp. Med. *126*:171, 1967.
157. Shorley, P. G., and Collier, H. O. J.: Nature *188*:999, 1960.
158. Skidmore, I. F., and Whitehouse, M. W.: Pharmacol. *15*:1965, 1966.
159. Skidmore, I. F., and Whitehouse, M. W.: J. Pharm. Pharmacol. *18*:558, 1966.
160. Skidmore, I. F., and Whitehouse, M. W.: Biochem. J. *99*:5P, 1966.
161. Skidmore, I. F., and Whitehouse, M. W.: Biochem. Pharmacol. *16*:737, 1967.
162. Smith, M. J. H.: J. Pharm. Pharmacol. *2*:705, 1959.
163. Smith, M. J., and Dawkins, P. D.: J. Pharm. Pharmacol. *23*:729, 1971.
164. Smith, J. L., and Forbes, J. J.: Nature *215*:538, 1967.
165. Smith, W. L., and Lands, W. E. M.: J. Biol. Chem. *21*:6700, 1971.
166. Smith, J. B., and Willis, A. L.: Nature (New Biol.) *231*:235, 1971:
167. Snider, D. A., Parker, C. W., and Jacobs, L.: Clin. Res. *21*:819, 1973.
168. Sonova, L.: In "Supplementum to Advances in the Biosciences," Vol 9, International Conference on Prostaglandins, Vienna, S. Bergström and S. Bernhart, eds. Pergamon Press Vieweg, Braunschweig, 1973, p. 53.
169. Spector, W. G., and Willoughby, D. A.: Bacteriol. Rev. *27*:117, 1963.
170. Spragg, J., Talamo, R. C., and Aasten, K. F.: In "Handbook of Experimental Pharmacology," Vol. 25, E. G. Erdös, ed. Springer-Verlag, Berlin, 1970.
171. Stuart, R. K.: J. Lab. Clin. Med. *75*:463, 1970.
172. Swyer, G. I. M.: Biochem. J. *42*:28, 1948.
173. Sykes, J. A., and Maddox, I. S.: Nature (New Biol.) *237*:59, 1972.
174. Takeguchi, C., and Sih, C. J.: Prostaglandins *2*:169, 1972.
175. Tan, L., Wang, H. M., and Le Houx, J. G.: Prostaglandins *4*:9, 1973.
176. Tanaka, K., and Tizuka, Y.: Biochem. Pharmacol. *17*:2023, 1968.
177. Tomlinson, R. V., Ringold, H. J., Aureshi, M. C., and Forchelli, E.: Biochem. Biophys. Res. Commun. *46*:552, 1972.
178. Tormey, D. C., Fudenberg, H. H., and Kamin, R. M.: Nature *213*:281, 1967.
179. Trethewie, E. R., and Morris, C. W.: Aust. J. Exp. Biol. Med. Sci. *29*:433, 1959.
180. Trnavská, Z., and Trnavsky, K.: Med. Pharmacol. Exp. *12*:167, 1965.
181. Trnavská, Z., Trnavsky, K., and Kühn, K.: Biochem. Pharmacol. *17*:1501, 1968.
182. Trnavsky, K., and Trnavská, Z.: J. Pharm. Pharmacol. *20*:564, 1968.
183. Trnavsky, K., and Trnavská, Z.: Pharmacology *6*:9, 1971.
184. Ulevitch, R. J., and Letchford, D. J.: Fed. Proc. *32*:845 (Abstr.), 1973.
185. Ungar, C.: Biochem. Pharmacol. *12* (Suppl. 10) : 173, 1963.
186. Van Arman, C. G. Carlson, R. P., Brown, W. R., and Itkin, A.: Proc. Soc.

Exp. Biol. Med. *134*:163, 1970.

187. Van Arman, C. G., Carlson, R. P., Risley, E. A., Thomas, R. H., and Nuss, G. W.: J. Pharmacol. Exp. Ther. *175*:459, 1970.
188. Van Arman, C. G., Risley, E. A., and Kling, P. J.: Pharmacologist *13*: 284, 1971.
189. Vane, J. R.: Nature (New Biol.) *231*:232, 1971.
190. Vane, J. R.: Hosp. Pract. *7*:61, 1972.
191. Vane, J. R., and Williams, K. I.: Br. J. Pharmacol. *45*:146 P, 1972.
192. Walters, M. N. L., and Willoughby, D. A.: J. Pathol. *90*:641, 1965.
193. Weiss, H. J., and Aledort, L. M.: Lancet *2*:495, 1967.
194. Weiss, H. J., and Aledort, L. M., Kochwas: J. Clin. Invest. *47*:2169, 1968.
195. Weissman, G.: Fed. Proc. *23*:1038, 1964.
196. Weissman, G.: N. Engl. J. Med. *286*:141, 1972.
197. Weissman, G., and Dingle, J. T.: Exp. Cell Res. *25*:207, 1961.
198. Weissman, G., and Thomas, L.: J. Exp. Med. *116*:433, 1962.
199. Weissman, G., and Thomas, L.: Recent Prog. Horm. Res. *20*:215, 1964.
200. Whitehouse, M. W.: Biochem. Pharmacol. *13*:319, 1964.
201. Whitehouse, M. W.: Prog. Drug Res. *8*:321, 1965.
202. Willis, A. L., and Cornelsen, M.: Prostaglandins *3*:353, 1973.
203. Willis, A. L., Davison P., Ramwell, P. W., Brocklehurst, W. E., and Smith, B.: In "Prostaglandins in Cellular Biology," P. W. Ramwell and B. B. Phariss, eds. Plenum Press, New York, 1972, p. 227.
204. Willoughby, D. A., Dunn, C. J., Yamamoto, S., Capasso, F., Deporter, D. A., and Giroud, J. P.: Agents Actions *5*:35, 1975.
205. Wono, P. Y. D., Bedwani, J. R., and Cuthbert, A. W.: Nature (New Biol.) *238*:27, 1972.
206. Wyllie, J. H., Hesselbo, T., and Black, J. W.: Lancet *2*:1117, 1972.
207. Zicha, L., and Bregulla, B.: Arzneim. Forsch. *12*:474, 1972.
208. Zucker, M. B., and Peterson, J.: Proc. Soc. Exp. Biol. Med. *127*:547, 1968.
209. Zucker, M. B., and Peterson, J.: J. Lab. Clin. Med. *76*:66, 1970.
210. Zweifach, B. W., Nagler, A. L., and Troll, W.: J. Exp. Med. *113*:437, 1961.

Chapter 15

Toxicity of Non-Steroidal Antiinflammatory Drugs

1. GENERAL CONSIDERATIONS

The laboratory assessment of the toxicity of a compound designed to be used for therapeutic purposes is to provide a set of guidelines for clinicans when they subsequently administer the latter to normal subjects and patients. These guidelines should deal with dosage relationships in respect to lethality, efficacy and physiological function. Some general directives for toxicity studies, depending on the phase of investigation in which the compound is being studied, i.e., phase I, II or III, have been suggested (61) (Table 39).

Any compound is toxic at some dose or another and, conversely, there exists a low dose of even the most toxic agent at which no toxicity can be found. Somewhere between these extremes most—if not all—synthetic chemicals exert their pharmacological effects. Therefore, a judgement concerning a certain compound can be formulated after the examination of two dose-responses curves cover-

TABLE 39. General guidelines for animal toxicity studies

Duration of Human Administration (Oral or parenteral)	Phase (1)	Duration of Animal Treatment
Several days	I, II, III, NDA	2 species, 2 weeks
Up to 2 week	I	2 species, 2 weeks
	II	2 species, up to 4 weeks
	III, NDA	2 species, up to 3 months
Up to 3 months	I, II	2 species, 4 weeks
	III	2 species, 3 months
	NDA	2 species, up to 6 months
6 months to unlimited	I, II	2 species, 3 months
	III,	2 species, 6 months or longer
	NDA	2 species, 12 months in non-rodents, 18 months in rodents

(1) Phase I   = Clinical studies of normal adult males, designed primarily for safety evaluation.

Phase II = Clinical studies on small number of patients, to determine safety and efficacy.

Phase III = Clinical studies on large number of patients, to determine safety and efficacy.

NDA   = New Drug Application - completion of all previous data submitted for the approval of the U.S. Food and Drug Administration.

ing the separation of desirable versus undesirable pharmacological effects. The desirable effect, in the case of antiinflammatory drug, is the inhibition, depression or modulation of the inflammatory process. The undesirable pharmacological effects can vary from simply an unpleasant taste or odor to lethality.

Basic to almost all other pharmacological data obtained in short-term animal studies is the single dose that is lethal to 50% of the animals within a specified period of time—the LD_{50}. To be of value for further investigations and to allow justifiable comparison with other laboratory values, the conditions under which the LD_{50} is obtained must be clearly defined. Because most acute pharmacological studies tend to place an animal under stress, it is of paramount importance to understand what this stress can do to the normal reaction to and biodisposition of the compound in question. This is particularly true for antiinflammatory drugs because the methods of testing their efficacy usually require the induction of some form of stressful situation: paw edema, granuloma or arthritis. It has, therefore, been suggested that, during the chronic administration of an investigational compound to animals with an experimentally induced disease or organ damage, it should be determined whether the disease itself plays a role in the compound's toxicity (110).

If a substance has the desired effect within a dosage range that appears to exclude adverse reactions (including lethality) in laboratory animals, it is nearly always a serious candidate for clinico-pharmacological trials. Not always, however, can accurate predictions be made. For example, the acute oral LD_{50} of indomethacin in mouse and rat is 50 and 12 mg/kg, respectively. The chronic oral LD_{50}, in rat and dog is 0.5 and 0.75 mg/kg, respectively. When these data are subsequently translated into human dosages, the recommended therapeutic dose of indomethacin becomes 1.5-4.0 mg/kg/day which is between 3-8 times the toxic dose for the two most common species of laboratory animals (130).

A quite comprehensive toxicological program has been recommended, including a number of biochemical tests, an extensive histological evaluation and tests for host defense, endocrine functions, and autonomic nervous system (180).

Other important considerations in conducting toxicity studies are the actual metabolic alterations of a compound in the various species of animals, the bioavailability of the compound even after it has been absorbed and is present in the blood stream and the induction of adapted metabolic enzymes. Even after all these studies have been performed, and a compound has also passed all the animal test there is still no guarantee that it is not harmful to man as demonstrated in the case of an antiinflammatory drug, fenclozic acid (3).

2. TOXIC EFFECTS ON GASTROINTESTINAL TRACT

One of the most common reason for rejecting a compound from further consideration, even though it has no major life-threatening side effect, is a high incidence of gastrointestinal disturbance (11). Most, if not all, of the drugs employed in the treatment of rheumatic disease tend to cause gastrointestinal problems ranging from subjective feelings of discomfort to hemorrhage and development or reactivation of mucosal lesions. In animals, there is obviously no possibility for evaluating subjective responses and more objective assessments must be made.

The most common method for determining if a compound produces gastrointestinal effects is to look for its ulcerogenic potential in animals. Usually drugs are administered by oral route and then, after a specified period of time, the animals are sacrificed and their stomachs examined for the presence of ulcerations (6). The parenteral route has also been used and stomach—and sometimes intestine—have been examined for ulcerations and petechial hemorrhages (167). These methods have been largely applied for the assessment of gastrointestinal damage induced by indomethacin (8, 18,19,97), flufenamic acid (26), acetylsalicylic acid (6,18,19,26, 166) and phenylbutazone (18,19,26), to mention only a few of the many available reports. The experimental data on animals are sometime confusing since the methods used have been mostly descriptive and the observations relate to different parts of the intestinal tract (4,33,103,133). Efforts have been made to introduce more quantitative parameters. Protein-bound vital dye has been injected to measure gastric plasma loss and to delineate the areas of hemorrhage in rats following the administration of antiinflammatory compounds (163). In other studies, red blood cells labeled with either ^{51}Cr or ^{59}Fe were used to quantitate gastrointestinal blood loss in rats and dogs (46,111,129,134). In comparable investigations in man, fecal blood loss induced by aspirin-like drugs has been demonstrated after their repeated administration over several days (22,66,101,109, 135,136,145). Other clinical studies have implicated aspirin and aspirin-like drugs as major causative agents in the development of gastric and duodenal ulcers (39,43,59,80,141). Several factors are implicated in the development of gastrointestinal damage following non-steroidal antiinflammatory drug administration.

The acidity of gastric content has a positive implication both in man and animals. In achlorhydric subjects (78,83) or when concurrently administered with antacids (100,109,136,161,164), aspirin produces less damage to gastric mucosa. The reduction of gastric acidity in animals by various treatments markedly decreases gastric damage by salicylates (6,16,17,62). The lowering of gastric acidity probably results in decreased absorption of the drug (158).

Gastroscopic examinations suggest that the particle size of the drug is of importance, with coarse particles being more harmful than are fine ones (68,152,164). Controversial results have been obtained in animals (4,5,77). It seems, however, that high concentrations of the acidic form of the drug must be present for damage to occur (5,138,140).

TABLE 40. Acute toxicity and acute ulcerogenic actions of some non-steroidal antiinflammatory drugs

Compound	LD_{50} Oral Rat mg/kg	ED_{50} Ulcerogenic 1 dose mg/kg	2 doses mg/kg	ED_{150}[1] Bleeding mg/kg
Aspirin	1435	315	48	240
Phenylbutazone	680	106	63	113
Oxephenylbutazone	980	>300	100	>300
Indomethacin	12	6	1	5
Flufenamic acid	708	34	47	—
Ibuprofen	1600	92	—	—
Naproxen	543	17	—	—
Diclofenac	482	12	—	17

[1]Dose required to produce blood loss of 150 μ l/72 hr estimated with [51] Cr-labeled erythrocyte technique (111).

A marked association between alcohol intake and gastric damage by aspirin-like drugs has been observed (15,63,123). A synergistic effect has also been found in animals (6,82).

Although extensive studies in laboratory animals have shown that tolerance toward aspirin-induced gastric damage develops after repeated administration of the drug (6,77,82), investigations in man show that the same amount of "blood loss," estimated with the ^{51}Cr technique, occurs regardless of the timing of administration (102).

A multifactorial cause is implicated in the mechanism of gastric damage by aspirin and related drugs. Immediate effects are the sloughing of the mucous protective layer (142,148,149), denaturation of the surface mucosal cells—leading to rapid cell death (34, 140,148,149)—and changes in permeability of gastric mucosa to ions and various molecules of different size (32,35,36,37,38,163), accompanied by a reduction in acid output (4,16,17,36,60). However, salicylates stimulate the production of histamine in the stomach (84,85) and indomethacin causes a dose-dependent increase of pentagastrin-stimulated acid secretion (108). Since the depression or block of vagal activity reduce aspirin damage to gastric mucosa, these results seem conflicting. They can be reconciled, supposing that aspirin-like drugs initially induce vagal stimulation of acid production and that this causes an overall depression in acid secretion, through activation of a feed-back control of acid production (149).

Among the secondary drug effects are (i) the reduction in the synthesis of gastric mucous components, which occurs with a wide variety of both steroidal and non-steroidal antiinflammatory agents with ulcerogenic potential (40,41,69,98,119,146) and, (ii) the increased hemorrhagic tendency following the inhibition of platelet aggregation and stickiness (55,115,155,170). Since prostaglandins prevent the development of many different types of experimentally induced ulcerations and decrease gastric acid production (98,147), the role of the inhibition of prostaglandin synthesis by non-steroidal antiinflammatory agents has been considered in gastric damage. It has been suggested that these drugs cause mucosal erosions through such a mechanism (12,108) but other drug action, e.g., on energy production and synthesis of cAMP (107,112) may be responsible for the observed effects.

3. TOXIC EFFECTS ON KIDNEY

Many non-steroidal antiinflammatory drugs have been reported to cause kidney damage after prolonged administration to laboratory animals. This damage—renal papillary necrosis—has been produced mainly in rats, occasionally in rabbits and dogs, and—rarely in monkeys.

The evaluation of renal toxicity in the animal is much more complicated than appears from just measuring renal function. In a study of a compound similar to flufenamic acid, the lesion was consistently produced in rats, but the animals, shedding 20% of their papillary apex, functionally adapted so that renal function tests could not detect this injury. Renal toxicity in rats also seems to vary with the strain of animals used (14) and, at least, in the case of a recently described antiinflammatory drug, sudoxicam (175), it can be sex dependent, the females being more susceptible than the males (176). It should be noted, however, that the plasma half-life of sudoxicam is sex-related in rats (T 1/2 in female = 27 hr, in male = 13 hr) but not in other animal species (73,175). Because dogs are commonly included in chronic toxicity studies, a renal clearance study can be performed at a number of points throughout the chronic toxicity trial, evaluating such items as renal clearance of compounds that have passed through the glomeruli and are not reabsorbed of those that are cleared through the tubuli without being reabsorbed and, finally, of those that are reabsorbed through the tubuli. Among the non-steroidal antiinflammatory drugs causing renal papillary necrosis in rats, the following may be cited: the pyrazolones (20,30), mefenamic acid (87,120), flufenamic acid (70,87), meclofenamic acid (187) and fenoprofen (48). High doses of indomethacin have also been reported to cause renal papillary necrosis (8). Similarly as in laboratory animals, when large doses of non-steroidal antiinflammatory drugs are administered to man over a prolonged period, they will cause renal papillary necrosis. The incidence of this syndrome is subject to argument and its estimate ranges from "rare" (95) to 3-12% in carefully selected populations (1,91). The lesion is often seen on autopsy of long-term sufferers from rheumatoid arthritis (21,23,121) but it is not clear whether this is an aspect of the disease or one of the consequences of the prolonged administration of antiinflammatory drugs. Nevertheless, it is practice of some clinicians to withdraw such drugs from subjects in whom kidney function is compromised (89).

Several reports describe the occurrence of renal papillary necrosis in both laboratory animals and man following prolonged ingestion of aspirin (27,39,49,57,65,67,71,88). A better case can be made for a complex induction incriminating salicylates, phenacetin and possibly caffeine (1,27,56,88,105,174). Phenacetin alone in rats (20,122,177) and dogs (177) failed to provoke renal papillary necrosis but prolonged administration of this compound—as well as of aspirin—did cause kidney damage in rabbits (28). Aspirin and aspirin-phenacetin-caffeine combination caused renal papillary lesions in rats (122).

Despite many investigations, a wealth of clinical observations and critical analysis (1,57), crucial details of analgesic nephropathy still remain uncertain. It is premature to impute or to absolve any of the components of the antipyretic-analgesic combinations as the causative factor. A more balanced view is that the prolonged abuse of these combinations may cause kidney damage in the susceptible subject or in concert with other variables as, for instance, concurrent bacterial infections whose role has been alleged, at least, in experimental animals (9,90).

4. MISCELLANEOUS TOXIC EFFECTS

In addition to the toxic effects on the gastrointestinal tract and kidney, several other adverse reactions have been described as being caused by non-steroidal antiinflammatory agents.

Therapeutic doses of salicylates produce definite changes in the acid-base balance and electrolyte pattern. The initial event is an extracellular and intracellular respiratory alkalosis for which, however, compensation promptly ensues (94). Alterations of water and electrolyte balance are usually observed when acid-base disturbances occur. The low plasma P_{CO_2} leads to decreased renal tubular reabsorption of bicarbonate, and increased renal excretion of sodium, potassium and water. Intrarenal factors, such as, for instance, the inhibition of the active system for Na-K transport in cells contribute to potassium depletion (24,94,99). Salicylates also stimulate respiration directly and indirectly: this effect contributes to the acid-base disturbances. Full therapeutic doses of salicylates increase oxygen consumption and CO_2 production in experimental animals and man. As the salicylate gains access to the medulla, it directly stimulates the respiratory center (132,153).

Salicylate medication does not ordinarily alter the leukocyte or erythrocyte count, or the hematocrit and hemoglobin content. It causes, however, a definite prolongation of the bleeding time at doses as small as 0.3 g. This is not due to hypothrombinemia, which occurs only after large doses of salicylates (over 6 g), but depends on the effects of these drugs on platelet function. They block the adhesion of platelets to connective tissue or collagen fibers, inhibit ADP release from platelets and the resultant aggregation induced by connective tissue or collagen and the synthesis of prostaglandins (114,162,171). It follows that care should be exercised in the use of salicylates (and of other non-steroidal antiinflammatory drugs) during long-term treatment with oral anticoagulant agents. This aspect will be discussed in the following paragraph. Moreover, it should be mentioned that the intentional use of salicylates and other drugs inhibiting platelet aggregation in conjunction with oral anticoogulants is being actively explored for the prophylaxis of coronary and cerebral arterial thrombosis.

The list of adverse reactions attributed to phenylbutazone, in addition to the gastrointestinal side effects, is quite impressive. It includes several types of sometimes fatal blood dyscrasias, fluid and electrolyte disturbances leading to water and sodium retention, kidney failure and anuria, cardiac decompensation and hypertension, optic neuritis, retinal hemorrhage, thyroid hyperplasia, toxic goiter, allergic reactions, and fatal and non-fatal hepatitis (29,64,106). The toxicity of phenylbutazone precludes its use in long-term therapy. It should be employed for short periods, primarily for relief of acute exacerbations of rheumatoid arthritis that are not relieved by other measures and after careful evaluation of the risk involved (44,58,64,160).

Approximately 35-50% of the patients receiving usual therapeutic doses of indomethacin experience untoward symptoms and about 20% must discontinue its use. The most frequent side effects are severe frontal headache, occurring in 25-50% of patients who take the drug chronically, dizziness, vertigo, mental confusion, hematopoietic reactions consisting of neutropenia and thrombocytopenia, and hypersensitivity sometimes manifested as an acute attack of asthma (13).

5. DRUG INTERACTIONS

The simultaneous use of several therapeutic agents has become commonplace, and some interactions between almost any two simultaneously administered drugs must be expected and are often clinically important.

Drug interactions with coumarin anticoagulants are of preeminent interest because an even moderate alteration of the hypothrombinemic effect of the anticoagulants may have serious consequences.

Drugs can modify the action of coumarins by a variety of mechanisms. They can alter the bioavailability of Vitamin K, the metabolic fate of coumarins, the prothrombin-complex concentration and the receptor affinity for coumarins (92).

Phenylbutazone and its hydroxy analog, oxyphenylbutazone, are among the most effective potentiators of coumarin anticoagulants. Excessive hypothrombinemia induced by these two drugs in patients chronically treated with coumarins has been responsible for many hemorrhages (2,47,51,55). Phenylbutazone is an acidic compound that competitevely inhibits the binding of warfarin to albumin. Clinical plasma concentrations displace up to 40% of bound warfarin from its binding site in vitro (2,126,159). The resultant increase of free warfarin is responsible for the markedly enhanced hypothrombinemic action (2,126,128). This enhancement may be seen after only one day of phenylbutazone therapy and may reduce warfarin requirement by 50-75% (2,126,157,165). The plasma half-life of warfarin is shortened by phenylbutazone (2, 126). This is the expected result of the increased displacement of warfarin from albumin which makes more of it available to liver metabolizing enzymes. In addition, phenylbutazone induces human drug-metabolizing enzymes (31). Since the net result of the warfarin-phenylbutazone interaction in man is increased hypothrombinemia, any enzyme induction appears quantitatively less important. In dogs whose albumin binds warfarin less than does human albumin, the effects of enzyme induction are predominant (125).

Present evidence indicates that therapeutic doses of aspirin or other salicylates have no major effects on the hypothrombinemic action of the coumarins (79,127,165,168). On the other hand, it is known that salicylates decrease the prothrombin-complex activity in normal subjects (137,143,154). The relatively slight potentiation of the action of coumarins suggests that their fate in the body may also be altered by salicylates. The increased risk of bleeding in patients on coumarin therapy who take aspirin is caused by its effects on platelet function (118).

Among the other antiinflammatory drugs, mefenamic acid (156,157) and indomethacin (72) have been shown to displace warfarin from human albumin in vitro. However, in controlled studies, indomethacin did not alter hypothrombinemia induced by coumarin anticoagulants (54,116). Conversely, mefenamic acid substantially prolonged the prothrombin time in subjects chronically maintained on warfarin (75). In a double-blind clinical trial, a recently described antiinflammatory drug—diclofenac—did not interact with coumarin anticoagulant (113). Ibuprofen also failed to alter the hypothrombinemia caused by warfarin.

Among the antigout agents, allopurinol has been described as interfering with hepatic inactivation of oral anticoagulants (144, 153). The effect is, however, variable and of clinical significance only in some patients.

Since two (or more) antiinflammatory drugs are often administered concurrently to rheumatic patients, the problem of interaction may be of clinical importance. The reported antagonism between indomethacin and acetylsalicylic acid in some laboratory tests for anti-inflammatory activity has provoked speculation that a similar antagonism may occur during therapy. Interaction studies of these two drugs have been carried out in man with divergent results (53,81,86,104,124). These investigations, however, cannot be immediately compared because of differences in dosing regimes and analytical methods. Subjects on indomethacin and aspirin exhibit unchanged serum levels of indomethacin as compared to those receiving indomethacin alone (53,104,124). According to the results of other investigations (81,86), the serum levels of indomethacin are reduced by concurrent teratment with acetylsalicylic acid. On the basis of experiments in rats (178,179), it has been suggested that the mechanism underlying the interaction is the reduced gastrointestinal absorption of indomethacin in presence of aspirin, causing an increased biliary excretion of the former. However, in man (45), in contrast to the findings in rat (76), only a minimal enterohepatic circulation of unmodified indomethacin has been found. Displacement of bound indomethacin from plasma proteins has not been determined.

A pharmacodynamic interaction between acetylsalicylic acid and the antiinflammatory agent, fenoprofen, has been observed. When subjects received both drugs, the concentrations of fenoprofen in plasma were lowered significantly, compared to those attained after fenoprofen alone. The latter, however, did not affect plasma salicylate levels (150). Similar to the results in man, fenoprofen plasma levels were lowered by aspirin in rat (167). Fenoprofen is extensively and firmly bound to human plasma albumin, however, but this binding is unaffected by aspirin in vitro at concentrations comparable to those observed in vivo (150,151). The mechanism of this interaction remains largely unexplained: probably different mechanisms are involved in rat and man (167). The competition for plasma albumin-binding sites explains the potentiation of sulfa drugs by aspirin and phenylbutazone (7). The displacement by these agents of methotrexate, with fatal consequences, has also been reported (42). A recently described antiinflammatory agent, Diftalone, increases the effect of tolbutamide on insulin secretion, possibly through interference at the level of albumin binding (52). Other different mechanisms of interaction have also been suggested. Phenylbutazone inhibits the metabolism of oral hypoglycemic agents—tolbutamide (25) and chlorpropamide (93)—and interferes with the renal handling of the active metabolite of acetohexamide (50). The interference with the renal elimination of other drugs and of acidic metabolic products provides an explanation for the divergent effects of low and high doses of salicylates on uric acid excretion (10), and for the hyperuricemic effect of salicylates and phenylbutazone given concurrently (30).

Table 41 summarizes some clinically relevant drug interactions.

TABLE 41. Clinically relevant drug interactions

Drug	May Interact with	Possible Result
Aspirin	Corticosteroids	Cumulation of salicylate with toxicity when chronic steroid therapy withdrawn
	Coumarins	Large doses of salicylate may increase coumarin activity
	Antidepressants	Serum levels and side effects of nortriptyline increased
	Methotrexate	Activity of methotrexate increased
	PAS	Increased risk of mutual toxicity
	Spironolactone	Inhibition of natriuretic activity
	Probenecid	Therapeutic effect of probenecid markedly increased
Indomethacin	Probenecid	Serum level and half-life of indomethacin increased
	Salicylates	Absorption of indomethacin impaired
Mefenamic acid	Coumarins	Activity of coumarins increased
Phenylbutazone	Methandrostenolone	Plasma levels of oxyphenbutazone increased
	Coumarins	Activity of coumarins increased
	Adrenergic neuron-blocking agents	Antihypertensive effect antagonized
	Hypoglycemic sulfonylurea	Hypoglycemic activity increased
Probenecid	Cephalosporins	Serum levels of cephalexin and cephalotin increased and prolonged
	Penicillins	Serum levels of penicillins increased and prolonged
	PAS	Serum levels of PAS increased
Allopurinol	Ampicillin	Increased incidence of ampicillin rash
	Mercaptopurine	Activity of mercaptopurine increased

REFERENCES

1. Able, J. A.: Clin. Pharmacol. Ther. *12*:583, 1971.
2. Aggelev, P. M., O'Reilly, R. A., and Leong, L.: N. Engl. J. Med. *276*:496, 1967.
3. Alcock, S. J.: Proc. Eur. Soc. Study Drug Toxicity *12*:184, 1971.
4. Anderson, K. W.: Arch. Int. Pharmacodyn. Ther. *152*:379, 1964.
5. Anderson, K. W.: Arch. Int. Pharmacodyn. Ther. *152*:392, 1964.
6. Anderson, K. W.: Arch. Int. Pharmacodyn. Ther. *157*:181, 1965.
7. Anton, A. H.: Clin. Pharmacol. Ther. *9*:561, 1968.
8. Arnold L., Lollins, C., and Starmer, G. A.: Pathology *6*:303, 1974.
9. Axelsen, R. A., and Burry, A. F.: Br. Med. J. *5*:784, 1973.
10. Azarnoff, D. L., and Hurwitz, A.: Pharmacol. Physicians *4*:2, 1970.
11. Bein, H. J., Eichenberger, E., Jung, G., Polzer, C., Stamm, W., and Toeschler, H.: Proc. Eur. Soc. Study Drug Toxicity *12*:179, 1971.
12. Bennett, A., Stamford, I. F., and Unger, W. C.: J. Physiol. (Lond.) *229*:349, 1973.
13. Boardman, P. L., and Hart, E. D.: Ann. Rheum. Dis. *26*:127, 1967.
14. Bokelman, D. L., Bagdon, W. J., Mattis, P. A., and Stoner, P. F.: Toxicol. Appl. Pharmacol. *19*:111, 1971.
15. Bouchier, I. A. D., and Williams, H. S.: Lancet *1*:178, 1969.
16. Brodie, D. A., and Chase, B. J.: Gastroenterology *53*:604, 1967.
17. Brodie, D. A., and Chase, B. J.: Gastroenterology *56*:206, 1969.
18. Brodie, D. A., Cook, P. G., Baner, B. J., and Dogie, G. E.: Toxicol. Appl. Pharmacol. *17*:615, 1970.
19. Brodie, D. A., Tate, C. L., and Hooke, K. F.: Science *170*:183, 1970.
20. Brown, M. D., and Hardy, T. L.: Br. J. Pharmacol. *32*:17, 1968.
21. Bulger, R. J., Healey, L. A., and Polinsky: Ann. Rheum. Dis. *27*:339, 1968.
22. Burne, J. A., Bianchine, J. R., Johnson, P. C., and Wortham, C. F.: Clin. Pharmacol. Ther. *16*:821, 1974.
23. Burry, H. C.: Rheum. Phys. Med. *11*:2, 1971.
24. Charnock, J. S., Opit, L. J., and Hetzel, B. S.: Metabolism *10*:874, 1961.
25. Christensen, L. K., Hansen, J. M., and Kristensen, M.: Lancet *2*:1298, 1963.
26. Cioli, V., Silvestrini, B., and Dordoni, F.: Exp. Mol. Pathol. *6*:68, 1967.
27. Clarkson, A. J. R., and Lawrence, J. R.: In "Renal Infection and Renal Scarring," P. Kincaid-Smith and K. F. Fairley, eds. Mercedes, Melbourne, 1971, p. 375.
28. Clausen, E.: Lancet *1*:123, 1964.
29. Clinicopathologic Conference: Am. J. Med. *30*:268, 1961.
30. Collier, J. C., and Flower, R. J.: Lancet *2*:852, 1971.
31. Conney, A. H.: Pharmacol. Rev. *19*:317, 1967.
32. Cooke, A. R., and Kienzle, M. G.: Gastroenterology *66*:56, 1974.
33. Cooper, G. N., Meade, R. C., and Ellison, E. M.: Arch. Surg. *93*:171, 1966.
34. Croft, D. N.: Br. Med. J.: *2*:897, 1963.
35. Davenport, H. W.: Gastroenterology *46*:245, 1964.
36. Davenport, H. W.: N. Engl. J. Med. *276*:1307, 1967.
37. Davenport, H. W.: Gastroenterology *56*:439, 1969.
38. Davenport, H. W., Cohen, B. J., Bree, M., and Davenport, V. D.: Gastroenterology *49*:189, 1965.

39. Dawborn, J. K., Fairley, I. F., Kincaid-Smith, P., and King, W. E.: Quart. J. Med. *35*:60, 1966.
40. Denko, C. W.: J. Lab. Clin. Med. *51*:174, 1958.
41. Denko, C. W.: J. Lab. Clin. Med. *63*:953, 1964.
42. Dixon, R. L., Hendersson, E. S., and Rall, D. P.: Fed. Proc. *24*:454, 1965.
43. Douglas, R. A., and Johnson, E. D.: Med. J. Aust. *2*:893, 1961.
44. Dudley Hart, F.: Br. Med. J. *4*:191, 1975.
45. Duggan, D. E., Hogans, A. F., Kwan, K. C., and McMahon, F. G.: J. Pharmacol. Exp. Ther. *181*:563, 1972.
46. Edelson, J., and Douglas, I. F.: J. Pharmacol. Exp. Ther. *184*:449, 1973.
47. Eisen, M. J.: J. Am. Med. Assoc. *189*:64, 1964.
48. Emmerson, J. L., Gibson, W. R., Pierce, E. C., and Kiplinger, G. F.: Toxicol. Appl. Pharmacol. *25*:444, 1973.
49. Fellner, S. K., and Tuttle, E. P.: Arch. Intern. Med. *124*:379, 1969.
50. Field, J. B., Ohta, M., Boyle, C., and Remer, A.: N. Engl. J. Med. *17*:889, 1967.
51. Fox, S. L.: J. Am. Med. Assoc. *188*:320, 1964.
52. Fritzsche, H., Scherak, O., Weissel, M., and Kolarz, G.: Scand. J. Rheumatol. *4* (Suppl. 8) : 43, 1975.
53. Garnham, J. C., Raymond, K., Shatton, E., and Turner, P.: In "33rd International Congress of Pharmaceutical Sciences, Abstracts. Stockholm, 1973, p. 169.
54. Gáspárdy, G., Bálint, G., and Gáspárdy, G., Jr.: Z. Rheumaforsch. *26*: 332, 1967.
55. Gast, L. F.: Ann. Rheum. Dis. *23*:500, 1964.
56. Gault, M. H.: Can. Med. Assoc. J. *107*:756, 1972.
57. Gault, M. H., Rudwal, T. C., Engles, W., and Dossetor, B.: Ann. Intern. Med. *68*:906, 1968.
58. Gifford, R. H.: Ration. Drug Ther. *7*:1, 1973.
59. Gilles, M., and Skyring, A.: Med. J. Aust. *2*:1132, 1968.
60. Glarborg Jørgensen, T., Kaplan, E. L., and Peskin, G. W.: Scand. J. Lab. Clin. Invest. *33*:31, 1974.
61. Goldenthal, E. I.: FDA Pap. *2*:13, 1968.
62. Gottschalk, A. M., and Menguy, R.: Surg. Forum *21*:300, 1971.
63. Goulston, K., and Cooke, A. R.: Br. Med. J. *4*:664, 1968.
64. Graham, W.: Can. Med. Assoc. J. *79*:634, 1958.
65. Grimlund, K.: Acta Med. Scand. *174* (Suppl. 405) : 1, 1963.
66. Grossman, M. J., Matsumoto, K. K., and Lichter, R. J.: Gastroenterology *40*:383, 1961.
67. Gsell, O., Dubach, U. C., and Raillard-Peucker, U.: Dtsch. Med. Wochenschr. *93*:101, 1968.
68. Györy, A. Z., and Stiel, J. J.: Lancet *2*:300, 1968.
69. Häkkinen, H., Johansson, R., Pautio, M.: Gut *9*:712, 1968.
70. Hardy, T. L.: Br. J. Exp. Pathol. *51*:348, 1970.
71. Harwald, B.: Am. J. Med. *35*:69, 1963.
72. Henry, R. A., and Wosilait, W. D.: Toxicol. Appl. Pharmacol. *33*:267, 1975.
73. Hobbs, D. C.: Pharmacologist *17*:268, 1975.
74. Hobbs, C. B., Miller, A. L., and Thornley, J. H.: Postgrad. Med. J. *41*: 563, 1965.

75. Holmes, E. L.:Ann. Phys. Med. (Suppl.) *8*:36, 1966.
76. Hucker, H. B., Zacchei, A. G., Cox, S. V., Brodie, D. A., and Cantwell, N. H. R.: J. Pharmacol. Exp. *153*:237, 1966.
77. Hurley, J. W., and Crandall, L. A.: In "Salicylates, an International Symposium," A. St. J. Dixon, B. K. Martin, M. J. H. Smith, and P. H. N. Wood, eds. Churchill, London, 1963, p. 213.
78. Jabarri, M., and Valberg, L. S.: Can. Med. Assoc. J. *102*:178, 1970.
79. Jarnum, S.: Scand. J. Lab. Clin. Invest. *6*:91, 1954.
80. Jennings, G. H.: Gut *6*:1, 1965.
81. Jeremy, R., and Towson, J.: Med. J. Aust. *2*:127, 1970.
82. John, D. J. B. St., Yeomans, N. D., McDermott, F. T., and de Boer, W. G. R.: Am. J. Dig. Dis. *18*:881, 1973.
83. John, D. J. B. St., and McDermott, F. T.: Br. Med. J. *2*:450, 1970.
84. Johnson, L. R.: Proc. Soc. Exp. Biol. Med. *121*:386, 1966.
85. Johnson, L. R., and Overholt, B. F.: Gastroenterology *52*:505, 1967.
86. Kaldestad, E., Hansen, T., and Brath, H. K.: Eur. J. Clin. Pharmacol. *9*: 199, 1975.
87. Kaump, D. H.: Ann. Phys. Med. *9*:16, 1966.
88. Kincaid-Smith, P.: Med. J. Aust. *2*:1131, 1969.
89. Kincaid-Smith, P.: Br. Med. J. *4*:618, 1970.
90. Kincaid-Smith, P., Naura, R. S., and Fairley, K. F.: In "Renal Infection and Renal Scarring," P. Kincaid-Smith and K. F. Fairley, eds. Mercedes, Melbourne, 1971, p. 385.
91. Kingsley, D. P. E., Goldberg, B., Abrahams, C., Meyers, A. J., Furman, K. J., and Cohen, I.: Br. Med. J. *4*:656, 1972.
92. Kock-Weser, J., and Sellers, E. M.: N. Engl. Med. *285*:487, 1971.
93. Kristensen, M., and Hansen, J. M.: Acta Med. Scand. *183*:83, 1968.
94. Lamont-Havers, R. W., and Wagner, B. M. (Eds.): "Proceedings of the Conference on Effect of Chronic Salicylate Administration." NIH, Bethesda, 1966.
95. Lawson, D. H.: J. Chron. Dis. *26*:39, 1973.
96. Lee, Y. H., Cheng, W. D., Bianchi, R. G., Mollison, K., and Hansen, J.: Prostaglandins *3*:29, 1973.
97. Lee, V. H., Mollison, K. W., and Cheng, W. D.: Arch. Int. Pharmacodyn. Ther. *191*:370, 1971.
98. Lev, R., Siegel, H. I., and Glass, G. B. J.: Gastroenterology *62*:970, 1972.
99. Levitan, H., and Barker, J. L.: Science *176*:1423, 1972.
100. Leonards, J. R., and Levy, G.: J. Pharm. Sci. *58*:1277, 1969.
101. Leonards, J. R., Levy, G.: Clin. Pharmacol. Ther. *14*:62, 1973.
102. Leonards, J. R., Levy, G., and Niemczura, R.: N. Engl. J. Med. *289*:1020, 1973.
103. Levrat, M., and Lambert, R.: Gastroenterologia *94*:273, 1960.
104. Lindquist, B., Møller Jensen, K., Johansson, H., and Hansen, T.: Clin. Pharmacol. Ther. *15*:247, 1974.
105. Linton, A. L.: Can. Med. Assoc. J. *107*:749, 1972.
106. Maner, E. F.: N. Engl. J. Med. *253*:404, 1955.
107. Mangla, J. C., Kim, Y. M., and Rubulis, A. A.: Biochem. Med. *11*:376, 1974.
108. Main, I. H. M., and Whittle, B. J. R.: Br. J. Pharmacol. *53*:217, 1975.
109. Matsumoto, K. K., and Grossman, M. J.: Proc. Soc. Exp. Biol. Med. *102*:

517, 1959.

110. Melmon, K. L.: N. Engl. J. Med. *284*:1361, 1971.

111. Menassé-Gdynia, R., and Krupp, P.: Toxicol. Appl. Pharmacol. *29*:389, 1974.

112. Menguy, R., Desbaillets, L., and Masters, Y. F.: Gastroenterology *64*:722, 1973.

113. Michot, F., Ajdacic, K., and Glans, L.: J. Int. Med. Res. *3*:153, 1975.

114. Mielke, C. H., Ramos, J. C., and Britten, A. F. H.: Am. J. Clin. Pathol. *59*:263, 1973.

115. Mills, D. G., Borda, I. T., Philp, R. B., and Eldridge, C.: Clin. Pharmacol. Ther. *15*:187, 1974.

116. Müller, H. K., and Herrmann, K.: Med. Welt *17*:1553, 1966.

117. Murray, T., and Goldberg, M.: Ann. Rev. Med. *26*:537, 1975.

118. Mustard, J. F., and Packham, M. A.: Pharmacol. Rev. *22*:97, 1970.

119. Narumi, S., and Kanno, M.: Jap. J. Pharmacol. *22*:675, 1972.

120. Naura, R. S., Chirawong, P., and Kincaid-Smith, P.: In "Renal Infection and Renal Scarring," P. Kincaid-Smith and K. F. Fairley, eds. Mercedes, Melbourne, 1971, p. 347.

121. Naura, R. S., Hicks, J. D., McNamara, J. H., and Kincaid-Smith, P.: Med. J. Aust. *1*:293, 1970.

122. Naura, R. S., and Kincaid-Smith, P.: Br. Med. J. *3*:559, 1970.

123. Needham, C. D., Kyle, J., Jones, P. F., Johnson, S. J., and Kerridge, D. F.: Gut *12*:819, 1971.

124. Okun, R., Pearson, C. M., and Sarkissian, E.: Clin. Pharmacol. Ther. *13*: 239, 1972.

125. O'Reilly, R. A.: Clin. Res. *18*:177, 1970.

126. O'Reilly, R. A., and Aggeler, P. M.: Proc. Soc. Exp. Biol. Med. *128*:1080, 1968.

127. O'Reilly, R. A., and Aggeler, P. M.: Pharmacol. Rev. *22*:35, 1970.

128. O'Reilly, R. A., and Levy, G.: J. Pharm. Sci. *59*:1258, 1970.

129. Owen, C. A., Bollman, J. L., and Grindlay, J. H.: J. Lab. Clin. Med. *44*: 238, 1974.

130. Peck, H. M.: In "Importance of Fundamental Principles in Drug Evaluation," D. H. Tedeschi and R. E. Tedeschi, eds. Raven Press, New York, 1968, p. 449.

131. Penner, J. B., and Abbrecht, P. H.: Curr. Ther. Res. *18*:862, 1975.

132. Pentiah, P., Reilly, F., and Borison, H. L.: J. Pharmacol. Exp. Ther. *154*: 110, 1966.

133. Pfeiffer, C. J., and Lewandowski, L. G.: Arch. Int. Pharmacodyn. Ther. *190*:5, 1971.

134. Phillips, B. M.: Toxicol. Appl. Pharmacol. *24*:181, 1973.

135. Phillips, B. M., Krans, P. J., Allen, J. L., and Buslea, R. M.: Toxicol. Appl. Pharmacol. *20*:515, 1971.

136. Pierson, R. N., Holt, P. R., Watson, R. M., and Keating, R. P.: Am. J. Med. *31*:259, 1961.

137. Quick, A. J., and Clesceri, L.: J. Pharmacol. Exp. Ther. *128*:95, 1960.

138. Rainsford, K. D.: Clin. Exp. Pharmacol. Physiol. *2*:45, 1975.

139. Rainsford, K. D.: Agents Actions *5*:326, 1975.

140. Rainsford, K. D.: Gut *16*:514, 1975.

141. Rainsford, K. D.: Aust. J. Pharmacol. *56*:373, 1975.

142. Rainsford, K. D., Watkins, J., and Smith, M. J. H.: J. Pharm. Pharmacol. *20*:941, 1968.
143. Rapaport, S., Wing, M., and Guest, G. M.: Proc. Soc. Exp. Biol. Med. *53*: *40*, 1943.
144. Rawhus, M. D., and Smith, S. E.: Br. J. Pharmacol. *48*:693, 1973.
145. Ridolfo, A. S., Rubin, A., Crobtree, R. E., and Gruber, C. M.: Clin. Pharmacol. Ther. *14*:226, 1972.
146. Robert A., and Nezamis, J. E.: Proc. Soc. Exp. Biol. Med. *114*:545, 1963.
147. Robert, A., Nezamis, J. E., and Phillips, J. P.: Gastroenterology *55*:481, 1968.
148. Roth, J. L. A., and Valdes-Dapena, A.: In "Salicylates: an International Symposium," A. St. J. Dixon, B. K. Martin, M. J. H. Smith, and P. H. N. Wood, eds. Churchill, London, 1963, p. 224.
149. Roth, J. L. A., Valdes-Dapena, A., Pieses, P., and Buchman, E.: Gastroenterology *44*:146, 1963.
150. Rubin, A., Rodda, B. E., Warrick, P., Gruber, C. M., Jr., and Ridolfo, A. S.: Arthritis Rheum. *16*:635, 1973.
151. Rubin, A., Warrick, P., Wolen, R. L., Chernish, S., Ridolfo, A. S., and Gruber, C. M., Jr.: J. Pharmacol. Exp. Ther. *183*:449, 1972.
152. Salter, R. H.: Am. J. Dig. Dis. *13*:38, 1968.
153. Samet, P., Fierer, E. M., and Bernstein, W. H.: J. Appl. Physiol. *15*:826, 1960.
154. Shapiro, S.: J. Am. Med. Assoc. *125*:546, 1944.
155. Schmid, F. R., and Green, D.: Clin. Res. *20*:790, 1972.
156. Sellers, E. M., and Koch-Weser, J.: Clin. Pharmacol. Ther. *11*:524, 1970.
157. Sellers, E. M., and Koch-Weser: Ann. N. Y. Acad. Sci. *179*:213, 1971.
158. Siurala, M., Mustala, O., and Jussila, J.: J. Gastroenterol. *4*:269, 1969.
159. Solomon, H. M., Schrogie, J. J., and Williams, D.: Biochem. Pharmacol. *17*:143, 1968.
160. Steinbrocker, O., and Argyros, T. G.: Arthritis Rheum. *3*:368, 1960.
161. Stubbé, E. L., Pietersen, J. H., and Van Heulen, C.: Br. Med. J. *1*:675, 1962.
162. Sutor, A. H., Bowie, E. J. W., and Owen, C. A.: Mayo Clin. Proc. *46*:178, 1971.
163. Takagi, K., and Kawashina, K.: Jap. J. Pharmacol. *19*:431, 1969.
164. Thorsen, W. B., Western, D., Tanaka, Y., and Morrissey, J. F.: Arch. Intern. Med. *121*:499, 1968.
165. Udall, J. A.: Clin. Med. *77*:20, 1970.
166. Walter, J. E., Drines, R. M., and Earl, A. E.: Toxicol. Appl. Pharmacol. *17*:314, 1970.
167. Warrick, P., and Rubin, A.: Proc. Soc. Exp. Biol. Med. *147*:599, 1974.
168. Watson, R. M., and Pierson, R. N., Jr.: Circulation *24*:613, 1961.
169. Wax, J., Clinger, W. A., Varner, P., Bass, P., and Winder, C. V.: Gastroenterology *58*:772, 1970.
170. Weiss, H. J., and Aledort, L. M.: Lancet *2*:495, 1968.
171. Weiss, H. J., Aledort, L. M., and Kochwa, S.: J. Clin. Invest. *47*:2169, 1968.
172. Welch, R. M., Harrison, Y. E., and Conney, A. H.: Clin. Pharmacol. Ther. *10*:817, 1969.
173. Wesell, E. S., Passananti, G. T., and Green, F. E.: N. Engl. J. Med. *283*:

1484, 1970.
174. Wilson, D. R.: Can. Med. Assoc. J. *107*:752, 1972.
175. Wiseman, E., and Chiaini, J.: Biochem. Pharmacol. *21*:2323, 1972.
176. Wiseman, E. H., and Reinert, H.: Agents Actions *5*:322, 1975.
177. Woodard, G., Post, K. F., Cockrell, K. O., and Cronin, M. T. J.: Toxicol. Appl. Pharmacol. *7*:503, 1965.
178. Yesair, D. W., Callahan, M., Remington, L., and Kenseler, C. J.: Biochem. Pharmacol. *19*:1579, 1970.
179. Yesair, D. W., Callahan, M., Remington, L., and Kenseler, C. J.: Biochem. Pharmacol. *19*:1591, 1970.
180. Zbinden, G.: Clin. Pharmacol. Ther. *5*:537, 1964.

Chapter 16

Non-Steroidal Antiinflammatory Agents

The development of antiinflammatory drugs has been an area of intensive research since the 1940s. The pyrazolones represented the main field of interest in the early forties; then, after a decade of research on corticosteroids, a large variety of aryl acids was prepared in the sixties. In more recent years, many laboratories have been engaged in the synthesis and evaluation of non-acidic derivatives belonging to different chemical classes.

It is convenient to define these compounds as being "antiinflammatory" since they depress generally accepted models of experimental inflammation and afford symptomatic relief in arthritic disorders. The term "antirheumatic" would qualify agents which are probably not antiinflammatory but do more than simply suppress symptoms and signs of the disease. The two terms may partially overlap but, more likely, are at the distant ends of the spectrum.

This chapter deals with antiinflammatory agents as defined before and it is intended to provide only a brief summary of the huge amount of research performed in this area: moreover, only compounds submitted to more extensive investigation are described here. Further information is provided in the following references: 4,63,71,87,88,91,163,209,221,222,243,259,273,280,286,287,297, 315,328,336,341,348.

1. ARYL- AND HETEROARYLCARBOXYLIC ACIDS

This group of compounds includes the N-arylanthranilic acids and their analogs, and the salicylic acids.

A. N-arylanthranilic acids

The N-arylanthranilic acids used in man have been given the generic name of "fenamic acids." The one first described as an antiinflammatory agent has been mefenamic acid, followed by flufenamic and meclofenamic acids. Their chemical structure is reported in Fig. 15, and their biological properties in Table 42.

Mefenamic acid is available as an antiinflammatory analgesic in several countries. In the United States, it can be obtained as an analgesic with a 7-day limitation on its use. Its efficacy as an analgesic has been supported by a large-scale multiagent trial at a dose level of 250 mg (208). However, its continued use has been discouraged (12): apparently, the possibility of allergic diarrhea is a factor limiting the period of its administration (344).

In multiple-dose trials in normal adult subjects receiving 1 g doses of mefenamic acid, q.i.d., the plasma levels of free unchanged drug reach a plateau of about 20 γ/ml on the second day and remain at that level for the duration of 4 days of dosing. In man, as in monkey, urine is the major route of excretion of the unchanged compound and of its metabolites (mainly dicarboxylic acid). In dogs, feces are the principal route of excretion. In both dogs and monkeys, there is an extensive enterohepatic cycling which is probably a toxicologically important aspect of this drug's metabolism (116).

Several clinical trials with *flufenamic acid* have been reported (104,251). The clinically recommended dose is in the 600 mg/day range. Flufenamic acid has a half-life of 2-4 hours in man but reaches the maximum blood level only at 6 hours. It is extensively metabolized, the main metabolite being the 4-hydroxy derivative. Both urine and feces are major routes of excretion of flufenamic acid and its metabolites in man (116).

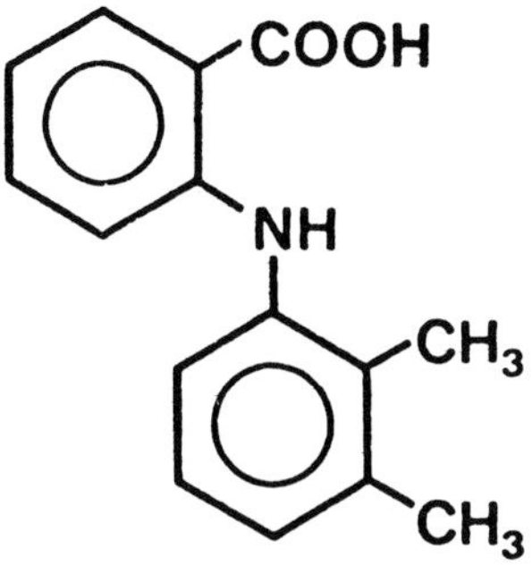

FIG. 15. Chemical structure of fenamic acids

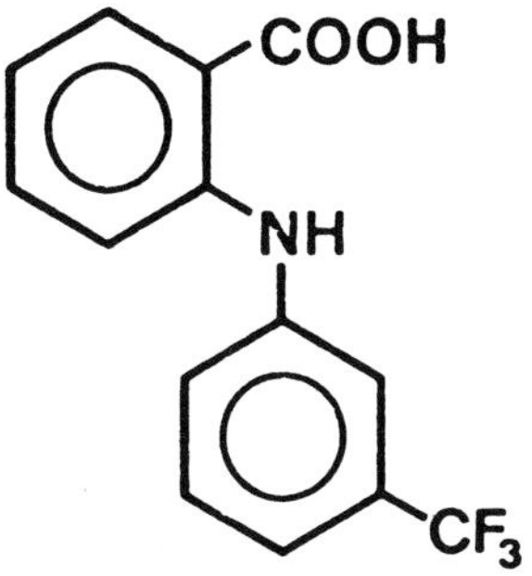

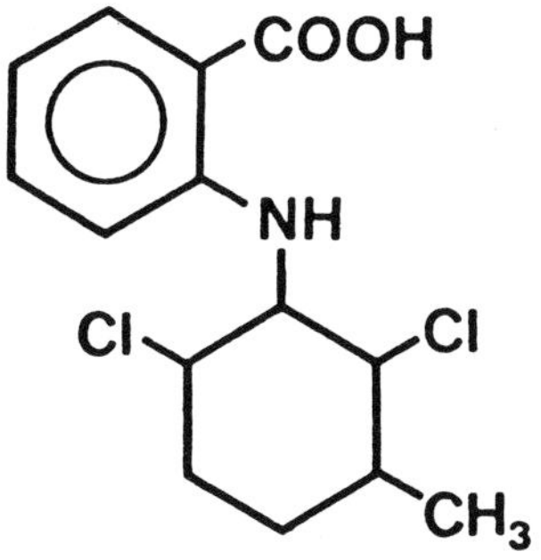

TABLE 42. Biological properties of fenamic acids

	Mefenamic Acid	Flufenamic Acid	Meclofenamic Acid	Indomethacin
		ED_{50} mg/kg p.os.		
U.V. erithema	12	4	0.5	2
Carrageenin edema	75	25	15	2.5
Adjuvant arthritis (therapeutic)	100	30	12	2
Acetylcholine-induced writhing	77	33	11	0.5
Acute LD_{50} rat	1420	430	126	12
Subacute LD_{50} rat, 14 days	415	107	38	6.5
		Antiinflammatory dose in man g/day		
	1.5-2.0	0.4-0.6	0.1-0.2	0.1-0.2

Data derived from: 9, 55, 64, 79, 108, 145, 185, 212, 340, 344

Meclofenamic acid is currently under clinical investigation. A double-blind clinical trial indicated efficacy at 100 mg/day in rheumatoid arthritic patients (81). In several animal models, it is the most potent of the three fenamates (347). It is particularly active as an in vitro inhibitor of prostaglandin-synthetase (108).

Among the heterocycles of N-arylanthranilic acid compounds clonixin and niflumic acid are of special interest. Their chemical structures and biological properties are reported in Fig. 16 and Table 43, respectively.

The activity of *clonixin* is of the order of flufenamic acid in most assays (335). It is especially active as an analgesic (62,335). In double-blind trials 600 mg of clonixin has been found equivalent to about 10 mg of morphine (106,128).

Niflumic acid, a nicotinic acid analog of flufenamic acid, showed an activity lower or comparable to that of flufenamic acid (30) in a variety of animal assays. It is of interest that the metabolic products (5- and 4-monohydroxyderivatives) of niflumic acid are also analogous to those of flufenamic acid (32,115).

An homolog of the N-arylanthranilic acid— *diclofenac sodium*

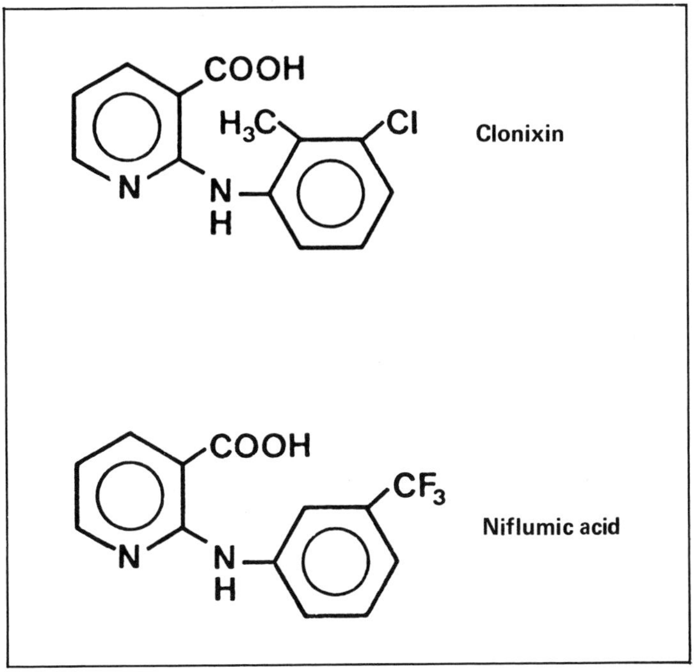

FIG. 16.   Chemical structures of anilinonicotinic acids

(Voltarene®), already marketed in several countries, has aroused great interest. This compound appears highly active in a variety of assays (159,160,162,329) : its potency is comparable to that of indomethacin and its therapeutic index, based on acute LD_{50}, is very favorable. In a large series of clinical trials, mostly performed according to a double-blind cross-over method, diclofenac proved to have significant antiinflammatory and analgesic effects at the dose of 25-50 mg. t.i.d. (60,97,193,204,207,330). The incidence of side effects appears not substantially different from that caused by indomethacin. It is rapidly absorbed from the gut, maximum blood level being reached within 2 hours and dropping to zero after 24 hours. About 60% of the administered dose is excreted in the urine (61) (Fig. 17).

B. Salicylic acids

Acetylsalicylic acid is the most investigated of all antiinflammatory agents in terms of its biological and biochemical propertes.

TABLE 43. Biological properties of anilinonicotinic acids

	Clonixin	Niflumic Acid	Phenylbutazone
	ED_{50} mg/kg p.os.		
Carrageenin edema	35	130	75
Cotton pellet granuloma	25	100	100
Adjuvant arthritis (therapeutic)	15	125	30
Acute LD_{50} rat	660		467

Data derived from: 29, 30, 31, 32, 62, 275, 334, 335

Fig. 18 presents a largely incomplete "reference list" of papers dealing with biological properties of this compound.

Some aspects of acetylsalicylic acid metabolism have recently received more attention.

After oral administration, salicylates are absorbed rapidly partly from the stomach but mostly from the upper small intestine. Appreciable plasma concentrations are found after 30 minutes and a peak value in about 2 hours. They are rapidly distributed throughout all body tissues and most transcellular fluid, mainly by pH-dependent passive processes. The biotransformation of salicylates occurs primarily in the liver. The three main metabolic products are: salicyluric acid (the glycine conjugate), ether or phenolic glucuronide, and ester or acyl glucuronide. In addition, small quantities of gentisic acid are formed. Excretion takes place mainly through the kidney. Studies in man indicate that salicylate is eliminated as free salicylic acid (10%), salicyluric acid (75%), salicylic phenolic- and acyl-glucuronide (15%), and gentisic acid (<1%) (76,180). It has also been shown (176,180,310) that the capacity of man to conjugate salicylic acid with glycine is limited. A consequence of this limited metabolic capacity is a quantitatively major change in the kinetics of elimination of salicylate from the body. Thus following a 250 mg dose, the elimination half-life is about 2 hours but is about 20 hours following a dose of several grams.

Considerable attention has been attracted by two derivatives of acetylsalicylic acid, benorylate and flufenisal (Fig. 19).

Benorylate is an ester of acetylsalicylic acid with acetomino-

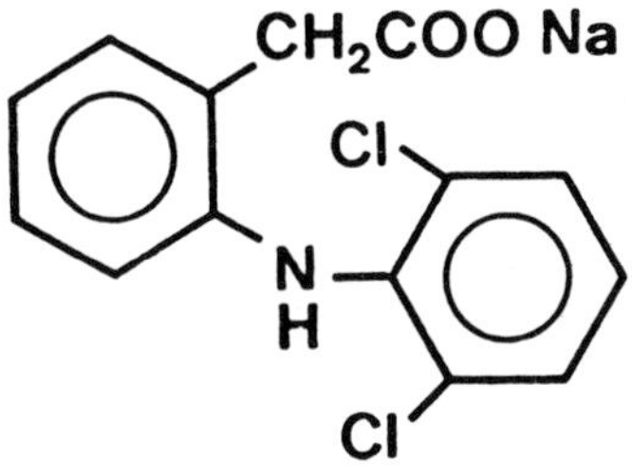

	Diclofenac Na	Indomethacin	Phenylbutazone
	Dose level mg/kg p.os. (ED_{50})		
Carrageenin edema	3.5	3.5	100
Adjuvant arthritis (therapeutic)	0.3-1	0.3	5-10
Phenylquinone writhing	4.3	2.7	95
Acute LD_{50} rat	390	50	1100

Data derived from: 160

FIG. 17. Chemical structure and biological properties of diclofenac sodium (Voltarene)

phen, whose hydrolysis leads to compounds with complementary activity. Its activity is comparable to that of acetylsalicylic acid (18). Lower incidence of gastrointestinal side effects has been reported (72).

Flufenisal was selected from more than 400 compounds related to acetylsalicylic acid (288). After an extensive evaluation, it was dropped for lack of sufficient superiority to aspirin (277).

2. ARYL- AND HETEROARYLALKANOIC ACIDS

This class of compounds is the most widely explored group of potential non-steroidal antiinflammatory agents. Only the most significant compounds will be outlined.

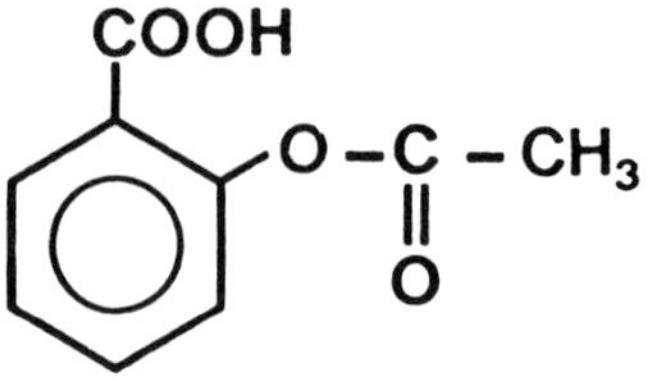

Toxicity	Antiinflammatory activity	Metabolism	Reviews
10, 42, 44, 52, 69, 102, 152, 154, 155, 157, 173, 178, 182, 188, 196, 217, 236, 243, 258, 279, 285, 296, 303, 317, 338, 339, 354	19, 28, 66, 76, 77, 80, 89, 92, 93, 95, 105, 123, 126, 213, 317, 320, 321, 324, 337, 343, 351	8, 36, 74, 75, 76, 137, 141, 177, 179, 180, 185, 210, 211, 242, 289, 295, 298, 299, 309, 310	4, 276, 297, 314, 315

FIG. 18. Chemical structure and reference list of biological properties of acetylsalicylic acid

A. Phenylacetic acids

In the early 1960's, extensive research on the antiinflammatory activity of these derivatives was initiated which led to the description of several compounds subsequently submitted to clinical trials.

One of them, *ibufenac* (Fig. 20) was found to be 2-4 times more potent than aspirin in several animal assays (3,5) and active in human inflammatory conditions (131). Its hepatotoxicity precluded further clinical use (11).

The α-methyl derivative of ibufenac, *ibuprofen* (Fig. 20)) is several times more potent than aspirin and the parent compound in acute experimental inflammations but is less active than phenylbutazone in adjuvant arthritis (6). The only significant pathological effect in animals after repeated administration, was gastric ulceration which appeared more evident in dogs than in rats; this difference in species susceptibility is probably due to the drug be-

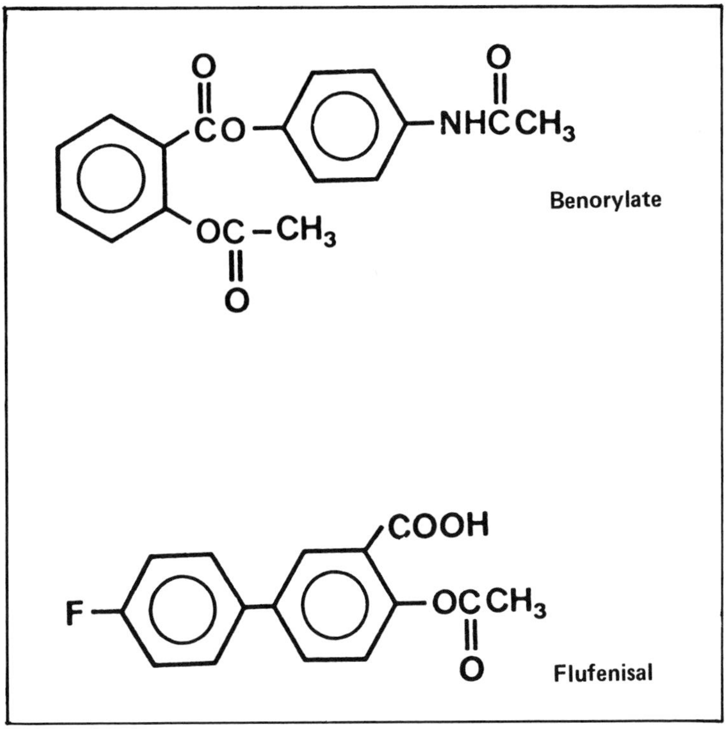

FIG. 19.   Derivatives of acetylsalicylic acid

ing more persistent in dog plasma (2). Many clinical studies have been reported on ibuprofen. Rheumatoid arthritis and allied conditions seem to improve on long-term treatment (119,270). A recent review suggests that ibuprofen is an active analgesic but definite proof of its antiinflammatory activity in man is still lacking (140).

Among the many other phenylacetic acid derivatives endowed with antiinflammatory activity, the following should be mentioned:
Alclofenac
Bufexamac
Fenoprofen
Ketoprofen

A short outline of their properties and the pertinent references as well as their chemical structure are presented in Fig. 21.

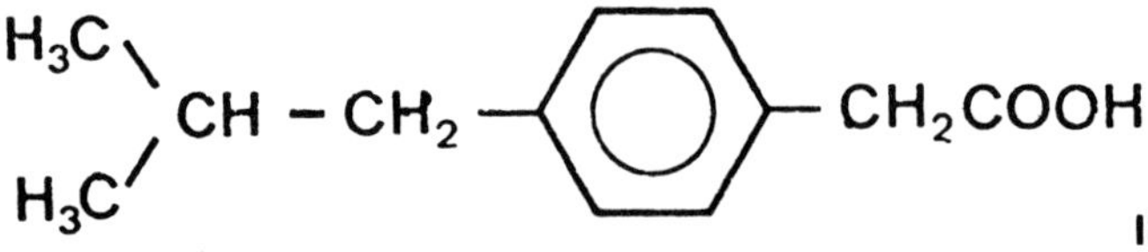

$$H_3C-CH-CH_2-\bigcirc-CH_2COOH$$

Ibufenac

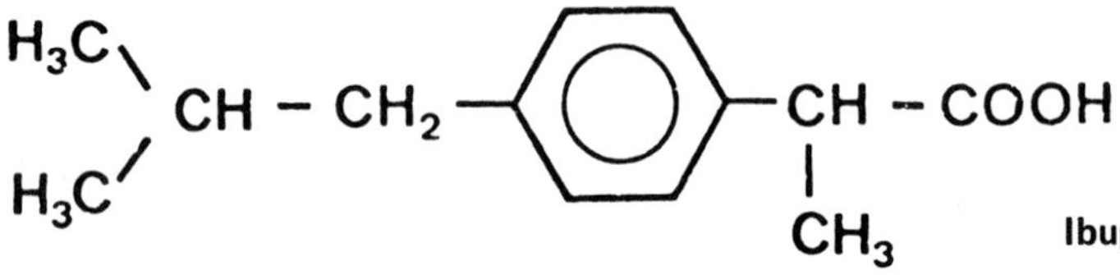

$$H_3C-CH-CH_2-\bigcirc-CH-COOH$$
$$CH_3$$

Ibuprofen

	Ibufenac	Ibuprofen
LD_{50} mg/kg Acute toxicity (mouse, oral)	1800	800
ED_{30} mg/kg: carrageenin edema	~100	~20
Cotton pellet granuloma	~300	~50
Adjuvant arthritis	~ 50	~40

FIG. 20.   Chemical structure and biological properties of ibufenac and ibuprofen

FIG. 21.   Phenylacetic acid derivatives

Alclofenac

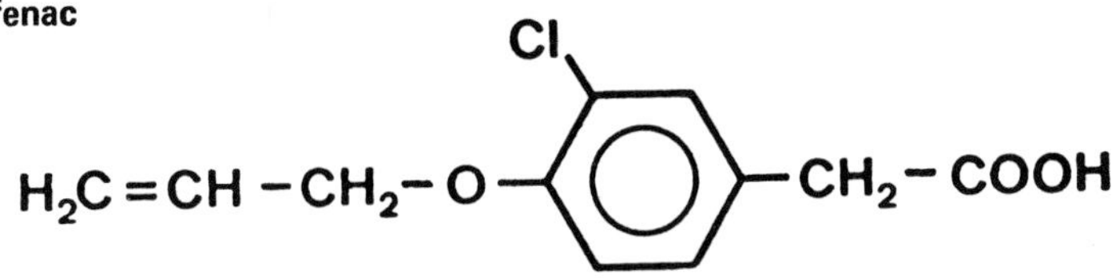

$$H_2C = CH - CH_2 - O - \text{(ring, Cl)} - CH_2 - COOH$$

Equipotent to phenylbutazone in animal assays and probably less toxic (51, 168, 169, 263). Effectiveness reported in rheumatoid arthritis and allied conditions at daily doses of 1.5-3.0 g, the drug being well tolerated (156, 170).

Bufexamac

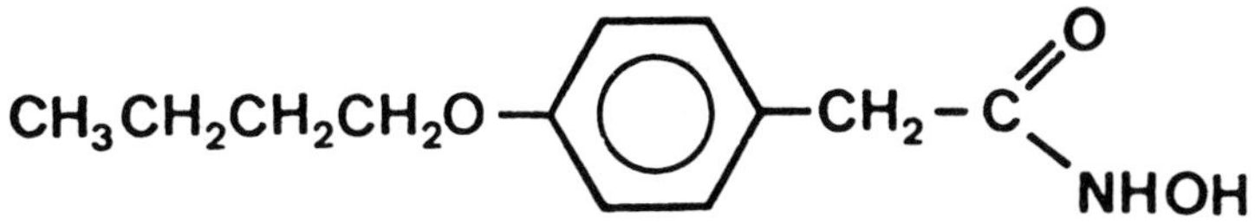

$$CH_3CH_2CH_2CH_2O - \text{(ring)} - CH_2 - C \overset{O}{\underset{NHOH}{\big\backslash}}$$

Equipotent to phenylvutazone in acute experimental inflammations (165, 167). Maximum tolerated dose in repeated administration to rat and dogs 125 mg/kg (166, 256). — Extensive conjugation with glucuronic acid (260, 261, 263). Reports of clinical efficacy in rheumatoid arthritis and osteo arthritis at daily doses of 1.0-1.5 g (25, 265).

Fenoprofen

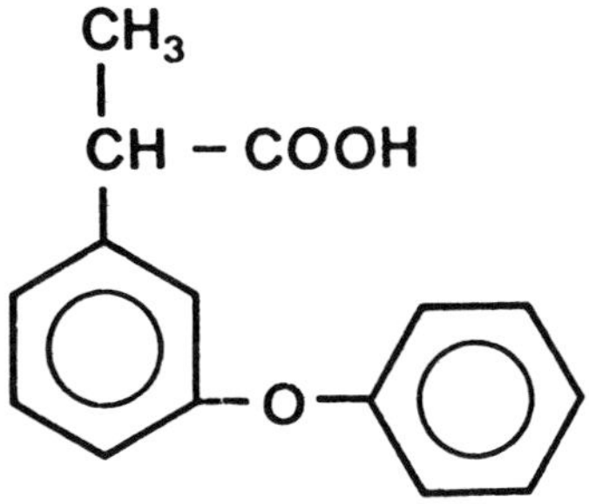

$$\begin{array}{c} CH_3 \\ | \\ CH - COOH \end{array}$$

(ring) - O - (ring)

After extensive studies in animals (20, 202, 223) and pharmacokinetic investigations — half life = 2 hrs - (73, 271, 272) clinical trials on rheumatoid patients showed symptomatic relief after 4 days treatment at daily dose of 250-750 mg (111, 255, 311).

Ketoprofen

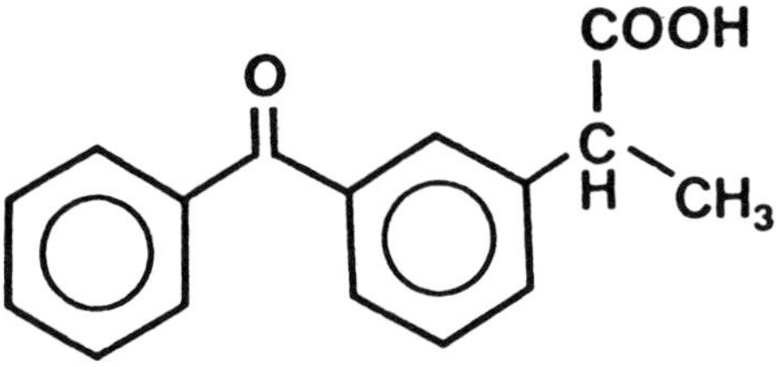

$$\text{(ring)} - C(=O) - \text{(ring)} - \underset{H}{\overset{COOH}{\underset{|}{C}}} - CH_3$$

Equipotent to indomethacin in animal assays (149) and in a clinical trial (43, 125). Incidence of side effects less than with indomethacin (43). Additional clinical investigations suggested it has superior antiinflammatory activity to ibuprofen (203).

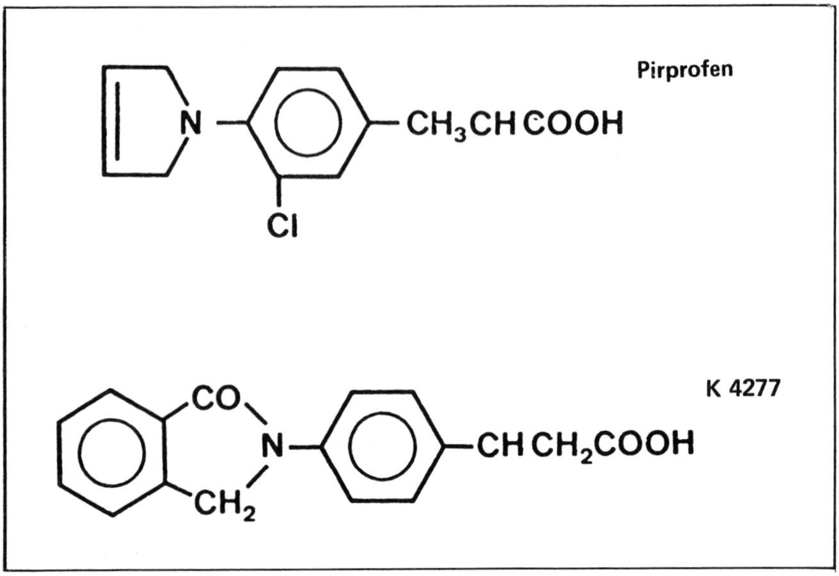

FIG. 22. Chemical structure of phenylpropionic acid derivatives

B. Phenylpropionic acids

A derivative of phenylpropionic acids, *pirprofen*, (Fig. 22) has been shown to be an effective antiinflammatory agent in animals and man. Subsequent clinical studies proved its efficacy at daily doses of 100-500 mg in rheumatoid arthritis. Side effects were not reported (167,249,250). Pirprofen has an apparent elimination half-life of about 7 hrs. It is excreted through the kidney, mainly as a labile conjugate (189).

A new phenylpropionic acid derivative *K 4277* (Fig. 22) has recently been reported as being approximately 20 times more potent than phenylbutazone (50,214). Its metabolism has been described (59,118) and it is now in clinical trial.

C. Phenylbutyric acids

The more extensively studied is *Bucloxic acid* (Fig. 23) whose antiinflammatory activity in acute inflammatory assays is 2-4 times

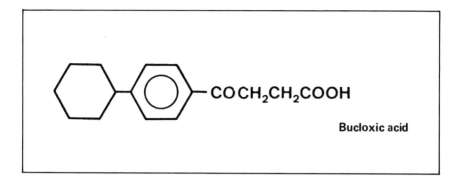

FIG. 23. Chemical structure of bucloxic acid

that of phenylbutazone and is comparable to the latter in adjuvant arthritis. Moreover, it exerts noticeable analgesic and antipyretic effects (158,218). Toxicological studies in rats and dogs revealed ulcerogenic activity at a dose level of 50 mg/kg on long-term treatment (194). It has also been reported to be active in experimental glomerulonephritis in rabbits (326) and, possibly, in human chronic glomerulonephritis (164). Clinical trials revealed its efficacy in rheumatoid patients at a daily dose of 1.0-2.0 g (82,184). In one clinical study, however, the drug has been withdrawn in 30% of the patients because of its side effects (82) (Fig. 23).

D. Naphthaleneacetic acids

A series of naphthaleneacetic acids was found to possess anti-inflammatory, analgesic and antipyretic activity (129). *Naproxen* (Fig. 24) proved to be more active. Subsequently, extensive evaluation in animals indicated that its activity is 20-50 times higher than that of aspirin (94,264,268). In a clinical trial, naproxen was effective in rheumatoid arthritis at daily doses of 300-500 mg (187). Its half-life in man is about 14 hours; it is excreted almost completely in urine, either unchanged or glucuronized and as its 6-desmethyl metabolite (35,274).

E. Indoleacetic acids

The erroneous belief that serotonin plays an important role as an inflammatory mediator in man led to a synthesis of a series of indole derivatives as potential antagonists. A few compounds

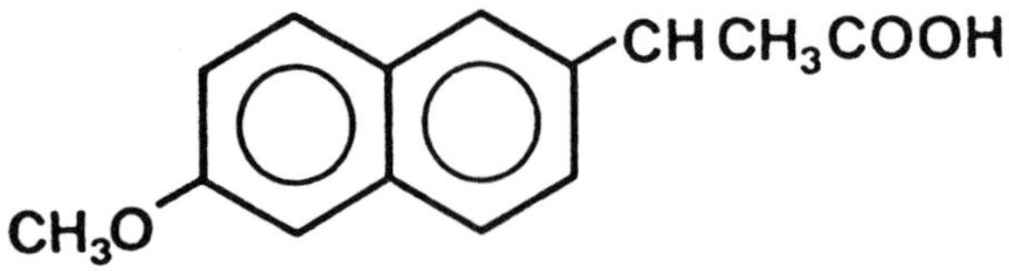

Assay	Relative activity of Naproxen	
	Phenylbutazone = 1	Indomethacin = 1
Carrageenin edema	11	0.7
Cotton pellet granuloma	10	0.2
Adjuvant arthritis	25	3
Antipyresis (yeast)	7	1.5
Analgesia (phenylquinone)	9	0.1

FIG. 24. Chemical structure and biological properties of naproxen

showed significant antiinflammatory activity and the search for optimal structural features led to the synthesis of *indomethacin.*

All the available evidence indicates its very high antiinflammatory potency in a number of animal assays: some data are reported in Fig. 25. Many reports have appeared on the clinical tests of this compound. Indomethacin has been found active in inflammatory disease, such as rheumatoid arthritis, osteoarthritis, ankylosing spondylitis and gout, at daily doses of 50-200 mg. Following a single oral dose of 25-50 mg, peak plasma levels of 1-2 μg/ml are reached within one hour. No accumulation seems to occur on a repeated dose schedule. The elimination half-life in human plasma is about 2 hours. Gross species differences exist in the route of excretion of indomethacin: in monkey, the prevalent route is the kidney, in dog —the intestine, rat and man occupying an intermediate position. The biliary elimination of a drug is likely to play an important role in intestinal toxicity. In contrast to earlier reports, indomethacin is now found to be extensively O-demethylated and N-deacylated in man. Approximately 35-50% of patients receiving usual therapeutic doses of indomethacin experience untoward symptoms and about 20% must discontinue its use. Gastrointestinal and central nervous

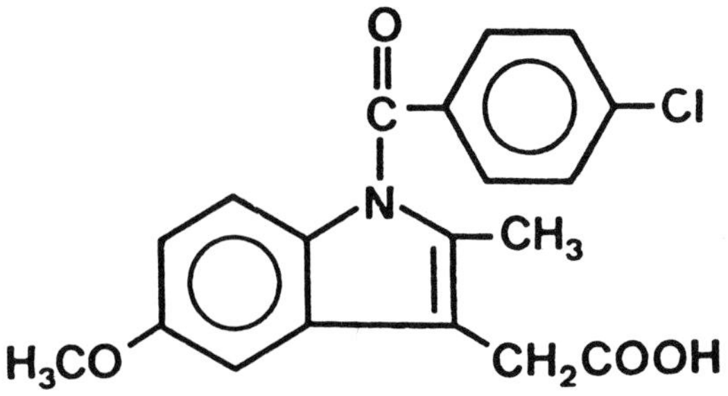

LD$_{50}$, mice p.os, mg/kg 25

LD$_{50}$, rats p.os, mg/kg 12

ED$_{30}$ carrageenin edema mg/kg p.os 2.5

ED$_{30}$ cotton pellet granuloma mg/kg p.os 1

ED$_{30}$ adjuvant arthritis mg/kg p.os 0.3

Antiinflammatory activity	Toxicology	Pharmacokinetic and metabolism
37, 96, 206, 207, 231, 232, 233, 245, 300, 304, 322, 323, 349, 351	16, 27, 39, 86, 107, 136, 151, 198, 302, 331, 332	15, 39, 98, 99, 128, 138, 150, 355, 356

FIG. 25. Indomethacin : chemical structure, biological properties and reference list

system side effects are the most common complaints.

Fig. 25 provides a summarized reference list.

F. Pyrroleacetic acids

Two compounds of this group have been developed and introduced into therapy.

Tolmetin (Fig. 26), approximately 0.4 times as potent as indomethacin in animal assays (56), has been found active in the treatment of rheumatic disorders at daily dose of 0.4-1.6 g. Gastrointestinal side effects have been reported (22).

Clopirac (Fig. 26) is at least equipotent to phenylbutazone (257). It is claimed to be devoid of ulcerogenic effects in the gastro-

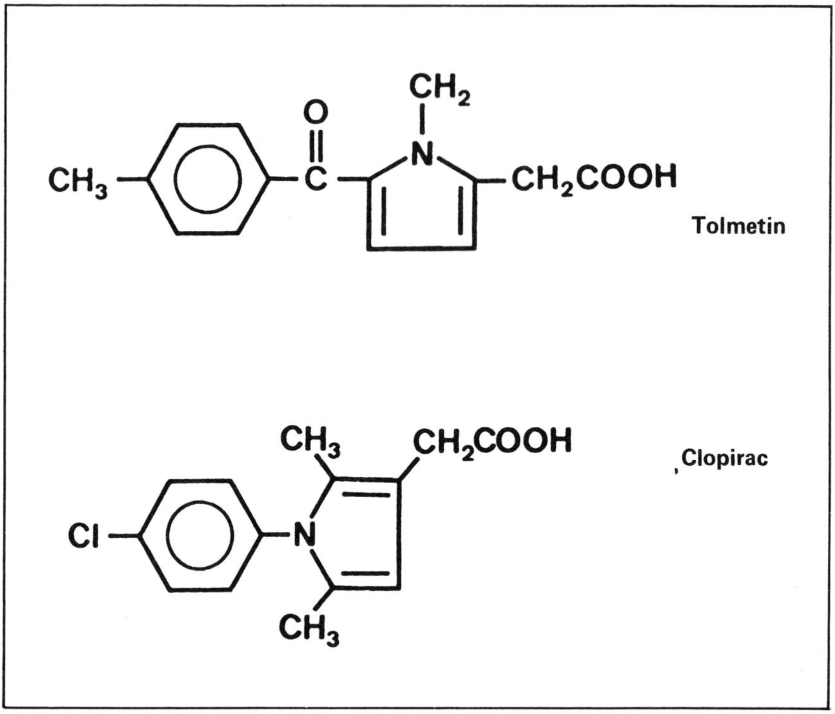

FIG. 26. Chemical structure of pyrroleacetic acid derivatives

intestinal tract of rats (139) and dogs (127). Clinical trials suggest it to be comparable, at daily doses of 0.3-0.6 g, to standard antiinflammatory drugs (24,67,117,135).

G. Thiazoleacetic acids

Fenclozic acid (Fig. 27) has a potency equal to phenylbutazone in acute assays. In adjuvant arthritis, however, it was several times more potent than phenylbutazone due to its much longer serum half-life (109,134,220,247). At a daily dose of 200-400 mg, its therapeutic effect was comparable to aspirin, at 3.6 g daily (58). Due to its hepatotoxicity, the drug was withdrawn from the clinical use (7,130).

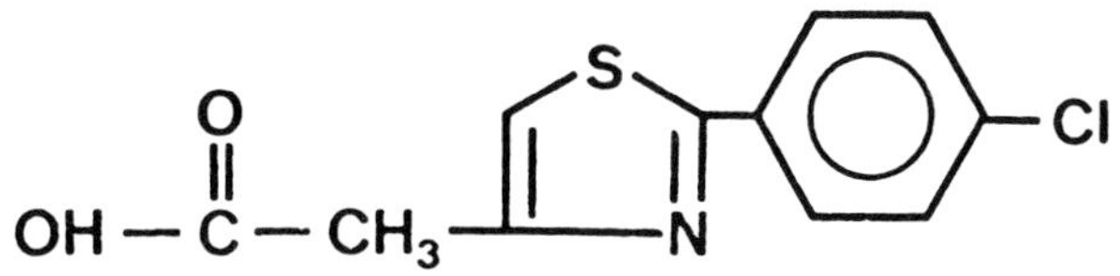

FIG. 27. Chemical structure of fenclozic acid

H. Phenothiazineacetic acids

The most potent compound of a large series of phenothiazine-acetic acids is *metiazinic acid* (201) whose structure and biological properties are reported in Fig. 28. Animal assays showed that, in addition to its antiinflammatory effect, metiazinic acid is also endowed with analgesic and antipyretic properties (146,147,148,248). In a clinical study, daily doses of 0.75-1.5 g have been of benefit in a variety of arthritic conditions (83,123).

I. Other recently described heteroarylalkanoic acid derivatives

Not long ago, the antiinflammatory activity of two arylalkanoic acid derivatives has been described. *Tianafac* (Fig. 29) is less active than indomethacin but more potent than phenylbutazone in several experimental assays (65).

Suprofen (Fig. 29) has been extensively studied in a number of animal assays. In addition to being highly active in several experimental models of inflammation, it is a potent inhibitor of platelet aggregation and of the early phases of protaglandin biosynthesis (13,14,225,226,227,228,229,230).

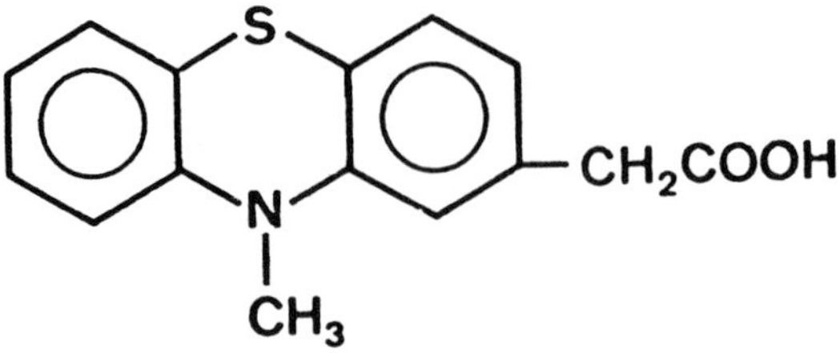

LD$_{50}$ mice p.os mg/kg 800

LD$_{50}$ rats p.os mg/kg 500

ED$_{50}$ carrageenin edema mg/kg p.os 62

ED$_{50}$ carrageenin abscess mg/kg p.os 30

ED$_{50}$ granuloma pouch mg/kg p.os 4.5

ED$_{50}$ adjuvant arthritis mg/kg p.os 100

FIG. 28. Chemical structure and biological properties of metiazinic acid

3. PYRAZOLIDINEDIONES

The oldest and most thoroughly studied drug for the treatment of inflammation is *phenylbutazone* (Fig. 30). Table 44 provides a list of selected bibliographic references which also includes its therapeutically active metabolites.

A number of derivatives of phenylbutazone has been synthetized and evaluated for antiinflammatory activity. Two of these deserve mention.

Prenazone (Fig. 31) was selected from several related terpene-substituted diphenylpyrazolidinediones (239). It has an antiinflammatory activity comparable to that of phenylbutazone but a lower ulcerogenicity (23,186). The half-life is shorter than that of phenylbutazone (45). No metabolites have been identified and its blood levels are considerably lower in man and animals than levels of phenylbutazone administered in comparable doses (70). Clinical ac-

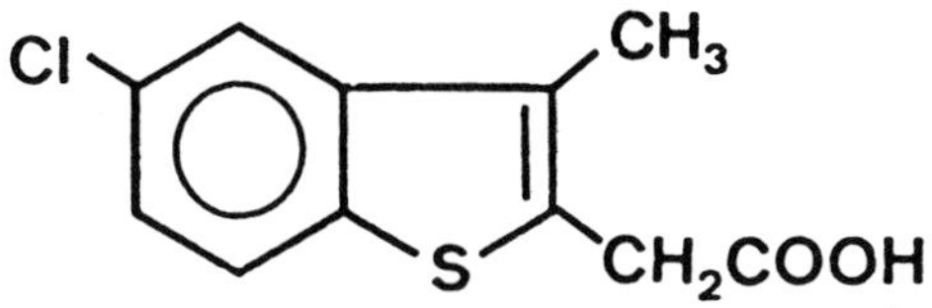

Tianafac

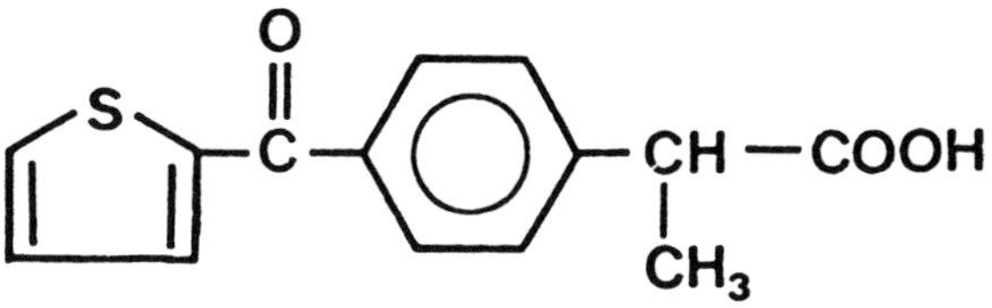

Suprofen

Biological properties of Suprofen

LD_{50} mice oral mg/kg 590

LD_{50} rats oral mg/kg 353

Ulcerogenic dose in rats (50%) mg/kg 200

ED_{50} analgesic (acetic acid writhing), mice, mg/kl oral 0.08

ED_{50} ultraviolet erithema, guinea pigs, mg/kg, oral 1.13

ED_{50} Nystatin edema, rats, mg/kg, oral 2.7

Minimal effective dose in cotton pellet granuloma, rats mg/kg oral 5.0

ED_{50} adjuvant arthritis, rats, mg/kg oral, 10.0

ED_{50} antipyretic (yeast fever), rats, mg/kg oral, 10.0

FIG. 29.   Other arylalkanoic acid derivatives

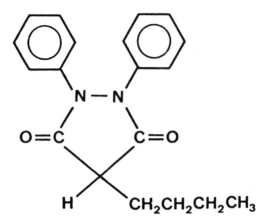

LD_{50} mg/kg mice oral 680

LD_{50} mg/kg mice i.p 355

LD_{50} mg/kg rats oral 467

LD_{50} mg/kg rats i.p 243

ED_{50} mg/kg oral ultraviolet erythema, guinea pig   18

ED_{50} mg/kg oral carrageenin edema, rats   75

ED_{50} mg/kg oral nystatin edema, rats   97

ED_{50} mg/kg oral cotton pellet granuloma, rats   95

ED_{50} mg/kg oral adjuvant arthritis, rats   90

ED_{50} mg/kg oral ulcerogenic activity, rats   150

Half life hrs man   72
Half life hrs dog   6
Half life hrs rabbit   3
Half life hrs rat   6
Half life hrs guinea pig   5
Half life hrs monkey   8

Plasma binding (24 hrs, pH 7.4) 98%

FIG. 30. Phenylbutazone

Metabolites =

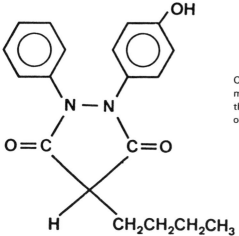

Oxyphenbutazone = active as antirheumatic, half life = 72 hrs, accumulate in the body after chronic administration of phenylbutazone

Weak antirheumatic, half life = 12 hr

TABLE 44. Phenylbutazone: selected references

Reviews:
26, 40, 114, 120, 244, 252, 254, 305, 341, 357

Toxicology:
17, 33, 34, 41, 53, 90, 132, 171, 175, 188, 199, 200, 279, 284

Antiinflammatory activity:
37, 100, 181, 197, 219, 266, 318, 333, 345, 346, 350

Pharmacokinetic and metabolism:
46, 47, 48, 49, 60, 78, 133, 173, 235, 238, 246, 325, 342, 358

Side effects:
40, 192, 195, 237, 254, 290, 306, 307, 353

tivity has been reported at daily doses of 400-600 mg (101,183,244).

When a pyrazolidinedione ring was fused to a benzotriazine system, the result was the antiinflammatory agent, *azapropazone* (Fig. 31). Extensive pharmacological and toxicological investigations support the conclusion that azapropazone possess an antiinflammatory potency similar to that of phenylbutazone but lower toxicity and ulcerogenicity (143,181). Metabolic pathways appear to be similar both in rat and man (141,153), and lead to a 6-hydroxylated metabolite (205). The half-life in man is 8-12 hours (153). Several clinical trials indicate that the effectiveness of optimal doses of azapropazone (600-1200 mg, daily) is equivalent to that of optimal doses of phenylbutazone and indomethacin (191, 278,283,327). Side effects seem fewer and less intense than with reference drugs (278,283).

4. 1,2-BENZOTHIAZINES

Several derivatives of this class of compounds have been reported as potent inhibitors of inflammation in animals (84,85,359). Among the N-heterocyclic amides derived from 1,2-benzothiazines, *sudoxicam* (Fig. 32) has been more extensively evaluated. Doses of 1-3 mg/kg significantly inhibit carrageenin edema, granuloma formation and the development of adjuvant arthritis. Plasma half-life

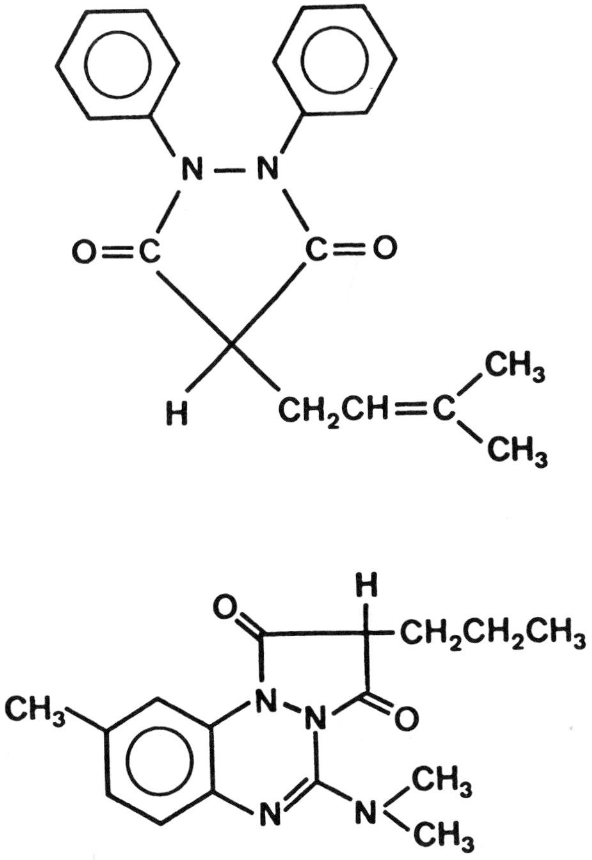

Prenazone

Azapropazone

FIG. 31. Phenylbutazone derivatives

of sudoxicam is long both in laboratory animals (60 hours in dogs) and in man (24-96 hours) (352). Clinical activity in rheumatoid arthritis, at a daily dose of 20 mg, has been reported (246). Sudoxicam strongly inhibits aggregation of rabbit, dog and human platelets induced by collagen and thrombus formation in dogs (68).

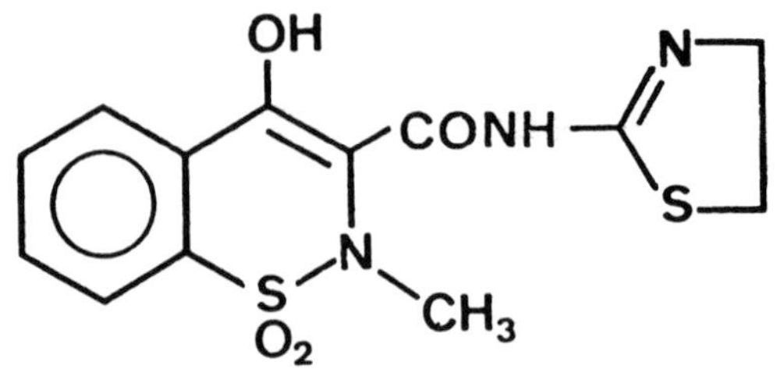

FIG. 32. Sudoxicam

5. FLUOROALKANESULFONANILIDES

This is a relatively new class of acidic antiinflammatory agents whose development led to the evaluation of diflumidone and triflumidate (Fig. 33).

Diflumidone is about 5 times more active than aspirin in acute experimental inflammation and is equipotent to phenylbutazone in adjuvant arthritis (312). Marked species differences were seen among rats, dogs, and man in the nature of urinary metabolites, extent of conjugation and in the plasma half-life (233).

Triflumidate is the ethoxycarbonyl derivative of diflumidone; its antiinflammatory activity is comparable to that of aspirin. It seem that the N-decarbethoxy metabolite is the active compound (313).

6. NON-ACIDIC ANTIINFLAMMATORY AGENTS

The few agents mentioned here were selected from a vast volume of literature (Fig. 34).

Benzydamine (Fig. 34) is an antiinflammatory analgesic which provides some benefit against inflammation of a primary type, such as occurs postoperatively and after a trauma. It is moderately active in animal assays (57,291,292,293, 294).

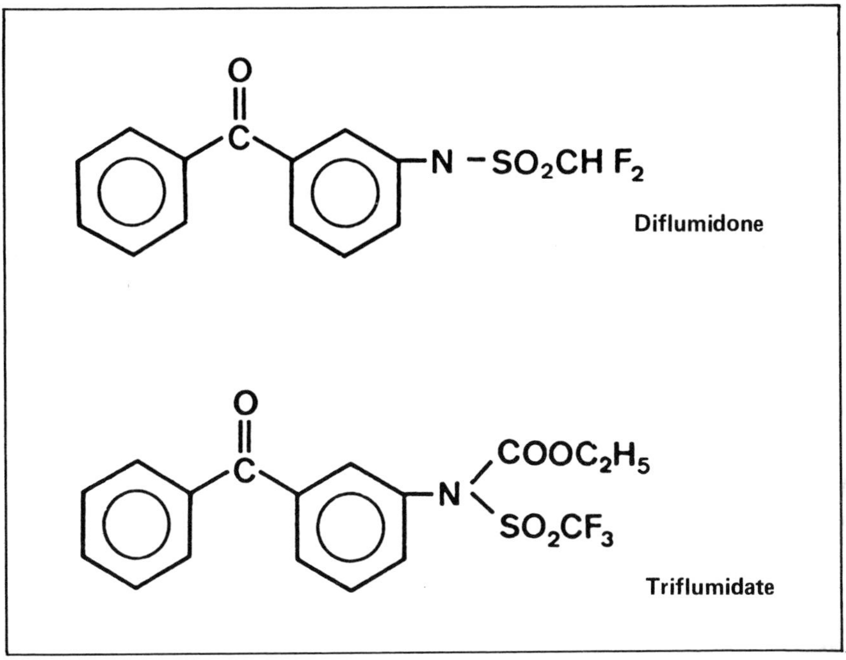

FIG. 33.   Fluoroalkane sulfonanilides

Bimetopyrol (Fig. 34) has been reported by Japanese investigators to be 2-5 times more potent than phenylbutazone in animal assays. It suppresses leukocyte migration in vivo and in vitro and appears to be well tolerated in dogs (142,316).

Tinoridine (Fig. 34) is a moderately active agent comparable to aminopyrine. Interestingly enough, it inhibits histamine release from rat mast cells (216).

PC 796 (Fg. 34) is an hydantoin derivative moderately active in antiinflammatory assays. It is, however, a potent inhibitor of the increased vascular permeability induced by bradykinin, histamine and serotonin, and of passive cutaneous anaphylaxis (215).

Seclazone (Fig. 34) is a cyclized salicylamide derivative, effective orally as an antiinflammatory analgesic and antipyretic in laboratory animals at doses where side effects are absent. In man, seclazone is also a uricosuric agent at its antiinflammatory dose. The major urinary metabolites are 5-chlorosalicylic acid and its

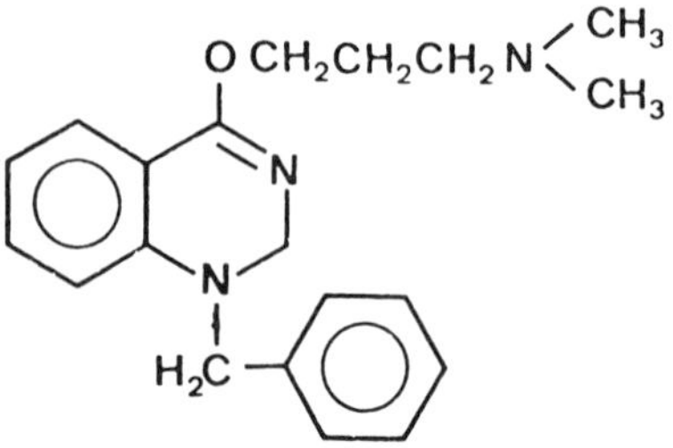

Benzydamine

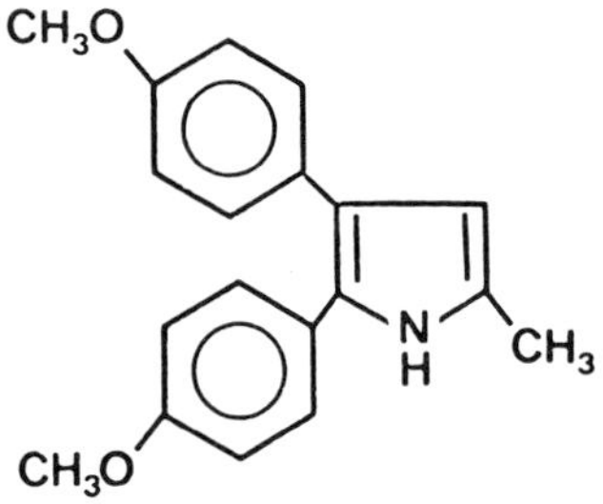

Bimetopyrol

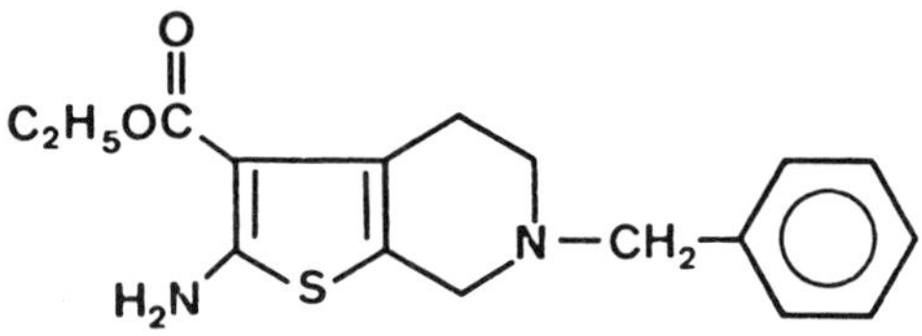

Tinoridine

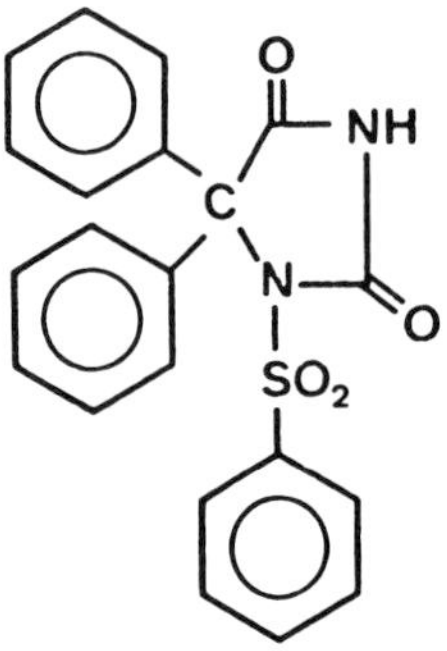

PC-796

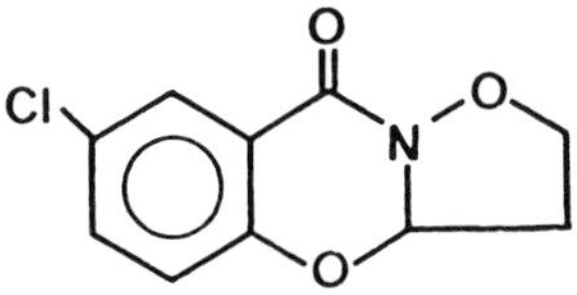

Seclazone

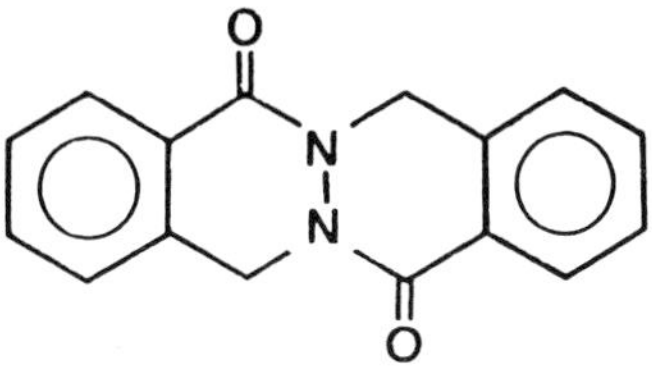

Diftalone

FIG. 34.   Non acidic antiinflammatory agents

glucuronide. It is likely that the metabolites contribute to the pharmacological action of seclazone (21,103,289,301).

Several reports have recently appeared on *diftalone* (Fig. 34). In animal assays, its antiinflammatory effects are less than those of phenylbutazone but exceed those of aspirin. The ulcerogenic activity is lower than that of equivalent antiinflammatory doses of phenylbutazone, aspirin and indomethacin (54,172,281). Several clinical trials showed that diftalone is effective in rheumatoid patients, at daily doses of 0.5-1.0 g. The incidence of side effects was lower than that observed with equipotent doses of indomethacin (121,190,224, 240,308). The main urinary metabolite is the 7-hydroxyderivative, present largely in conjugated form (113). It has been reported that diftalone combined with tolbutamide may increase the effect of the latter on insulin secretion, possibly through an interference at the level of albumin binding (112).

REFERENCES

1. Abdel-Galil, A. A. M., and Marshall, P. B.: Br. J. Pharmacol. *33*:1, 1968.
2. Adams, S. S., Bough, R. C., Clifte, E. E., Lessel, B., and Mills, R. F. N.: Toxicol. Appl. Pharmacol. *15*:310, 1969.
3. Adams, S. S., Cliffe, E. E., Lessel, B., and Nicholson, J. S.: Nature *200*: 271, 1963.
4. Adams, S. S., and Cobb, R.: Prog. Med. Chem. *5*:59, 1967.
5. Adams, S. S., Hebborn, P., and Nicholson, J. S.: J. Pharm. Pharmacol. *20*:305, 1968.
6. Adams, S. S., McCullough, K. F., and Nicholson, J. S.: Arch. Int. Pharmacodyn. Ther. *178*:115, 1969.
7. Alcock, S. J.: Proc. Eur. Soc. Study Drug Toxic. *12*:184, 1971.
8. Ali, M. A., and Routh, J. I.: Clin. Chem. *15*:1027, 1969.
9. Alpermann, H. G.: Arzneim. Forsch. *20*:293, 1970.
10. Anderson, K. W.: Arch. Int. Pharmacodyn. Ther. *152*:379, 1964.
11. Anonymous: Drug Ther. Bull. *6*:48, 1968.
12. Anonymous: Med. Lett. *14*:31, 1972.
13. Awouters, F., Niemegeers, C. J. E., Lenaerts, P. M. H., and Janssen, P. A. J.: Arzneim. Forsch. *25*:1509, 1975.
14. Awouters, F., Niemegeers, C. J. E., Lenaerts, F. M., and Janssen, P. A. J.: Arzneim. Forsch. *25*:1526, 1975.
15. Baer, J. E.: J. Pharm. Sci. *61*:1674, 1972.
16. Barron, D. I., Copley, A. R., and Vallance, D. K.: Br. J. Pharmacol. *33*: 396, 1968.
17. Barroy, J. P., Willems, G., Verbeustel, S., and Gerard, A.: Acta Gastroenterol. Belg. *33*:469, 1970.
18. Beales, D. L., Burry, H. C., and Grahame, R.: Br. Med. J. *2*:483, 1972.
19. Benitz, K. F., and Hall, L. M.: Arch. Int. Pharmacodyn. Ther. *144*:185, 1963.
20. Benslay, D. N.: Fed. Proc. *30*:563, 1971.
21. Berger, F. M.: Pharmacology *9*:164, 1973.
22. Berkowitz, S. S.: Curr. Ther. Res. *16*:442, 1974.
23. Bianchi, G., Lumachi, B., and Marazzi Uberti, E.: Arzneim. Forsch. *22*: 183, 1972.
24. Bloch-Michel, H.: Scand. J. Rheumatol. *4* (Suppl. 8) : 503-03, 1975.
25. Bloch-Michel, H., and Parrot, M.: Thérapie *25*:969, 1970.
26. Bloom, B. M., and Lanbach, G. D.: Annu. Rev. Pharmacol. *2*:92, 1962.
27. Boardman, P., and Hart, E. D.: Ann. Rheum. Dis. *26*:127, 1967.
28. Boardman, P. L., and Hart, E. D.: Br. Med. J. *4*:264, 1967.
29. Boissier, J. R., Fichelle-Pagny, J., and Horakova, S.: Thérapie *22*:157, 1967.
30. Boissier, J. R., Lwolf, J. M., and Hertz, F.: Thérapie *25*:43, 1970.
31. Boissier, J. R., Tillement, J. P., Frossard, C., and Fabiani, P.: Ann. Pharm. Fr. *26*:707, 1968.
32. Boissier, J. R., Tillement, J. P., and Larousse, C.: Thérapie *26*:211, 1971.
33. Bonfils, S., Loefooghe, G., Rossi, G., and Lambling, A.: C. R. Soc. Biol. *151*:1149, 1957.
34. Bonfils, S., Hardoun, J. P., and Delbarre, F.: C. R. Soc. Biol. *148*:881, 1954.

35. Boost von G.: Arzneim. Forsch. *25*:281, 1975.
36. Boreham, D. R., and Martin, B. K.: Br. J. Pharmacol. *37*:294, 1969.
37. Boris, A., and Stevenson, R. H.: Arch. Int. Pharmacodyn. Ther. *153*:205, 1965.
38. Boulos, B. M., Davis, L. E., Larks, S. D., Larks, G. G., Sirtori, C. R., and Almond, C. H.: Arch. Int. Pharmacodyn. Ther. *194*:403, 1971.
39. Brodie, D. A., Cook, P. G., Bauer, B. J., and Dagle, G. E.: Toxicol. Appl. Pharmacol. *17*:615, 1970.
40. Brodie, B. B., Lowman, E. W., Burns, J. J., Lee, P. R., Chenkin, T., Goldman, A., Weiner, M., and Steel, J. M.: Am. J. Med. *16*:181, 1954.
41. Brodie, D. A., Marshall, R. W., and Moreno, O.: Gastroenterology *43*:675, 1962.
42. Brodie, D. A., Tate, C. L., and Hooke, K. F.: Science *170*:183, 1970.
43. Brogden, R. N., Splight, T. M., and Avery, G. S.: Drugs *8*:168, 1974.
44. Brown, R. A., and West, G. B.: J. Pharm. Pharmacol. *16*:563, 1964.
45. Buniva, G., Gatto, G., Chierichetti, S., Granata, D., and Maniery, G.: Arzneim. Forsch. *22*:258, 1972.
46. Burns, J. J.: Ann. N. Y. Acad. Sci. *151*:959, 1968.
47. Burns, J. J.: Proc. Eur. Soc. Study Drug Toxic. *11*:9, 1970.
48. Burns, J. J., Rose, R. K., Chenkin, T., Goldman, A., Schulert, A., and Brodie, B. B.: J. Pharmacol. Exp. Ther. *109*:346, 1953.
49. Burns, J. J., Rose, R. K., Goodwin, S., Reichenthal, J., Horning, E. C., and Brodie, B. B.: J. Pharmacol. Exp. Ther. *113*:481, 1955.
50. Buttinoni, A., Cuttica, A., Franceschini, J., Mandelli, V., Orsini, G., Passerini, N., Turba, C., and Tommasini, R.: Arzneim. Forsch. *23*:1100, 1973.
51. Buu Hoi, N. P., Lambelin, G., and Gillet, C.: Naturwissenschaften *56*:330, 1969.
52. Calder, I. C., Funder, C. C., Green, C. R., Ham, K. N., and Tange, J. D.: Br. Med. J. *4*:518, 1971.
53. Carlisle, C. H., Penny, R. H. C., Prescott, C. W., and Davidson, H. A.: Br. Vet. J. *124*:560, 1968.
54. Carminati, P., and Lerner, L. J.: Proc. Soc. Exp. Biol. Med. *148*:455, 1975.
55. Carvano, R. A., and Malbica, J. O.: J. Pharm. Sci. *61*:1450, 1971.
56. Carson, J. R., McKinstry, D. N., and Wong, S: J. Med. Chem. *14*:646, 1971.
57. Catanese, B., Grasso, A., and Silvestrini, B.: Arzneim. Forsch. *16*:1354, 1966.
58. Chalmers, T. M., and Pohl, J. E. F.: Ann. Rheum. Dis. *28*:590, 1969.
59. Chasseaud, L. F., Fry, B. J., Valzelli, G., and Tosolini, G. P.: Arzneim. Forsch. *24*:1606, 1974.
60. Chignell, C. F., and Starkweather, D. K.: Pharmacology *5*:235, 1971.
61. Ciccolunghi, S. N., Levi, B., and Chaudri, H. A.: Wien. Med. Wochenschr. *125*:66, 1975.
62. Ciofalo, V. B., Patel, J., and Taber, R. J.: Jap. J. Pharmacol. *22*:749, 1972.
63. Collier, H. O. J.: Adv. Pharmacol. Chemother. *7*:333, 1969.
64. Collier, H. O. J., Dinneen, L. C., Johnson, C. A., and Schneider, C.: Br. J. Pharmacol. *32*:295, 1968.
65. Colot, M., Damme van M., Dirks, M., Bersaerts, J., and Chalier, R.: Arch. Int. Pharmacodyn. Ther. *208*:328, 1974.
66. Combined Rheumatic Fever Study Group: N. Engl. J. Med. *272*:63, 1965.

67. Commandre, F., and Viani, J. L.: Scand. J. Rheumatol 4 (Suppl. 8): 503-04, 1975.

68. Constantine, J. W., and Purcell, I. M.: J. Pharmacol. Exp. Ther. 187:653, 1973.

69. Cooke, A. R.: Am. J. Dig. Dis. 18:225, 1973.

70. Coppi, G., Bonardi, G., and Perego, R.: Arzneim. Forsch. 22:234, 1972.

71. Coyne, W. E.: In "Medicinal Chemistry," A. Burger, ed. Wiley (Interscience), New York, 1970, p. 953.

72. Croft, D. N., Cuddigan, J. H. P., and Sweetland, C.: Br. Med. J. 2:546, 1972.

73. Culp, H. W.: Fed. Proc. 30:564, 1971.

74. Cummings, A. J., and Martin, B. K.: Biochem. Pharmacol. 13:767, 1964.

75. Cummings, A. J., and Martin, B. K.: J. Pharm. Sci. 57:891, 1968.

76. Davison, C.: Ann. N. Y. Acad. Sci. 179:249, 1971.

77. Davison, C., and Rensselaer, N. Y.: Drug Intell. Clin. Pharm. 4:349, 1970.

78. Davies, D. S., and Thorgeirsson, S. S.: Drug Intell. Clin. Pharm. 4:350, 1970.

79. De Marchi, F., Torrielli, M. V., and Tamagnone, G. F.: Clin. Ther. 3:43, 1968.

80. Deodhar, S. D., Dick, W. G., Hodgkinson, R., and Buchanan, W. W.: Quart. Med. J. 42:387, 1973.

81. De Salcedo, I., Carrington, M. D., Santos, J. A., and Silva, J. L.: Hormones 1:193, 1970.

82. de Séze, S., Dryll, A., and Dreiser, R.: Arzneim. Forsch. 24:1425, 1974.

83. Deshayes, P., and Gogny, J. C.: Rheumatologie 22:29, 1970.

84. Di Pasquale, G., Rassert, C., Richter, R., and Tripp, C. V.: Arch. Int. Pharmacodyn. Ther. 203:92, 1973.

85. Di Pasquale, G., Rassaert, C., Richter, R., Welai, P., Gingold, J., and Singer, R.: Agents Actions 5:256, 1975.

86. Djahanguiri, B.: Scand. J. Gastroenterol. 4:265, 1965.

87. Doebel, K. J., Graeme, M. L., Gruenfeld, N., Ignarro, L. J., Piliero, S. J., and Wasley, J. W. F.: Annu. Rep. Med. Chem. 1968:207 (1969); Annu. Rep. Med. Chem. 1969: 225 (1970).

88. Doebel, K. J.: Pure Appl. Chem. 19:49, (1969).

89. Domenjoz, R.: Arch. Exp. Pathol. Pharmacol. 225:14, 1955.

90. Domenjoz, R.: Ann. N. Y. Acad. Sci. 86:263, 1960.

91. Domenjoz, R.: Adv. Pharmacol. 4:143, 1966.

92. Domenjoz, R., and Wilhelmi, G.: Arzneim. Forsch. 1:151, 1951.

93. Done, A. K.: Pediatrics 26:800, 1960.

94. Dorfman, R. I.: Arzneim. Forsch. 25:278, 1975.

95. Du Boistesselin, R., and Porcile, E.: Thérapie 18:177, 1963.

96. Dudley Hart, F.: Br. Med. J. 4:191, 1975.

97. Duerrigl, T., Vitaus, M., Pucar, I., and Miko, M.: J. Int. Med. Res 3: 139, 1975.

98. Duggan, D. E., Hogans, A. F., Kwan, K. C., and McMahon, F. G.: J. Pharmacol. Exp. Ther. 181:563, 1972.

99. Duggan, D. E., Lamp, A. L., McMahon, F. G., and Kwan, K. C.: Fed. Proc. 30:391, 1971.

100. Dorfman, R. I., and Dorfman, A. S.: Proc. Soc. Exp. Biol. Med. 119:859, 1965.

101. Dotti, F., Ongari, R., Carazzi, R., and Chierichetti, S.: Arzneim. Forsch.

22:265, 1972.

102. Earley, P. A., and Hayden, J.: Lancet *1*:763, 1964.
103. Edelson, J., Schuster, E., Shahinian, S., and Douglas, J. F.: Arch. Int. Pharmacodyn. Ther. *209*:66, 1974.
104. "Fenamates in Medicine": Ann. Phys. Med. *23* (Suppl.) : 7, 1967.
105. Ferreira, S. H., and Vane, J. R.: Annu. Rev. Pharmacol. *14*:57, 1974.
106. Finch, J. S., and De Kornfeld, J. J.: J. Clin. Pharmacol. New Drugs *11*: 371, 1971.
107. Fleming, J. S., Bierwagen, M. E., Pircio, A. W., and Pindell, M. H.: Arch. Int. Pharmacodyn. Ther. *178*:423, 1969.
108. Flower, R., Gryglewski, R., Herbaczynska-Cedro, K., and Vane, J. R.: Nature (New Biol.) *238*:104, 1972.
109. Foulkes, D. M.: J. Pharmacol. Exp. Ther. *172*:115, 1970.
110. Fox, A. E., Gingold, J. L., and Freedman, H. H.: Infect. Immun. *8*:549, 1973.
111. Fries, J. F., and Britton, M. C.: Arthritis Rheum. *16*:629, 1973.
112. Fritzsche, H., Shera, K. O., Weissel, M., and Kolarz, G.: Scand. J. Rheumatol. *4* (Suppl. 8) : 43-07, 1975.
113. Gallo, G. G., Rimorini, N., Zerilli, L. F., and Radaelli, P.: J. Chromatogr. *101*:163, 1974.
114. Gifford, R. M.: Ration. Drug Ther. *7*:1, 1973.
115. Glasson, B., Benakis, A., and Strolin-Benedetti, M.: Biochem. Pharmacol. *18*:663, 1969.
116. Glazko, A. I.: Ann. Phys. Med. *23* (Suppl.) : 25, 1967.
117. Goddeeris, T., and Dequeker, J.: Scand. J. Rheumatol. *4* (Suppl. 8) : 503-02, 1975.
118. Goldaniga, C. C., Pianezzolo, E., and Valzelli, G.: Arzneim. Forsch. *24*: 1603, 1974.
119. Goldberg, A. A. J., Hall, J. E., Buckler, J. W., Dodsworth, P. G., and Agar, J.: Practitioner *207*:343, 1971.
120. Graham, W.: Can. Med. Assoc. J. *76*:634, 1958.
121. Grimaldi, M. G., and Luvara, A.: J. Int. Med. Res. *3*:333, 1975.
123. Gross, F.: Schweiz. Med. Wocherschr. *80*:697, 1950.
124. Gross, D.: Praxis *60*:1334, 1971.
125. Gyory, A. N., Bloch, M., Burry, M. C., and Grahame, R.: Br. Med. J. *4*: 398, 1972.
126. Haberland, G. L., Busch, L., Fink, W., and Friedrich, H.: Z. Rheumaforsch. *18*:220, 1959.
127. Hardy, T. L.: Scand. J. Rheumatol. *4* (Suppl. *8*) : 40-14, 1975.
128. Harman, R. E., Meisinger, M. A. P., Davis, G. E., and Kuehl, F. A.: J. Pharmacol. Exp. Ther. *143*:215, 1964.
129. Harrison, I. T., Lewis, B., Nelson, P., Rooks, W., Roszkowski, A., Tomolonis, A., and Fried, J. H.: J. Med. Chem. *13*:203, 1970.
130. Hart, F. D., Bain, L. S., Huskisson, E. C., Littler, T. R., and Taylor, R. T.: Ann. Rheum. Dis. *29*:684, 1970.
131. Hart, F. D., and Boardman, P. L.: Ann. Rheum. Dis. *24*:61, 1965.
132. Hazleton, L. W., Tusing, T. W., and Holland, E. G.: J. Pharmacol. Exp. Ther. *109*:387, 1953.
133. Hegermann Nielsen, G., and Holmen-Christensen, H.: Acta Pharmacol. Toxicol. (Kbh.) *25* (Suppl. 4) : 42, 1967.
134. Hepworth, W., Newbould, B. B., Platt, D. S., and Stacey, G. J.: Nature

221:582, 1969.

135. Heynen, G., and Franchimont, P.: Scand. J. Rheumatol. *4* (Suppl. 8): 503-01, 1975.
136. Hitchens, J. T., Goldstein, S., Sambuca, A., and Shemano, I.: Pharmacologist *9*:242, 1967.
137. Hogben, C. A. M., Tocco, D. J., Brodie, B. B., and Schanker, L. S.: J. Pharmacol. Exp. Ther. *125*:275, 1959.
138. Hucker, M. B., Zacchei, A. G., Cox, S. V., Brodie, D. A., and Cantwell, N. H. R.: J. Pharmacol. Exp. Ther. *153*:237, 1966
139. Hughes, B.: Scand. J. Rheumatol. *4* (Suppl. *8*) : 40-13, 1975.
140. Huskisson, E. C., Hart, F. D., Shenfield, G. M., and Taylor, R. T.: Practitioner *207*:639, 1971.
141. Howes, J. F., and Hunter, W. H.: J. Pharm. Pharmacol. *20*:107, 1968.
142. Iizuka, Y., and Tanaka, K.: J. Pharm. Soc. Jap. *92*:11, 1972.
143. Jahn, U., and Adrian, R. W.: Arzneim. Forsch. *19*:36, 1969.
144. Jahn, U., Reher, J., and Schatz, F.: Arzneim. Forsch. *23*:660, 1973.
145. Juby, P. F., Hudyama, T. W., and Brown, M.: J. Med. Chem. *11*:111, 1968.
146. Julou, L., Ducrot, R., Fournel, J., Ganter, P., Populaire, P., Durel, J., Myron, J., Pascal, S., and Pasquet, J.: Arzneim. Forsch. *19*:1207, 1969.
147. Julou, L., and Guyonnet, J. C.: C. R. Acad. Sci. (D) (Paris) *265*:1007, 1967.
148. Julou, L., Guyonnet, J. C., Ducrot, R., Bardone, M. C., Detaille, J. Y., and Laffargue, B.: Arzneim. Forsch. *19*:1198, 1969.
149. Julou, J., Guyonnet, J. C., Ducrot, R., Garvet, C., Bardone, M. C., Maignan, G., and Pasquet, J.: J. Pharmacol. *2*:259, 1971.
150. Kendall, M. J., Nutter, S., and Hawkins, C. F.: Br. Med. J. *1*:533, 1971.
151. Kent, T. H., Cardelli, R. M., and Stamler, F. W.: Am. J. Pathol. *54*:237, 1969.
152. Kirsner, J. B.: Ann. Intern. Med. *47*:666, 1957.
153. Klatt, C., and Koss, F. W.: Arzneim. Forsch. *23*:913, 1973.
154. Klein Obbink, H. I., and Dalderup, L. M.: Lancet *1*:565, 1964.
155. Klein Obbink, H. J., and Dalderup, L. M.: Lancet *2*:151, 1964.
156. Klemm, C., Frickle, R., Schattenkirchner, M., Treiber, W., and Mathies, H.: Z. Rheumaforsch. *30*:17, 1971.
157. Koutsaimanis, K. G., and De Wardener, H. E.: Br. Med. J. *4*:131, 1970.
158. Krausz, F., Brélieve, J. C., Vaillant, J., Brunand, M., and Navano, J.: Arzneim. Forsch. *24*:1364, 1974.
159. Krupp, P., Exer, B., Menassé-Gdynia, R., and Ziel, R.: Schweiz. Med. Wochenschr. *105*:646, 1975.
160. Krupp, P. J., Menassé-Gdynia, R., Sallmann, A., Wilhelmi, G., Ziel, R., and Jaques, R.: Experientia *29*:450, 1973.
161. Ku, E. C., Wasvary, J. M.: Biochim. Biophys. Acta *384*:360, 1975.
162. Ku, E. C., Wasvary, J. M., and Cash, W. D.: Biochem. Pharmacol. *24*:641, 1975.
163. Kuzell, W.: Annu. Rev. Pharmacol. *8*:357, 1968.
164. Lagrue, E., Masbernard, A., Giudicelli, C., and Hirbee, G.: Arzneim. Forsch. *24*:1434, 1974.
165. Lambelin, G., Buu-Hoi, N. P., Mees, G., Thiriaux, J., and Huriaux, M.: Med. Pharmacol. Exp. *15*:307, 1966.
166. Lambelin, G., Buu-Hoi, N. P., Mees, G., Thiriaux, J., and Huriaux, M.:

Med. Pharmacol. Exp. *15*:545, 1966.
167. Lambelin, G., and Mees, G.: Naturwissenschaften *53*:157, 1966.
168. Lambelin, G., Roba, J., Gillet, C., and Buu-Hoi, N. P.: Arzneim. Forsch. *20*:610, 1970.
169. Lambelin, G., Roba, J., Gillet, C., Gautier, M., and Buu-Hoi, N. P.: Arzneim. Forsch. *20*:618, 1970.
170. Lambotte, F.: Arzneim. Forsch. *20*:569, 1970.
171. Larsen, V., and Bredahl, E.: Acta Pharmacol. Toxicol. (Kbh.) *24*:443, 1966.
172. Lerner, L. J., Carminati, P., and Schiatti, P. F.: Proc. Soc. Exp. Biol. Med. *148*:329, 1875.
173. Levi, A. J., and Sherlock, S.: Gastroenterology *54*:159, 1968.
174. Levitan, H., and Barker, J. L.: Science *176*:1423, 1972.
175. Levrat, M., and Lambert, R.: Gastroenterologia *91*:182, 1959.
176. Levy, G.: Ann. N. Y. Acad. Sci. *179*:32, 1971.
177. Levy, G.: J. Pharm. Sci. *54*:959, 1965.
178. Levy, M.: N. Engl. J. Med. *290*:1158, 1974.
179. Levy, G., and Angelino, N. J.: J. Pharm. Sci. *57*:1449, 1968.
180. Levy, G., Tsuchiya, T., and Amsol, L. P.: Clin. Pharmacol. Ther. *13*:258, 1972.
181. Lewis, D. A., Capstick, R. B., and Ancill, R. J.: J. Pharm. Pharmacol. *23*: 931, 1971.
182. Lewis, R. B., and Schulman, J. D.: Lancet *2*:1159, 1973.
183. Liquiére, G. G., Colombo, B., Carrabba, M., Ferrari, P., and Robotti, E.: Arzneim. Forsch. *22*:253, 1972.
184. Louvat, P., Tamisier, J. M., and Pourel, J.: Arzneim. Forsch. *24*:1428, 1974.
185. Lowenthal, W., Borzelleca, J. F., and Corder, C. D.: J. Pharm. Sci. *59*: 1353, 1970.
186. Lumachi, E.: Arzneim. Forsch. *22*:204, 1972.
187. Lussier, A., MacCannell, K. L., Alexander, S. J., Multz, C. V., Boost, G., and Segre, E. J.: Clin. Pharmacol. Ther. *13*:146, 1972.
188. Maffii, G., Schott, G., and Serralunga, M. G.: In "Research Progress in Organic, Biological and Medicinal Chemistry," Vol. 2. North-Holland, Amsterdam, 1970, p. 255.
189. Maggio-Cavaliere, M. B., Luders, R. C., and Gum, O. B.: J. Clin. Pharmacol. *15*:563, 1975.
190. Marchetti, M., Vignati, E., and Nicolis, F. B.: Curr. Ther. Res. *16*:742, 1974.
191. Matthies, H.: Z. Rheumaforsch. *30*:246, 1971.
192. Mauer, E. F.: N. Engl. J. Med. *253*:404, 1955.
193. Mauracher, E., and Dannhorn, R.: Praxis *64*:1254, 1975.
194. Mazue, G., Vallée, E., Genett, P., and Navano, J.: Arzneim. Forsch. *24*: 1398, 1974.
195. McCarthy, D. D., and Chalmers, T. M.: Can. Med. Assoc. J. *90*:1061, 1964.
196. McColl, J. D., Robinson, S., and Globus, M.: Toxicol. Appl. Pharmacol. *10*: 244, 1967.
197. Meli, A., Smith, C. R., and Wolff, A.: Proc. Soc. Exp. Biol. Med. *117*:34, 1964.
198. Menguy, R., and Desbaillets, L.: Am. J. Dig. Dis. *12*:862, 1967.

199. Menguy, R., and Desbaillets, L.: Proc. Soc. Exp. Biol. Med. *125*:1108, 1967.
200. Meyers, H. G., and Wetzels, E.: Arzneim. Forsch. *14*:369, 1964.
201. Messer, M., Farge, D., Guyonnet, J. C., Jeanmart, C., and Julau, L.: Arzneim. Forsch. *19*:1193, 1969.
202. Miller, J. A., and Bromstrup, T. A.: Fed. Proc. *30*:564, 1971.
203. Mills, S. B., Bloch, M., and Bruckner, F. E.: Br. Med. J. *4*:82, 1973.
204. Miura, T.: J. Int. Med. Res. *3*:145, 1975.
205. Mixich, G.: Helv. Chim. Acta *55*:1031, 1972.
206. Mizushima, Y., and Sakai, S.: J. Pharm. Pharmacol. *21*:327, 1969.
207. Mizushima, Y., Sakai, S., and Yamaura, M.: Biochem. Pharmacol. *19*:227, 1970.
208. Moertel, C. G., Ahmann, D. L., Taylor, W. F., and Schwartau, N.: N. Engl. J. Med. *286*:813, 1972.
209. Moll, W.: Prog. Drug Res. *12*:165, 1968.
210. Moran, C. J., and Walker, W. H. C.: Biochem. Pharmacol. *17*:153, 1968.
211. Morris, C. H., Christian, J. E., Miya, T. S., and Hansen, W. G.: J. Pharm. Sci. *59*:325, 1970.
212. Mörsdorf, K., and Wolf, G.: Arzneim. Forsch. *22*:2105, 1972.
213. Multz, C. V., Bernhard, G. C., Blechman, W. C., Zane, S., Restifo, R. A., and Varady, J. C.: Clin. Pharmacol. Ther. *15*:310, 1974.
214. Nannini, G., Giraldi, P. N., Molgora, G., Biasioli, G., Spinelli, F., Logemann, W., Dradi, E., Zanni, G., Brettnoni, A., and Tommasini, R.: Arzneim. Forsch. *23*:1090, 1973.
215. Nakamura, H., Kadokawa, T., Nakatsuji, K., and Nakamura, K.: Arzneim. Forsch. *20*:1032 and 1579, 1970.
216. Nakanishi, M., Imamura, H., and Maruyania, Y.: Arzneim. Forsch. *20*: 998 and 1003, 1970.
217. Nanra, R. S., and Kincaid-Smith, P.: Br. Med. J. *3*:559, 1970.
218. Navano, J., Stoliaroff, M., Savy, J. M., Beruy, L., and Brunaud, M.: Arzneim. Forsch. *24*:1368, 1974.
219. Newbould, B. B.: Br. J. Pharmacol. *21*:127, 1963.
220. Newbould, B. B.: Br. J. Pharmacol. *35*:487, 1969.
221. Nicholson, J. S.: Rep. Prog. Appl. Chem. *49*:192, 1964.
222. Nicholson, J. S.: Rep. Prog. Appl. Chem. *53*:208, 1968.
223. Nickander, R. C., Kraay, R. J., and Marshall, W. S.: Fed. Proc. *30*:563, 1971.
224. Nicolis, F. B., Schiavctti, L., Porzio, F., Manzini, A., Marchetti, M., and Acocella, G.: Int. J. Clin. Pharmacol. Ther. Toxicol. *10*:239, 1974.
225. Niemegeers, C. J. E., Awouters, F., Lenaerts, P. M. H., and Janssen, P. A. I.: Arzneim. Forsch. *25*:1516, 1975.
226. Niemegeers, C. J. E., Bruggen van M., Awouters, F., and Janssen, P. A. I.: Arzneim. Forsch. *25*:1524, 1975.
227. Niemegeers, C. J. E., and Janssen, P. A. I.: Arzneim. Forsch. *25*:1512, 1975.
228. Niemegeers, C. J. E., Lenaerts, F. M., Awouters, F., and Janssen, P. A. I.: Arzneim. Forsch. *25*:1537, 1975.
229. Niemegeers, C. J. E., Lenaerts, P. M. H., and Janssen, P. A. I.: Arzneim. Forsch. *25*:1519, 1975.
230. Niemegeers, C. J. E., Bruggen van, J. A. A., and Janssen, P. A. I.: Arzneim. Forsch. *25*:1505, 1975.

231. Niemegeers, C. J. E., Verbruggen, F. J., and Janssen, A. J.: J. Pharm. Pharmacol. *16*:810, 1964.
232. Northover, B. J., and Richards, I. S.: Br. J. Pharmacol. *32*:426 P, 1968.
233. Ober, R. E., Chang, S. F., Miller, A. M., Funk, M. L., and Holmes, E. L.: Pharmacologist *13*:295, 1971.
234. O'Brien, W. M.: Clin. Pharmacol. Ther. *9*:94, 1968.
235. O'Malley, K., Crooks, J., Duke, E., and Stevenson, I. H.: Br. Med. J. *3*: 607, 1971.
236. O'Reiley, R. A.: Ann. N. Y. Acad. Sci. *179*:173, 1971.
237. O'Reiley, R. A., and Levy, G.: J. Pharm. Sci. *59*:1258, 1970.
238. Ottin-Pecchio, P. J., Bessin, P., and Thuillier, J.: Chim. Thér. *3*:46, 1968.
239. Palo, G., Mantegani A., Donetti, B., Lumachi, B., Marazzi-Uberti, E., and Casadio, S.: Arzneim. Forsch. *22*:174, 1972.
240. Pasquariello, G., Mainardi, L., and Luvara, A.: Curr. Med. Res. Opin. *3*: 109, 1975.
241. Passotti, C., Barbieri, C., Buniva, G., and Chierichetti, S.: Arzneim. Forsch. *22*:262, 1972.
242. Paulus, H. E., Siegel, M., Mongan, E., Okun, R., and Calabro, J. J.: Arthritis Rheum. *14*:527, 1971.
243. Paulus, H. E., and Whitehouse, M. W.: Annu. Rev. Pharmacol. *13*:107, 1973.
244. Perel, J. M., Snell, M. M., Chen, W., and Dayton, P. G.: Biochem. Pharmacol. *13*:1305, 1964.
245. Phelps, P., and McCarty, D. J.: J. Pharmacol. Exp. Ther. *158*:546, 1967.
246. Piperno, E., Ellis, D. J., Getty, S. M., and Brody, T. M.: J. Am. Vet. Med. Assoc. *153*:195, 1968.
247. Platt, D. S.: J. Pharm. Sci. *60*:366, 1971.
248. Populaire, P., Terlain, B., Pascal, S., Lebreton, G., and Decouvelaere, B.: Arzneim. Forsch. *19*:1214, 1969.
249. Proctor, J. D., Evans, E. F., Velandia, J., and Wasserman, A. J.: Clin. Pharmacol. Ther. *14*:143, 1973.
250. Proctor, J. R., Evans, E. F., Velandia, J., and Wasserman, A. J.: Clin. Res. *21*:97, 1973.
251. "Profile of an Antirheumatic Compound": Ther. Woche *19*:1765, 1969.
252. Randall, L. O.: Physiol. Pharmacol. *1*:369, 1963.
253. Rau, R., and Gross, D.: In "Abstracts." 13th International Congress of Rheumatology, Excerpta Medica, 1973, p. 117.
254. Rechenberg, von H. K.: "Phenylbutazone." Arnold, London, 1962.
255. Ridolfo, A. S., Gruber, C. M., and Mikulaschek, W. M.: Clin. Pharmacol. Ther. *12*:300, 1971.
256. Roba, J., Lambelin, G., and Buu-Hoi, N. P.: Arzneim. Forsch. *20*:565, 1970.
257. Roba, J., Roncucci, R., Gillet, C., and Lambelin, G.: Scand. J. Rheumatol. *4* (Suppl. *8*) : 503-08, 1975.
258. Robinson, M. J., Nichols, E. A., and Taitz, L.: Arch. Pathol. *84*:224, 1967.
259. Rodnan, G. P., and Benedek, P. G.: Arthritis Rheum. *13*:145, 1970.
260. Roncucci, R., Lambelin, G., Simon, M. J., Thiriaux, J., and Buu-Hoi, N. P:. Med. Pharmacol. Exp. *15*:460, 1966.
261. Roncucci, R., Simon, M. J., Lambelin, G., Buu-Hoi, N. P., and Thiriaux, J.: Biochem. Pharmacol. *15*:1563, 1966.

262. Roncucci, R., Simon, M. J., Lambelin, G., Thiriaux, J., and Buu-Hoi, N. P.: Biochem. Pharmacol. *17*:187, 1968.
263. Roncucci, R., Simon, M. J., Lambelin, G., Staquet, M., Gillet, C., Van Cauwenberge, H., Lefebvre, P., Daubresse, J. C., and Buu-Hoi, N. P.: Eur. J. Clin. Pharmacol. *3*:176, 1971.
264. Rooks, W. H.: Fed. Proc. *30*:386, 1971.
265. Rose, B. S., Isdale, I. C., and Conlon, P. W.: Curr. Ther. Res. *12*:150, 1970.
266. Rosenthale, M. E., and Nagra, C. L.: Proc. Soc. Exp. Biol. Med. *125*:149, 1967.
267. Rossi, F. A., and Baroni, L.: J. Int. Med. Res. *3*:267, 1975.
268. Roszkowski, A. P., Rooks, W. H., Tomolonis, A. J., and Miller, L. M.: J. Pharmacol. Exp. Ther. *179*:114, 1971.
269. Rowland, M., and Riegelman, S.: J. Pharm. Sci. *57*:1313, 1968.
270. Royer, G. L., Moxley, T. E., Hearron, M. S., Miyara, A., and Donovan, J. F.: Curr. Ther. Res. *17*:234, 1975.
271. Rubin, A., Rodda, B. E., Warrick, P., Ridolfo, A., and Gruber, C. M.: J. Pharm. Sci. *60*:1797, 1971.
272. Rubin, A., Warrick, P., Wolen, R. L., Ridolfo, A. S., and Gruber, C. M.: Clin. Pharmacol. Ther. *13*:151, 1972.
273. Rundles, R. W., Wyngaarden, J. B., Hitchings, G. H., and Elion, G. B.: Annu. Rev. Pharmacol. *9*:345, 1969.
274. Runkel, L., Chaplin, M., Boost, V. M. G., Segre, E., and Forchielli, E.: J. Pharmacol. Sci. *61*:703, 1972.
275. Sabin, C., Nevi, R. O., Tischler, C. D., and Watnick, A. S.: Fed. Proc. *30*: 386, 1971.
276. "Salicylates: An International Symposium." Churchill, J. A., London, 1963.
277. Sarett, L. H.: Arzneim. Forsch. *21*:1759, 1971.
278. Sausgruber, H.: Arzneim. Forsch. *21*:1230, 1971.
279. Schardein, J. L., Blatz, A. T., Woosley, E. T., and Kaump, D. H.: Toxicol. Appl. Pharmacol. *15*:46, 1969.
280. Scherrer, R. A., Annu. Rep. Med. Chem. 1965:224 (1966).
281. Schiatti, P., Selva, D., Arrigoni-Martelli, E., Lerner, C. J., Diena, A., Sardi, A., and Maffii, G.: Arzneim. Forsch. *24*:2003, 1974.
282. Schlosstein, L. H., Kippen, I., Whitehouse, M. W., Bluestone, R., Paulus, H. E., and Klinenberg, F. R.: J. Lab. Clin. Med. *82*:412, 1973.
283. Schmoekel, W.: Praxis *60*:1114, 1971.
284. Schwartz, J. C., Cohen, Y., and Valette, G.: Biochem. Pharmacol. *15*:2122, 1966.
285. Segal, H. L.: Am. J. Med. *29*:780, 1960.
286. Shen, T. Y.: In "Topics in Medicinal Chemistry," Vol. 1, J. L. Rabinowitz and R. M. Myerson, eds. Wiley (Interscience), New York, 1967, p. 29.
287. Shen, T. Y.: Annu. Rep. Med. Chem. 1966: 217 (1967); Annu. Rep. Med. Chem. 1967: 215 (1968).
288. Shen, T. Y.: Angew. Chem. (Engl.) *11*:460, 1972.
289. Sholkoff, S. D., Rowland, M., Eyring, E. J., and Riegelman, S.: Arthritis Rheum. *10*:312, 1967.
290. Siegmeth, W.: Wien. Med. Wochenschr. *121*:784, 1971.
291. Silvestrini, B.: Boll. Chim. Farm. *105*:12, 1966.
292. Silvestrini, B., Garau, A., Pozzatti, C., and Cioli, V.: Arzneim. Forsch. *16*:

59, 1966.

293. Silvestrini, B., Garau, A., Pozzatti, C., Cioli, V., and Catanese, B.: Arch. Int. Pharmacodyn. Ther. *163*:61, 1966.

294. Silvestrini, B., Scorza Barcellona, P., Garau, A., and Catanese, B.: Toxicol. Appl. Pharmacol. *10*:148, 1967.

295. Smith, M. J. H.: J. Pharm. Pharmacol. *3*:409, 1951.

296. Smith, M. J. H., and Dawkins, P. O.: J. Pharm. Pharmacol. *23*:729, 1971.

297. Smith, M. J. H., and Smith, P. K.: "The Salicylates, A Critical, Bibliographic Review." Wiley (Interscience), New York, 1966.

298. Smith, P. K.: Ann. N. Y. Acad. Sci. *86*:38, 1960.

299. Smith, P. K., Gleason, H. L., Stoll, G. B., and Ogorzalek, S.: J. Pharmacol. Exp. Ther. *87*:237, 1946.

300. Smyth, C. J.: Arthritis Rheum. *8*:921, 1965.

301. Sofia, R. D.: Eur. J. Pharmacol. *26*:51, 1974.

302. Somogyl, A., Koväcs, K., and Selye, H.: J. Pharm. Pharmacol. *21*:122, 1969.

303. Spector, W. S. (ed).: "Handbook of Toxicology," Vol. 1. Saunders, Philadelphia, 1956, Chapt. 43, p. 10.

304. Stenlake, J. B., Williams, W. D., Davidson, A. G., and Downie, W. W.: J. Pharm. Pharmacol. *23*:145, 1971.

305. Steinbrocker, O., and Arggros, T. G.: Arthritis Rheum. *3*:368, 1960.

306. Stevenson, A. C., Bedford, J., Hilie, A. G. S., and Hill, H. F. H.: Ann. Rheum. Dis. *30*:487, 1971.

307. Strandberg, B.: Acta Rheumatol. Scand. *10* (Suppl.) : 5, 1965.

308. Stroescu, V., Georgeseu, C., and Voiosu, R.: J. Int. Med. Res. *2*:338, 1974.

309. Sturman, J. A., Dawkins, P. D., McArtur, N., and Smith, M. J. H.: J. Pharm. Pharmacol. *20*:58, 1968.

310. Sturman, J. A., and Smith, M. J. H.: J. Pharm. Pharmacol. *19*:621, 1967.

311. Sunshine, A., and Laska, E.: Clin. Pharmacol. Ther. *12*:302, 1971.

312. Swingle, K. F., Hamilton, R. R., Harrington, J. K., and Kvam, D. C.: Arch. Int. Pharmacodyn. Ther. *189*:129, 1971.

313. Swingle, K. F., Hamilton, R. R., Harrington, J. K., and Kvam, D. C.: Arch. Int. Pharmacodyn. Ther. *192*:16, 1971.

314. Symposium "Aspirin and Salicylates": Clin. Toxicol. *1*:379, 1968.

315. Tainter, M. L., and Ferris, A. J.: "Aspirin in Modern Therapy. A Review." Bayer Co., New York, 1969.

316. Tanaka, K., Iizuka, Y., Yoskida, N., Tomita, K., and Masuda, H.: Experientia *28*:937, 1972.

317. Theobald, W., and Domenjoz, R.: Arzneim. Forsch. *8*:18, 1958.

318. Trnavsky, K., and Trnavská, Z.: Pharmacology *6*:9, 1971.

319. Tsuchiya, T., and Levy, G.: J. Pharm. Sci. *61*:800, 1972.

320. Ungar, G., Damgaard, E., and Hummel, F. P.: Am. J. Physiol. *171*:545, 1952.

321. Ungar, G., Kobrin, S., and Sezesny, B. R.: Arch. Int. Pharmacodyn. Ther. *123*:71, 1959.

322. Van Arman, C. G., Carlson, R. P., Brown, W. R., and Itkin, A.: Proc. Soc. Exp. Biol. Med. *134*:163, 1970.

323. Van Arman, C. G., Carlson, R. P., Risley, E. A., Thomas, R. H., and Nuss, G. W.: J. Pharmacol. Exp. Ther. *175*:459, 1970.

324. Van Cauwenberge, H., and Lecomte, J.: C. R. Soc. Biol. *151*:405, 1957.

325. Vesel, E. S., and Page, J. G.: Science, *159*:1479, 1968.
326. Vindel, J. A., Richer, G., Khoury, B., and Hirbee, G.: Arzneim. Forsch. *24*:1378, 1974.
327. Vokner, J.: Praxis *59*:1756, 1970.
328. Von Rechenberg, H. K.: "Phenylbutazone." Edward Arnold, Ltd., London, 1962.
329. Wagenhauser, F.: Scand. J. Rheumatol. *4*, Suppl. *8*:505, 1975.
330. Wagenhauser, F., and Narozna, H.: Schweiz. Med. Wochenschr. *105*:652, 1975.
331. Walter, J. E., Diener, R. M., and Earl, A. E.: Toxicol. Appl. Pharmacol. *17*:314, 1970.
332. Walter, J. E., and Diener, R. M.: Toxicol. Appl. Pharmacol. *19*:376, 1971.
333. Ward, J. R., and Cloud, R. S.: J. Pharmacol. Exp. Ther. *152*:116, 1966.
334. Watnick, A. S., Taber, R. J., and Tabachnick, I. I. A.: Fed. Proc. *27*:533, 1968.
335. Watnick, A. S., Taber, R. J., and Tabachnick, I. I. A.: Arch. Int. Pharmacodyn. *190*:78, 1971.
336. Weiner, M., and Piliero, S. J.: Annu. Rev. Pharmacol. *10*:171, 1970.
337. Weiss, J.: Med. Exp. *8*, 1, 1963.
338. Weiss, A., Pitman, E. R., and Graham, E. C.: Am. J. Med. *31*:266, 1961.
339. West, G. B.: J. Pharm. Pharmacol. *16*:788, 1964,
340. Westby, T. R., and Barfknet, C. F.: J. Med. Chem. *16*:40, 1973.
341. Whitehouse, M. W.: Prog. Drug Res. *8*:321, 1965.
342. Whittaker, J. A., and Price Evans, D. A.: Br. Med. J. *4*:323, 1970.
343. Wilhelmi, G.: Schweiz, Med. Wochenschr. *80*:936, 1950.
344. Winder, C. V., Kaump, D. H., Glazko, A. J., and Holmes, E. L.: Ann. Phys. Med. *7* (Suppl.) : 131, 1967.
345. Winder, C. V., Lembke, L. A., and Stephens, M. D.: Arthritis Rheum. *12*: 472, 1969.
346. Winder, C. V., Wax, J., Burr, V., Been, M., and Rosiere, C. E.: Arch. Int. Pharmacodyn. Ther. *116*:261, 1958.
347. Winder, E. V., Wax, J., and Welford, M.: J. Pharmacol. Exp. Ther. *148*: 422, 1965.
348. Winter, C. A.: Annu. Rev. Pharmacol. *6*, 157, 1966; Prog. Drug. Res. *10*: 139, 1966.
349. Winter, C. A.: Arzneim. Forsch. *21*:1805, 1971.
350. Winter, C. A., and Nuss, G. W.: Arthritis Rheum. *9*:394, 1966.
351. Winter, C. A., Risley, E. A., and Nuss, G. W.: J. Pharmacol. Exp. Ther. *141*:369, 1963.
352. Wiseman, E. H., and Chiaini, J.: Biochem. Pharmacol. *21*:2323, 1972.
353. Wissmuller, H. F.: Arzneim. Forsch. *21*:1738, 1971.
354. Wright, H. N.: Toxicol. Appl. Pharmacol. *11*:280, 1967.
355. Yesair, D. W., Callahan, M., Remington, L., and Kensler, C. J.: Biochem. Pharmacol. *19*:1579, 1970.
356. Yesair, D. W., Remington, L., Callahan, M., and Kensler, C.: Biochem. Pharmacol. *19*:1591, 1970.
357. Yu, T. F.: Am. J. Med. *56*:676, 1974.
358. Yu, T. F., Burns, J. J., Paton, B. C., Gutman, A. B., and Brodie, B. B.: J. Pharmacol. Exp. Ther. *123*:63, 1958.
359. Zinnes, H., Lindo, N. A., Sirear, J. C., Schwartz, M. L., Shavel, J., and Di Pasquale, G.: J. Med. Chem. *16*:44, 1973.

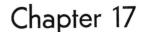

Chapter 17

Immunosuppressive Agents

1. IMMUNOPATHOLOGICAL MECHANISMS

Immunological responsiveness is one of the fundamental mechanisms by which higher organisms react to their environment.

The principal complication here is that most immune responses are the result of elaborate interactions between different subpopulations of lymphocytes, and between these and accessory non-lymphoid cells (macrophages). It appears that, in many immune responses, a preparatory step may be required where certain antigens are initially phagocytized and processed by macrophages. Following this reaction, macrophages produce a mediator (either a RNA or RNA-antigen complex) which serves to stimulate a receptive population of uncommitted lymphocytes. Stimulated cells then undergo a morphological transformation into large immunoblasts, complete a series of repetitive mitotic divisions and ultimately mature into immune effectors. Some lymphocytes derived from the immunoblasts appear to enter the recirculating pool as the immunological memory cell. Upon re-exposure to the inciting antigen, these memory cells are capable of an accelerated or anamnestic response.

Two distinct cellular pathways are recognized in immune reactions, namely those of T or B cells.

The thymus-derived lymphocytes (T-cells) are the specific initiator cells in cell-mediated immunity. Mature T cells can be subdivided into at least three different subclasses in regard to their functions:

1. Effector cells of cell-mediated immunity, which (a) release a variety of non-antibody soluble products—the limphokines—that can be regarded as mediators of inflammation (see Chapter 10), and (b) kill other cells selectively.
2. Helper cells which undergo proliferation in response to antigens and then help—by unknown mechanisms—other specific T and or B lymphocytes to become effector cells.
3. Suppressor cells of T- and B-cell function. This is a new, largely unexplored area of immunology on which the interest of many laboratories is currently focused.

When the effector T cell encounters antigen, it is triggered to proliferate and differentiate under the opposing influences of helper and suppressor T cells. The result is the destruction of cells bearing the activating antigen or the release of lymphokines—the typical inflammatory response of cell-mediated immunity in which macrophages are involved.

The activation of B cells by antigens is quite comparable to that of T cells, except that the products secreted are antibodies, not lymphokines.

Several pathogenetic mechanisms are implicated in immunological disorders; they have been subdivided into the following four different types:

Type I: Initiated by antigen reacting with basophils or mast cells passively sensitized by antibody produced elsewhere, leading to the release of vasoactive amines. Disorders of this type include cutaneous anaphylaxis, generalized anaphylaxis, allergic rhinitis, asthma, angioneurotic edema and gastrointestinal allergies (Fig. 35).

Type II: Initiated by antibody reacting with antigen on cell surfaces or with an antigenic component of a cell or tissue element, usually with the participation of complement. Disorders of this type include transfusion reactions, hemolytic disease, immune thrombocytopenia and leukopenia, and, probably, thyrotoxicosis (the role

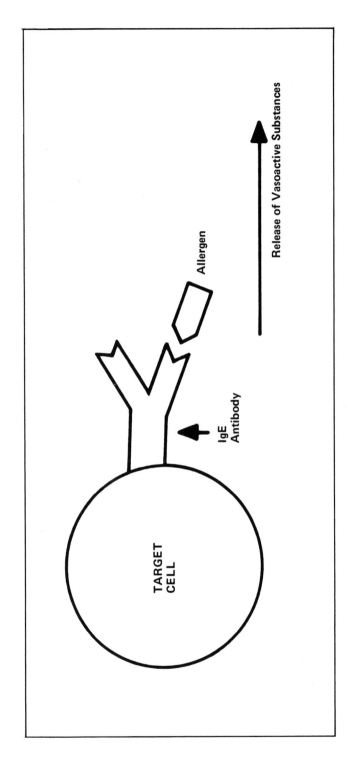

FIG. 35. Pathogenetic mechanisms of immunological disorder: Type I

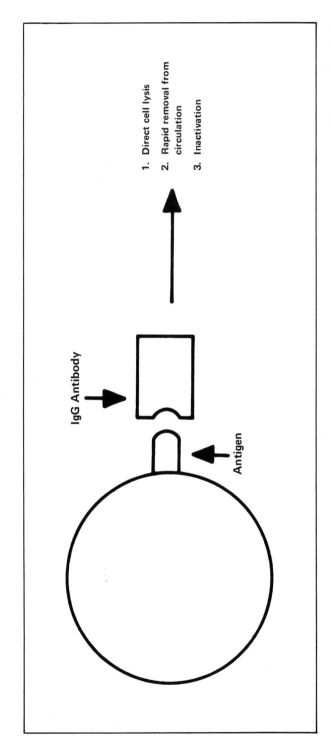

FIG. 36. Pathogenetic mechanisms of immunological disorders: Type II

of complement in the pathogenesis of this disease is not established) (Fig. 36).

Type III: Initiated when antigen reacts in the tissue spaces with potentially precipitating antibody, and forms microprecipitates in and around the small vessels, causing cell damage secondarily, or being precipitated in and interfering with the functions of membranes; or when excess antigen reacts in the blood stream with potentially precipitating antibody, it forms soluble circulating complexes which are deposited in the blood vessel walls or in the basement membrane and cause local inflammation or massive complement activation. Disorders of this type include serum sickness, systemic lupus erythematosus, nephrotic syndrome due to malaria and leprosy, extrinsic allergic alveolitis, lepromatous leprosy, many types of drug sensitivity and, probably, rheumatoid arthritis (Fig. 37).

Type IV: Initiated essentially by the reaction of actively sensitized thymus-derived lymphocytes, responding specifically to antigen by the release of lymphokines that are toxic and promote the local accumulation of macrophages. Active lymphocytes can also directly damage cells against which they are reacting by a little understood mechanism requiring cell contact. Disorders of this type are also classified as delayed or cell-mediated immune response which includes among its manifestations graft rejection, graft versus host reaction, contact sensitivity, some kinds of autoimmunity, immunity to tuberculosis, fungi and viruses and, probably, immune surveillance against tumors (Fig. 38).

Since the above section is intended to provide a schematic outline of the immunopathological mechanisms and not to review the enormous volume of research performed in this field, only a few handbooks are mentioned as a possible source of further information (35,86,91,114,158,234,254).

2. PRINCIPAL IMMUNOSUPPRESSIVE AGENTS: CLASSIFICATION AND MODE OF ACTION

By definition, immunosuppressive agents are able to prevent or suppress the immune response to some extent. They are of great interest in basic immunological research and are of considerable importance in clinical therapy as the most effective means of diminishing immune responsiveness. A vast literature on these agents has appeared (for reviews see 4,20,40,77,84,108,112,174,195,211). There

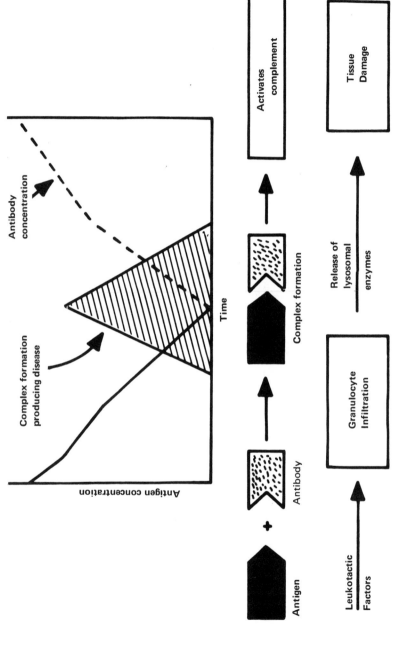

FIG. 37. Pathogenetic mechanisms of immunological disorders: Type III

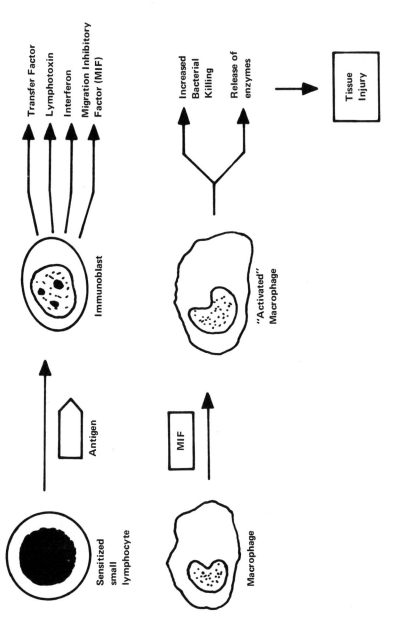

FIG. 38. Pathogenetic mechanisms of immunological disorders: Type IV

is no immunosuppressive agent in clinical use whose actions are perfectly understood. In respect to those that are being widely studied, a picture of remarkable complexity is beginning to emerge (25,45, 236). Further complications arise from the fact that immunosuppressive agents may inhibit two or more cooperative populations of cells (1,24) or, by selectively inhibiting suppressor populations, they may paradoxically enhance the immune response (107,128,132,186).

Immunosuppression can be exerted by physical agents (whole or local body irradiation), living organisms (viruses, parasites, microbial exo- and endo-toxins), and chemical and biological substances. Immunosuppression can also be achieved by surgical procedures, such as removal of lymphoid tissues or thoracic duct drainage, or by the administration of antilymphocyte serum. Only the compounds listed in Table 45 will be discussed in some detail.

A. Alkylating agents

Alkylating agents interact with the nucleophile centers of molecules, especially with the amino-carboxylic-, thio-, and phosphate groups, and with tertiary nitrogen. Their main site of action is located on N^7 of the guanine residue of DNA (62,84,258). Active alkylating agents cross-link native DNA together, DNA with proteins, RNA with RNA, or with proteins, or with DNA, labilize the glucoside bridge between base and deoxyriboside, and interfere with nucleic acid and protein synthesis (100,231,258). They act on rapidly dividing cells, such as small sensitized lymphocytes, but do not affect long-lived lymphocytes (100,160).

Alkylating agents used in immunosuppression are: cyclophosphamide, chlorambucil, melphalan, busulfan, and thioTEPA. These compounds act mainly through their lymphocytotoxic effect. Cyclophosphamide suppresses the primary immune response if administered before, during or after antigenic stimulation in mice and rats (37,63,206,231). In man, it impairs immunoglobulin production (6). Secondary immune response is also inhibited (206). When administered simultaneously with high doses of antigen, it causes immune tolerance (3,100,151). Delayed hypersensitivity reactions are inhibited by cyclophosphamide: graft survival is prolonged in mice, rats, rabbits and man, but not in dogs and guinea pigs (33,189,214). In many models of experimental autoimmune disease, cyclophosphamide was found to have an inhibitory effect (138,176,177,178, 179,204).

The action of other alkylating agents is similar to that of cyclo-

TABLE 45. Principal immunosuppressive agents

Alkylating agents	ThioTEPA
	Cyclophosphamide
	Chlorambucil
	Melphalan
	Busulfan
Antimetabolites	
Antipurines	6-Mercaptopurine
	Azathioprine
	6-Thioguanine
Antipyrimidine	5-Fluorouracil
	Cytosine arabinoside
Folic acid antagonists	Methotrexate
Antibiotics	Actinomycins C and D
	Chloramphenicol
Miscellaneous compounds	Vincristine
	Vinblastine
	Procarbazine
	L-Asparaginase

phosphamide (17,28,42), with some differences concerning the time of peak, optimal dosing regimens, and the sensitivity of different animal species to the effects of these drugs.

It should be noted that, in certain experimental conditions, cyclophosphamide (231) and busulfan (213) enhance antibody formation in rat. It has also been reported that cyclophosphamide had a selective effect in depleting the B-lymphocyte area of lymphoid tissue of both mice and guinea pigs (192,236), and enhanced delayed hypersensitivity in these two species (129,136,187,188). It also reversed the immunological tolerance (186). These findings have been interpreted as being the consequence of the inhibition of a population of suppressor cells by cyclophosphamide (186). Among the other alkylating agents tested, only melphalan was found to have similar effects (235).

Cyclophosphamide is inactive in vitro (124) and it is believed to be transformed in vivo into the active substance norchloretamine by tissue phosphoraminidase (205). Other possible metabolic transformations have been suggested; the hypothesis of an in vivo activation of cyclophosphamide has been, however, questioned (31,216).

B. Antimetabolites

Antimetabolites are synthetic substances that have structural analogies with nucleic acid precursors and can, therefore, interfere with nucleic acid synthesis. Purine and pyrimidine analogs, and folic acid antagonists are the most frequently used antimetabolites in immunosuppressive therapy.

Antipurines

6-Mercaptopurine, a structural analog of adenine and hypoxantine, is a powerful antimetabolite (65). In entering a cell, 6-mercaptopurine undergoes a series of transformations, giving rise to 6-methylthiopurine ribonucleotide which can be incorporated into DNA and RNA (16,64,174). Competing for specific enzymes, it blocks the de novo purine synthesis, thus essentially interfering with DNA formation (31,62,64,214). In vivo, 6-mercaptopurine is catabolized by xantine oxidase into thiouric acid, with consequent reduction of its activity. The imidazole-substituted 6-mercaptopurine—azathioprine, one of the most widely used immunosuppressive drug—is split in vivo to liberate 6-mercaptopurine.

6-Mercaptopurine and other purine analogs strongly inhibit antibody formation in several animal species, including man, when administered together with or after the antigen (80,81,102,110,121, 140,147,168,206,212,218,228,245). The antipurines also depress cellular immune responses and prolong graft survival in rabbit, goldfish, dog and man (133,140,141,156,217,227). The pronounced antiinflammatory effect of 6-mercaptopurine (113,171,172) has been thought to be responsible for this (117), however, it is not able to prevent a passive tuberculine reaction in guinea pigs even after massive pretreatment (34).

Antipyrimidines

The pyrimidine analogs include the structural analogs of cytosine and cytidine, of which cytosine arabinoside is an example.

5-Fluorouracil inhibits thymidilate synthetase, thus acting through a depletion of thymidine (31). 5-Fluorouracil and other analogs of uracil show relatively poor immunosuppressive activity in animals (29,84,157). In man, 5-fluorouracil exhibits good immunosuppressive activity (163). According to other investigations (30), this compound enhanced delayed hypersensitivity reactions in cancer patients.

Cytosine arabinoside inhibits DNA polymerase and the formation of deoxycytidine from cytosine diphosphate (95,105). Cytosine arabinoside inhibits primary antibody response in several animal species most of all when given after antigen (67,70,71,97,164) ; it prevents the induction of delayed hypersensitivity (126,127,165) and prolongs skin allograft survival in mice (96).

Folic acid antagonists

Methotrexate and aminopterin, the most common members of this class, bind firmly to dihydrofolate reductase, inhibiting the conversion of dihydrofolic into tetrahydrofolic acid (31). This step is necessary for the synthesis of several compounds, including DNA, RNA and many coenzyme species. The effects of folic acid antagonists can be totally reversed by the administration of large amounts of folic or folinic acid. This observation led to the introduction of the "rescue" technique in therapy, consisting of the administration of methotrexate in high doses and folinic acid in sequence in order to kill the most rapidly dividing cells, without damaging others (27).

Both primary and secondary responses are inhibited by methotrexate if it is injected early after antigenic stimulation in mice, rats, guinea pigs and dogs (18,50,78,149,189,214,242). It also prevents delayed hypersensitivity (50,84,189), and prolongs skin graft survival in mice (90,227) and guinea pigs (19) but not in rabbits (156). Methotrexate inhibits experimental autoimmune encephalomyelitis (38), experimental autoimmune thyroiditis (221) and adjuvant arthritis in rats (253), and antibody formation (109,206, 228) and delayed hypersensitivity reaction (228) in man. This latter finding has not, however, been confirmed (109,165).

C. Antibiotics

Actinomycin D inhibits DNA-dependent RNA synthesis, especially that of messenger RNA (62,104,263). When administered in vivo after the antigen (87,168), or in in vitro experiments (226), actinomycin D inhibits the primary response. However, the 19S reaction in mice immunized with sheep red blood cells has been found to be enhanced following actinomycin D treatment (59). The latter also inhibits delayed hypersensitivity in vitro (41,51) but, in vivo, it has little immunosuppressive effect in transplantation (150) *Actinomycin C* is similar in its action to actinomycin D (88).

Chloramphenicol blocks the binding of messenger RNA to

ribosome or the availability of template RNA, thus inhibiting protein synthesis (255). It prevents antibody synthesis (255) and limits the number of plaque-forming cells in cell culture (241); it does not inhibit delayed hypersensitivity but postpones allograft rejection (51).

D. Miscellaneous compounds

The Vinca alkaloids, vincristine and vinblastine, are mitotic-spindle inhibitors and block mitosis in metaphase (182,229,182). In rats, they inhibit antibody production and delayed hypersensitivity (2,5). In mice, they are effective if administered after the antigen (18), while they have no activity at all in rabbits (76). Although their immunosuppressive potential is relatively poor, vincristine and vinblastine have been extensively used for cytokinetic studies of immune response.

L-Asparaginase hydrolyzes L-asparagine. As the asparagine synthetase level is low in mammalian tissues, this disturbs cell metabolism and thymidine incorporation into DNA drops (257). L-Asparaginase is able to suppress the primary response in mice and rabbits, regardless of the time of administration: the best immunosuppressive effect occurs when drug and antigen are injected simultaneously (22,130,166,193,215). The exact mode of action of L-asparaginase is uncertain, but it seems to affect antigen recognition before cellular multiplication. It certainly acts on lymphoid tissue directly. Lymph-node lymphocytes do not migrate normally and the size of lymph nodes, spleen and thymus are reduced (257). The enzyme also inhibits delayed hypersensitivity (130), markedly prolongs skin graft survival (36,196) and blocks the onset of experimental autoimmune encephalomyelitis (131). In man, antibody production and delayed hypersensitivity are suppressed (169).

Procarbazine influences a number of enzymes and it has been suggested that its effect depends on alkylation of DNA (256). This agent is lymphocytotoxic (223) and it has been found to depress antibody production in mice, rats and rabbits (194,223,224). Allograft survival is prolonged when the drug is given after grafting (72,73).

3. TESTING OF IMMUNOSUPPRESSIVE AGENTS

The principal methods used to evaluate compounds expected to interfere with immunological processes have been reviewed in Chapter 12. Some of the more important factors should be emphasized here that are involved in assaying agents for immunosuppressive activity. The immune response is heterogenous, and a number of elements can influence or reverse the qualitative and quantitative aspects of a bioassay. A rigid control of experimental conditions is essential to achieve reproducible results.

The more important factors are:

1. Form and composition of the antigen influencing both the immunological response and the immunosuppressive effects of the drugs in question.
2. Route of administration and dose of antigen—also in relation to the dose of the immunosuppressive agents.
3. Timing of drug administration: most alkylating agents are active when given before antigen, whereas folic acid antagonists, antipurine and antipyrimidine agents are active when given after antigen.
4. Host factors: age, nutrition, endocrine status, species, strain, and sex are very important.

Extensive discussion of these factors can be found in general reviews on immunosuppressive agents (4,20,40,77,84,108,112,174, 195,211) (Table 46).

4. "ANTIINFLAMMATORY" ACTIVITY OF IMMUNOSUPPRESSANTS

Interference with one or more discrete phases in the sequence of events leading to an immunopathologic response is not necessarily the mechanism by which immunosuppressive agents modify inflammatory processes. Little evidence exists, in fact, that correlates clinical and experimental antiinflammatory activity with immunosuppression (34,49,54,228). Among the several mechanisms of action proposed are: interference with synthesis of enzymes necessary for the release of inflammatory mediators (134), interference with pharmacological mediators of the inflammatory response (237), reduction of complement levels (260), and inhibition of mononuclear cell exudation (8).

Antiinflammatory, as distinct from immunosuppressant activity has been described in several models of experimental inflammation for many immunosuppressive agents (9,39,117,171,203,222, 232,253). A number of data suggests that their antiflammatory activity depends on an effect of these drugs on macrophages or their

TABLE 46. Effects of cyclophosphamide, methotrexate and azathioprine on several immunological models - reference list

	Cyclo-phosphamide	Methotrexate	Azathioprine
Adjuvant arthritis	9, 10, 39, 49, 183, 202, 251	202, 250, 253	49, 183, 202, 259
Allergic encephalomyelitis	43, 135, 175, 201, 248	38, 43, 201	201, 135
Homograft response	20	20, 180	66, 180, 190, 246
Passive hemagglutination	26, 52, 63	26, 52, 70	26, 70
Antibody-forming cells	21, 152, 243, 244	21, 243, 244	23
Rosette inhibition test	13	13	13, 14
Active systemic anaphylaxis	106, 148, 200	200	20
Cellular hypersensitivity "in vitro"		44	252, 261, 262
Contact dermatitis	146, 148, 233	148, 233	
Graft versus host reaction	15, 32, 170, 142	32, 142, 170	15, 32, 142

precursors. It has been shown that 6-mercaptopurine inhibits the multiplication of bone-marrow monocytes (117), thus preventing the participation of macrophages in delayed hypersensitivity and their infiltration into an inflammatory site (173). The treatment of guinea pigs with high doses of 6-mercaptopurine completely inhibits in vivo the delayed hypersensitivity response to tuberculin. However, in vitro, lymphocytes of treated animals were able to undergo the normal blastogenic reaction to tuberculin. This suggested that a non-lymphoid feature of delayed hypersensitivity was affected, the macrophage being a good candidate in this respect (266). It has been shown subsequently that the non-specific inflammatory response was inhibited in guinea pigs by 6-mercaptopurine treatment (184). Also in man does this drug block the mononuclear phase of the inflammatory response, even when the total leukocyte count is not reduced (113). Other agents, including methotrexate, cyclophosphamide, chlorambucil and actinomycin D, also suppress the mononuclear phase of the inflammatory response (111).

It should be recalled, however, that established delayed hypersensitivity reactions usually persist during therapy with immuno-suppressive agents, suggesting that chronic inflammatory responses can occur. Furthermore, it has been clearly established in direct experimentation with several immunosuppressive agents that they have little effect on chronic inflammatory reactions while they abolish acute inflammations (222). In this context, the term "chronic inflammation" is used to indicate a granulomatous reaction; therefore, this finding is not in conflict with others previously mentioned indicating that immunosuppressive agents are able to inhibit development of the primary lesions of adjuvant arthritis (9,39,203).

Since the altered immunological reactions responsible for most autoimmune diseases have not yet been elucidated, it is very difficult to ascribe beneficial therapeutic effects specifically to immunosup-pression. Yet it would be equally tenous to state that the beneficial effects produced by this group of drugs are solely due to a suppression of inflammation.

5. TOXICITY

Immunosuppressive compounds used in the treatment of rheu-matoid arthritis and in a number of other chronic inflammatory conditions have generally been derived from antitumor studies, and are rather powerful cytotoxic-antiproliferative agents. Their toxicity profile should, therefore, be somewhat different from that of the conventional non-steroidal antiinflammatory drugs. Considerable information is available concerning the manner in which to evaluate the toxic effects of immunosuppressive or cytotoxic agents, and the qualitative toxicity of a large number of these drugs (57,75,207). Using the concept of "maximum tolerated dose" in man, monkey and dog (i.e., the dose causing mild to moderate toxic effects in a significant percentage of subjects), a reasonable correlation of toxicity data in man and animals has been established (75). A similar analogy has been found when the maximum tolerated dose in man was plotted against the LD_{10} in smaller animals (LD_{10} = the dose of drug which when administered to an animal kills 10% of that species within 3 weeks after cessation of daily dosing for 1-5 days) (75). In evaluating the comparative qualitative toxicity of 25 anti-cancer compounds of diverse chemical and functional character in dog and monkey, it was found that the screening of large animals served to predict a significant proportion of unwanted drug effects later encountered in clinical use (207). The dog and monkey trials correctly predicted bone marrow depression, gastrointestinal disturbances and hepatotoxicity for each drug producing these effects in man. However organ-specific toxicity has been observed in animals but not in man as far as the respiratory, lymphoid, neuromuscular and renal systems are concerned (207).

There are four general problems, probably applicable to all cytotoxic and immunosuppressant agents, which require more detailed consideration; these are: mutagenic and dismorphogenic effects, sterility induction, intercurrent infection, and neoplasia facilitation.

A. Mutagenic and dismorphogenic effects

Any drug that affects DNA structure should be suspected of producing late genetic damage and conception during their use should be prevented. Information on these effects is obtained largely from animal studies (11,12,74,85,167). Clinical reports have been more conflicting but leave little doubt about the potential dismorphogenic effects in humans (11,55,98,139,210,220).

B. Sterility induction

Animal experiments have demonstrated the damaging effect of these agents on the gonads, even if the results have not been uniform because they have been influenced by variables, such as the drugs and dose used, their distribution and other physiological factors (74,118,119,120,161). Several reports have described ovarian suppression or premature menopause in roughly 10% of patients given cyclophosphamide and chlorambucil (79,82,162). Azoospermia has been reported in men receiving alkylating agents (53,69,159, 199).

C. Intercurrent infections

There is little doubt that the major immediate complication of antiproliferative drug therapy is infection, even if it must be recognized that most human data are derived from extremely complex clinical situations. Great variety of organisms, some common and some exotic, can give trouble in the course of routine management with little or no leukopenia (83,94,153,155,208). It is likely that intercurrent infections are primarily due to an impairment of the cellular immune response.

D. Neoplasia facilitation

The potential threat of neoplasia is the most difficult of all the problems related to cytotoxic agents. The increased incidence of malignancies in immunosuppressed patients after organ transplantation is, however, an unequivocal fact (58,61,68,115,181,209,249). Neoplastic disease in patients undergoing prolonged immunosuppression occurs with an incidence about 100 times greater than in the general population. The most common tumor reported is reticulum cell sarcoma of an unusual intracerebral origin. Most of the others are epithelial in origin and include squamous carcinoma of the lip, squamous or basal cell carcinoma of the skin, and carcinoma of the colon, testis, ovary, and stomach. This increased risk of neoplasia does not appear related to the use of any one agent (48,103, 249,164). In animals, increased incidence of neoplasms has been observed after prolonged treatment with actinomycin D (56) or antilymphocyte serum (137). A greater number of "takes" of isotransplanted tumors has also been found in mice pretreated with cytotoxic agents (198). The most commonly expressed view is that, in the immunosuppressed state, immune surveillance is defective and that mutant or perhaps virus-transformed cell that would be promptly destroyed in the normal individual are instead permitted to survive and multiply (61,68) (Fig. 39).

6. IMMUNOSUPPRESSIVE AGENTS FOR RHEUMATOID ARTHRITIS

The use of cytotoxic or immunosuppressive therapy in rheumatoid arthritis goes back to the early 1950s when aminopterin (101) and nitrogen mustard (123) were first tried. It has only been over the past decade, however, that immunosuppressant drugs have been widely used in severe forms of this disease and reports of controlled studies have appeared. These drugs were initially used to treat rheumatoid arthritis on theoretical grounds, with the object of achieving significant immunosuppression since it has postulated that autoimmune mechanisms were implicated in the pathogenesis of rheumatoid arthritis. As previously discussed, however, conventional parameters of immune responsiveness are not predictably depressed by cytotoxic drugs and the clinical improvement observed need not necessarily be accounted for by their immunosuppressive effects (34,49,54,228). Furthermore, the improvement is rarely

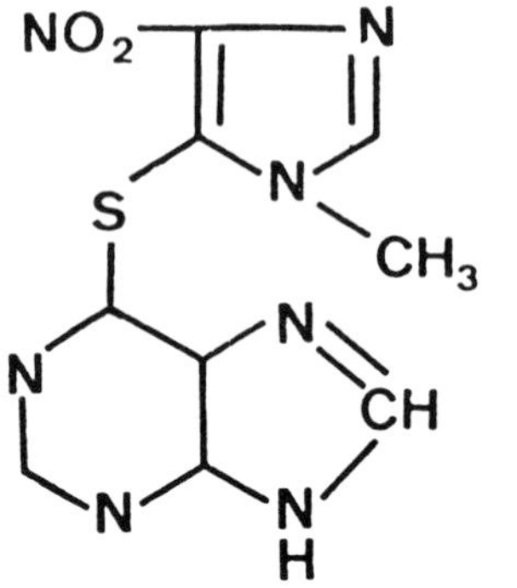

Azathioprine

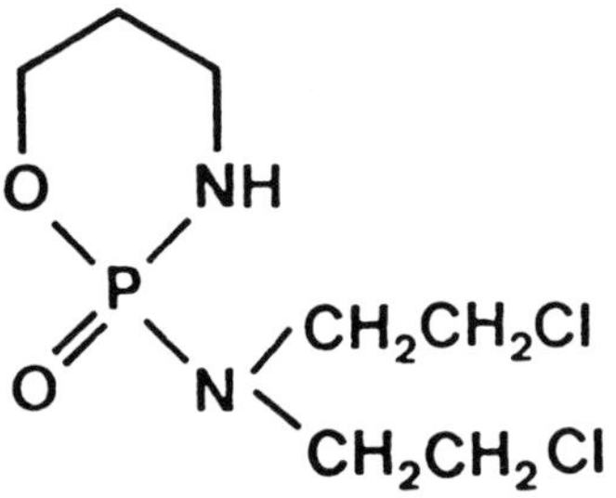

Cyclophosphamide

FIG. 39. Chemical structure of immunosuppressants used in the treatment of rheumatic diseases

dramatic, has not been obtained universally, is not maintained after treatment is discontinued and is achieved at a heavy price in morbidity, while the long-term risks are as yet unknown.

Despite the large number of immunosuppressive agents currently available, only cyclophosphamide and azathioprine have been submitted to extensive and controlled clinical trials in rheumatoid patients.

Cyclophosphamide appeared to be a promising drug in controlling both adult and childhood forms of rheumatoid arthritis (82, 83,122,197,219). Two major trials of this drug were reported by the Cooperating Clinics Committee of the American Rheumatism Association. The first trial (46) lasted 32 weeks with up to 150 mg/

day of cyclophosphamide being given versus a presumed homeo-pathic dose, 15 mg/day, in patients with definite or classical rheumatoid arthritis. A total of 48 patients completed the trial. A significant improvement in objective criteria assessing disease activity was reported. In the second 64-week long trial (47) 75 mg/day was administered, compared to the 150 mg/day given in the first study. The trial did not show that low doses were as effective as were high ones. The low-dose group showed only minimal and insignificant improvement and demonstrated nearly as many adverse effects as the high-dose patients. These findings have been confirmed in subsequent studies (145). Although cyclophosphamide offers substantial benefits, the high incidence of adverse effects indicates its use only when more standard forms of therapy have failed.

After a possible usefulness of azathioprine in rheumatoid arthritis was suggested (60), this drug has been evaluated by three different groups in well-controlled studies (144,154,238). These trials have shown that azathioprine, at doses 2-3 mg/kg body weight per day, is effective in suppressing the activity of severe rheumatoid arthritis. Long-term follow-up studies have revealed that azathioprine continues to suppress the disease when administered over a prolonged period of time (284) and that a reduced dosage (1-1,25 mg/kg body weight, day) is still fully effective (239). There is, however, no indication that a lasting remission of the disease process is induced, since discontinuation of therapy usually results in a recrudescence of disease activity (92).

Although possible antiinflammatory effects of both cyclophosphamide and azathioprine have been considered in explaining their mechanism of action (see point 4 above), in rheumatoid arthritis, the latter has been supposed to involve the inhibition or modification of one or more of the steps in the immune response. Disparity between clinical responses and modifications of immune parameters in rheumatoid patients treated with immunosuppressive drugs has been repeatedly observed (7,93,144,228). Nevertheless, rheumatoid factor titers, and IgA and IgM serum levels have been found to be significantly reduced by prolonged treatment with azathioprine, cyclophosphamide and chlorambucil (54,93,143). Cyclophosphamide also significantly reduced IgG serum levels (143). Effects on cell-mediated immunity have been described for these agents (61,225, 265,267). However, in rheumatoid patients, cyclophosphamide was found to inhibit the lymphocyte mitogen response (143) while azathioprine and chlorambucile failed to do so (54).

It seems that both azathioprine and cyclophosphamide are efficacious in the treatment of a minority of patients not sufficiently benefitted by other therapeutic measures. The cost in toxicity and long-term effects in patients whose disease though incapacitating and life-long is not itself lethal appears very high (238).

REFERENCES

1. Addison, I. E. Br. J. Exp. Pathol. *55*:487, 1974.
2. Aisenberg, A. C.: Nature *200*:484, 1963.
3. Aisenberg, A. C.: J. Exp. Med. *125*:833, 1967.
4. Aisenberg, A. C.: Adv. Pharmacol. Chemother. *8*:38, 1970.
5. Aisenberg, A. C., and Wilkes, B.: J. Clin. Invest. *43*:2394, 1964.
6. Alepa, F. P., Zvaifler, N. J., and Sliwinski, A. J.: Arthritis Rheum. *13*: 754, 1970.
7. Alepa, F. P., Zvaifler, N. J., and Sliwinski, A. J.: Arthritis Rheum. *18*: 754, 1970.
8. Arinoviche, R., and Loewi, G.: Ann. Rheum. Dis. *29*:32, 1970.
9. Arrigoni-Martelli, E., and Bramm, E.: Agents Actions *5*:264, 1975.
10. Arrigoni-Martelli, E., Schiatti, P., and Selva, D.: Pharmacol. Res. Commun. *3*:239, 1971.
11. Ashtone, H.: Adverse Drug React. Bull. *28*:80, 1971.
12. Auerbach, C.: Ann. N. Y. Acad. Sci. *68*:731, 1958.
13. Bach, J. F., Dardenne, M., and Fourmier, C.: Nature *222*:998, 1969.
14. Bach, J. F., and Dardenne, M.: Rev. Eur. Etud. Clin. Biol. *16*:770, 1971.
15. Beck, F. J., Levy, C., and Whitehouse, M. W.: Br. J. Pharmacol. *49*:293, 1973.
16. Bennett, L. L., and Allan, P. W.: Cancer Res. *31*:152, 1971.
17. Berenbaum, M. C.: Biochem. Pharmacol. *11*:29, 1962.
18. Berenbaum, M. C.: Nature *196*:384, 1962.
19. Berenbaum, M. C.: Nature *198*:606, 1963.
20. Berenbaum, M. C.: Br. Med. Bull. *21*:140, 1965.
21. Berenbaum, M. C.: Br. J. Cancer *23*:426, 1969.
22. Berenbaum, M. C.: Nature *225*:550, 1970.
23. Berenbaum, M. C.: Clin. Exp. Immunol. *8*:1, 1971.
24. Berenbaum, M. C.: Prog. Immunol. *5* (II) : 233, 1974.
25. Berenbaum, M. C.: In "Clinical Aspects of Immunology," P. G. H. Gell, R. R. A. Coombs, and P. J. Lachmann, eds. Blackwell, Oxford, 1975, p. 689.
26. Berenbaum, M. C., and Brown, I. N.: Immunology *7*:65, 1964.
27. Berenbaum, M. C., and Brown, I. N.: Immunology *8*:251, 1965.
28. Berenbaum, M. C., Timmis, G. M., and Brown, I. N.: Immunology *13*:517, 1967.
29. Bieber, S., Elion, G. B., Hitchings, G. H., Hooper, D. C., and Nathan, H. C.: Proc. Soc. Exp. Biol. Med. *111*:334, 1962.
30. Blomgren, S. E., Wolberg, W. H., and Kisken, W. A.: Cancer Res. *25*: 977, 1965.
31. Boesen, E., and Davis, W.: "Cytotoxic Drugs in the Treatment of Cancer." E. Arnold, London, 1969.
32. Bonney, W. W., Feldbush, T. L., and Neufeld, S. E.: J. Pharmacol. Exp.

Ther. *190*:576, 1974.
33. Borek, F.: Int. Arch. Allergy Appl. Immunol. *34*:479, 1968.
34. Borel, Y., Fauconnet, M., and Miescher, P. A.: Int. Arch. Allergy Appl. Immunol. *33*:583, 1968.
35. Boyd, W. C.: "Fundamentals of Immunology." Interscience, New York, 4th edition, 1966.
36. Brambilla, G.: Cancer Res. *30*:2665, 1970.
37. Brandner, G., and Kröger, H.: Biochem. Pharmacol. *17*:13, 1968.
38. Brandriss, M. W., Smith, J. W., and Friedman, R. M.: Ann. N. Y. Acad. Sci. *122*:356, 1965.
39. Brown, J. H., Schwartz, N. L., MacKey, H. K., and Murray, H. L.: Arch. Int. Pharmacodyn. Ther. *183*:1, 1970.
40. Bruce, W. R.: Can. Cancer Conf. *7*:53, 1967.
41. Brumer, K. T., Mauel, J., Cerottini, J. C., and Chapuis, B.: Immunology *14*:181, 1968.
42. Buskirk, H. H., Crim, J. A., Petering, H. G., Merritt, K., and Johnson, A. G.: J. Natl. Cancer Inst. *34*:747, 1965.
43. Calne, D. B., and Leibowitz, S.: Nature *197*:1309, 1963.
44. Caron, G. A.: In "Proceedings, 3rd Annual Leucocyte Culture Conference," W. O. Rieke, ed. Appleton, New York, 1969, p. 287.
45. Claman, H. N.: N. Engl. J. Med. *287*:388, 1972.
46. Cooperating Clinics Committee of the American Rheumatism Association: N. Engl. J. Med. *283*:883, 1970.
47. Cooperating Clinics Committee of the American Rheumatism Association: Arthritis Rheum. *15*:434, 1972.
48. Craig, S. R., and Rosenberg, E. W.: Arch. Dermatol. *103*:505, 1971.
49. Currey, H. L. F.: Clin. Exp. Immunol. *9*:879, 1971.
50. d'Arcy Hart, P., Rees, R. I. W., and Niven, J. S. F.: Clin. Exp. Immunol. *3*:91, 1968.
51. David, J. R.: J. Exp. Med. *122*:1125, 1965.
52. Davies, G. E.: Immunology *14*:396, 1968.
53. De Vita, V. T., Serpick, A. A., and Carbone, P. P.: Ann. Intern. Med. *73*: 881, 1970.
54. Denman, E. J., Denman, A. M., Greenwood, B. M., Gall, D., and Heath, R. B.: Ann. Rheum. Dis. *29*:220, 1970.
55. Deuschle, K. W., and Wiggins, W. S.: Blood *8*:576, 1953.
56. Di Paolo, J. A., and Elis, J.: Teratology *3*:53, 1970.
57. Dixon, R. O.: Cancer Chemother. Rep. *2*:61, 1971.
58. Doak, P. B., Montgomeric, J. Z., North, J. D. K., and Smith, F.: Br. Med. J. *4*:746, 1968.
59. Dobbs, J., Riviero, I., Sabb, F., and Lee, S. L.: Immunol. *14*:213, 1968.
60. Dodson, W. H., and Bennett, J. C.: J. Clin. Pharmacol. *9*:251, 1969.
61. Doll, R., and Kinlen, L.: Br. Med. J. *4*:420, 1970.
62. Dowling, M. D., Krakoff, I. H., and Karnofsky, D. A.: In "Chemotherapy of Cancer," H. E. Cole, ed. Lea and Febiger, Philadelphia, 1970, p. 1.
63. Dukor, P., and Dietrich, F. M.: Int. Arch. Allergy Appl. Immunol. *34*:32, 1968.
64. Elion, C. B.: Fed. Proc. *26*:918, 1967.
65. Elion, G. B., Burgi, E., and Hitchings, G.: J. Am. Chem. Soc. *74*:411, 1952.
66. Etheridge, E. E., Shons, A., Harris, N., and Najavian, J. S.: Transplanta-

tion *11*:353, 1971.

67. Evans, J. S., Musser, E. A., Bostwick, L., and Mengel, G. D.: Cancer Res. *24*:1293, 1964.
68. Fahey, J. C.: Ann. Intern. Med. *75*:310, 1971.
69. Fairley, K. F., Barvie, J. U., and Johnson, W.: Lancet *1*:568, 1972.
70. Fischer, D. S., Cassidy, E. P., and Welch, A. D.: Biochem. Pharmacol. *15*: 1013, 1966.
71. Fischer, D. S., and Gershon, R. K.: Clin. Res. *14*:331, 1966.
72. Florsheim, G.: Experientia *19*:546, 1963.
73. Florsheim, G.: Helv. Physiol. Pharmacol. Acta *22*:241, 1964.
74. Fox, B. W., and Fox, M.: Pharmacol. Rev. *19*:21, 1967.
75. Freireich, E. J., Gehan, E. A., Rall, D. P., Schmidt, L. H., and Skipper, H. E.: Cancer Chemother. Rep. *50*:219, 1966.
76. Frenger, W., Witte, S., and Stafilidis, S.: Med. Exp. *7*:45, 1962.
77. Frenkel, E. P., and Stone, M. J.: Adv. Intern. Med. *17*:21, 1971.
78. Friedman, R. M., Buckler, C. E., and Baron, S.: J. Exp. Med. *114*:173, 1961.
79. Fries, J. F., Sharp, G. C., and McDevitt, H. O.: Clin. Res. *18*:134, 1970.
80. Frisch, A. W., and Davies, G. H.: J. Immunol. *88*:269, 1962.
81. Frisch, A. W., Davies, G. H., and Melstein, V.: J. Immunol. *89*:300, 1962.
82. Fosdick, W. M., Parson, J. L., and Hill, D. F.: Arthritis Rheum. *11*:151, 1968.
83. Fosdick, W. M., Parson, J. L., and Hill, D. F.: Arthritis Rheum. *12*:663, 1969.
84. Gabrielsen, A. E., and Good, R. A.: Adv. Immunol. *6*:91, 1967.
85. Gebhardt, D. O. E.: Teratology *3*:273, 1970.
86. Gill, P. G. H., Coombs, R. R. A., and Cachmann, P. J.: "Clinical Aspects of Immunology," 3rd edition. Blackwell, Oxford, 1975.
87. Geller, B. D., and Speirs, R. S.: Immunology *15*:707, 1968.
88. Gilsenbach, H., Rübner, H., and Albers, P.: Z. Immunitaetsforsch. *141*: 223, 1971.
89. Glenn, E. M., and Rohloff, N.: Am. J. Vet. Res. *26*:1180, 1965.
90. Glynn, J. P., Bianco, A. R., and Goldin, A.: Nature *198*:1003, 1963.
91. Glynn, L. E., and Holborow, E. J.: "Antoimmunity and Disease," 2nd edition. Blackwell, Oxford, 1974.
92. Goebel, K. M., Goebel, F. D., Gassell, W. D., Neitzert, A., and Mueller, K.: Klin. Wochenschr. *52*:916, 1974.
93. Goebel, K. M., Janzen, R., Joseph, K., and Börngen, U.: Eur. J. Clin. Pharmacol. *9*:405, 1976.
94. Goodell, B. W., Jacobs, J. B., and Powell, R. D.: Ann. Intern. Med. *72*:337, 1970.
95. Gray, C. D., and Mickelson, M. M.: Immunology *19*:417, 1970.
96. Gray, C. D., and Mickelson, M. M.: Transplantation *9*:176, 1970.
97. Gray, C. D., Mickelson, M. M., and Crim, J. A.: Transplantation *6*:805, 1968.
98. Greenberg, L. H., and Tanaka, K. R.: J. Am. Med. Assoc. *188*:423, 1964.
99. Greig, M. E., Gibbons, A. J., and Elliot, G. A.: J. Pharmacol. Exp. Ther. *173*:85, 1970.
100. Gordon, R. O., Wade, M. E., and Mitchell, M. S.: J. Immunol. *103*:233, 1969.

101. Gubner, R., August, S., and Ginsberg, V.: Am. J. Med. Sci. *221*:176, 1951.
102. Hansen, H. J., Vandevoorde, J. P., Bennett, K. J., Giles, W. G., and Nadler, S. B.: J. Lab. Clin. Med. *63*:801, 1964.
103. Harris, C. C.: Arch. Dermatol. *103*:501, 1971.
104. Harris, G.: J. Exp. Med. *127*:675, 1968.
105. Harris, J. E., and Hersh, E. M.: Cancer Res. *28*:2432, 1968.
106. Harrison, E. F., and Fuquay, M. E.: Proc. Soc. Exp. Biol. Med. *139*:957, 1972.
107. Heppner, G. H., and Calabresi, P.: J. Natl. Cancer Inst. *48*:1161, 1972.
108. Hersh, E. M., and Bodey, G. P.: Transplant. Proc. *5*:1155, 1973.
109. Hersh, E. M., Carbone, P. P., and Freireich, E. J.: Cancer Res. *25*:997, 1965.
110. Hersh, E. M., Carbone, P. P., and Freireich, E. J.: J. Lab. Clin. Med. *67*: 566, 1966.
111. Hersh, E. M., and Freireich, E. J.: In "Methods in Cancer Research," Vol. 4, H. Bush, ed. Academic Press, New York, 1968, p. 355.
112. Hersh, E. M., and Freireich, E. J.: Meth. Cancer Res. *4*:356, 1968.
113. Hersh, E. M., Wong, V. G., and Freireich, E. J.: Blood *27*:38, 1966.
114. Hobart, M. J., and McConnelly, I.: "The Immune System," Blackwell, Oxford, 1975.
115. Hoover, R., and Fraumeni, J. F.: Lancet *2*:57, 1973.
116. Hunter, T., Urowitz, M. B., Gordon, D. A., Smythe, H. A., and Ogryzlo, M. A.: Arthritis Rheum. *18*:15, 1975.
117. Hurd, E. R., and Ziff, M.: J. Exp. Med. *128*:785, 1968.
118. Jackson, S.: Pharmacol. Rev. *11*:135, 1959.
119. Jackson, S.: Br. Med. Bull. *20*:107, 1964.
120. Jackson, H., Fox, B. W., and Craig, A. W.: J. Reprod. Fertil. *2*:447, 1961.
121. Janssen, R. J., Marshall, R. G., Gerone, P. J., and Cheville, N. F.: J. Infect. Dis. *111*:155, 1962.
122. Jarlov, N. V., and Sorensen, K.: Ugeskr. Laeger. *133*:587, 1971.
123. Jimenez-Diaz, C., Lopez-Garcia, E., and Merchante, M.: J. Am. Med. Assoc. *147*:1418, 1951.
124. Johnson, J. M., and Bergel, F.: In "Metabolic Inhibitors." Academic Press, New York, 1963.
125. Kalliomäki, J. L., Saarimaa, H. A., and Towanen, P.: Ann. Rheum. Dis. *23*:78, 1964.
126. Kaplan, S., and Calabresi, P.: Clin. Res. *13*, 543, 1965.
127. Kaplan, S., Northrup, J., De Conti, R. C., and Calabresi, P.: Clin. Res. *14*:483, 1966.
128. Katz, S. I., Parker, D., Somer, G., and Turk, J. L.: Nature *248*:612, 1974.
129. Kerckhaert, J. A. M., van den Berg, C. J., and Willers, J. M. N.: Ann. Immunol. *125C*:415, 1974.
130. Khan, A., and Hill, J. M.: J. Immunol. *104*:679, 1970.
131. Khan, A., Hill, J. M., and Adachi, M.: J. Immunol. *105*:256, 1970.
132. Kilshaw, P. J., Brent, L., and Pinto, M.: Nature *255*:489, 1975.
133. Kiskin, W. A.: Arch. Surg. *92*:386, 1966.
134. Koltai, M., and Minker, E.: Eur. J. Pharmacol. *6*:175, 1969.
135. Komarek, A., and Dietrich, F. M.: Arch. Int. Pharmacodyn. Ther. *193*: 249, 1971.
136. Lagrange, P. H., Mackaness, G. B., and Miller, T. E.: J. Exp. Med. *139*:

1529, 1974.

137. Law, L. W.: Fed. Proc. *29*:171, 1970.

138. Lemmel, E., Hurd, E. R., and Ziff, M.: Clin. Exp. Immunol. *8*:355, 1971.

139. Lenz, W.: Am. J. Dis. Child. *112*:99, 1966.

140. Levin, R. H., Landy, M., and Frei, E.: N. Engl. J. Med. *271*:16, 1964.

141. Levy, L.: Proc. Soc. Exp. Biol. Med. *114*:47, 1963.

142. Levy, D.: Arch. Int. Pharmacodyn. Ther. *211*:8, 1974.

143. Levy, J.: In "Immunopharmacology," M. E. Rosenthale and H. C. Hansmann, Jr., eds. Spectrum Publication, Inc., New York, 1976, p. 205.

144. Levy, J., Paulus, H. E., Barnett, E. V., Sokoloff, M., Pearson, C. M., and Bangert, R.: Arthritis Rheum. *15*:116, 1972.

145. Lidsky, M. D., Sharp, J. T., and Biling, S.: Arthritis Rheum. *16*:148, 153.

146. Maguire, H. C., and Ettore von L.: J. Invest. Dermatol. *48*:39, 1967.

147. Maibach, H. I., and Epstein, W. L.: Int. Arch. Allergy Appl. Immunol. *27*:102, 1965.

148. Maibach, H. I., and Maguire, H. C.: Int. Arch. Allergy Appl. Immunol. *29*:209, 1966.

149. Malmgren, R. A., Bennison, B. E., and McKinley, T. W., Jr.: Proc. Soc. Exp. Biol. Med. *79*:484, 1952.

150. Mannick, J. A.: Surgery *67*:711, 1970.

151. Many, A., and Schwartz, R. S.: Clin. Exp. Immunol. *6*:87, 1970.

152. Many, A., and Schwartz, R. S.: Proc. Exp. Biol. Med. *133*:754, 1970.

153. Marz, H. J., Dinsdale, H. B., and Marvin, P. A. F.: Ann. Intern. Med. *75*: 77, 1971.

154. Mason, M., Currey, H. L. F., Barnes, C. G., Dume, J. F., Hazaleman, B. L., and Strickland, I. D.: Br. Med. J. *1*:420, 1969.

155. Meadow, S. R., Weller, R. O., and Archibald, R. W. R.: Lancet *2*:876, 1969.

156. Meeker, W. R., Condie, R. M., Good, R. A., and Varco, R. L.: Ann. N. Y. Ac. Sci. *87*:203, 1960.

157. Merritt, K., and Johnson, A. G.: J. Immunol. *91*:266, 1963.

158. Miescher, P. A.: In "6th International Symposium on Immunopathology." Schwabe, Basel, 1971.

159. Miller, D. G.: J. Am. Med. Assoc. *217*:1662, 1971.

160. Miller, J. J., and Cole, L. J.: J. Exp. Med. *125*:109, 1967.

161. Miller, J. J., and Cole, L. J.: Proc. Soc. Exp. Biol. Med. *133*:190, 1970.

162. Miller, J. J., Williams, G. F, and Leissiring, J. C.: Am. J. Med. *50*:530, 1971.

163. Mitchell, M. S., and De Conti, R. S.: *Cancer* 26:884, 1970.

164. Mitchell, M., Kaplan, S., Robb, B., De Conti, R. C., and Calabresi, P.: Proc. Am. Assoc. Cancer Res. *8*:47, 1967.

165. Mitchell, M., Wade, M. E., De Conti, R. C., Bertino, J. R., and Calabresi, P.: Ann. Intern. Med. *70*:535, 1969.

166. Miuro, M.: Cancer Res. *31*:114, 1971.

167. Murphy, M. L., Del Moro, A., and Lacon, C.: Ann. N. Y. Ac Sci. *68*:762, 1958.

168. Nathan, H. C., Bieber, S., Elion, G. B., and Hitchings, G. H.: Proc. Soc. Exp. Biol. Med. *107*:796, 1961.

169. Ohno, R., and Hersh, E. M.: Cancer Res. *30*:1605, 1970.

170. Owens, A. H., and Santos, G. W.: Transplantation *2*:378, 1971.

171. Page, A. R., Condie, R. M., and Good, R. A.: Am. J. Pathol. *40*:519, 1962.
172. Page, A. R., Condie, R. M., and Good, R. A.: Blood *20*:118, 1962.
173. Page, A. R., Condie, R. M., and Good, R. A.: Am. J. Med. *36*:200, 1964.
174. Parker, C. W., and Vavra, J. D.: Prog. Hematol. *6*:1, 1969.
175. Paterson, P. Y.: J. Immunol. *106*:1473, 1971.
176. Paterson, P. Y., and Drobish, D. G.: Science *165*:191, 1969.
177. Paterson, P. Y., Drobish, D. G., and Biddick, A. S.: J. Immunol. *106*:570, 1971.
178. Paterson, P. Y., and Hanson, M. A.: J. Immunol. *103*:795, 1969.
179. Paterson, P. Y., Hanson, M. A., and Gerner, E. W.: Proc. Soc. Exp. Biol. Med. *124*:928, 1967.
180. Patkowski, J.: J. Pharm. Pharmacol. *20*:957, 1968.
181. Penn, I., Halgrimson, C. G., and Starzl, T. E.: Transplant, Proc. *3*:773, 1971.
182. Perkins, E. H., Sado, T., and Makinodan, T.: J. Immunol. *103*:668, 1969.
183. Perper, R. J., Alvarez, B., Colombo, C., and Schroder, H.: Proc. Soc. Exp. Biol. Med. *137*:506, 1971.
184. Phillips, S. M., and Zweiman, B.: Fed. Proc. *29*:701, 1970.
185. Piliero, S. J., Graeme, M. L., Sigg, E. B., Chinea, G., and Colombo, C.: Life Sci. *5*:1057, 1966.
186. Polak, L., and Turk, J. L.: Nature *249*:654, 1974.
187. Polak, L.: Clin. Exp. Immunol. *19*:543, 1975.
188. Polak, L., Geleick, H., and Turk, J. L.: Immunology *28*:939, 1975.
189. Polak, L., and Turk, J. L.: Clin. Exp. Immunol. *4*:423, 1969.
190. Porter, K. A., Calne, R. Y., and Zukoski, C. G.: Lab. Invest. *13*:809, 1964.
191. Possanza, G. J., and Stewart, P. B.: Clin. Exp. Immunol. *6*:291, 1970.
192. Poulter, L. W., and Turk, J. L.: Nature (New Biol.) *238*:17, 1972.
193. Prager, M. D., and Derr, I.: Nature *225*:952, 1970.
194. Quagliata, F., Phillips-Quagliata, J. M., and Florsheim, G.: Fed. Proc. *30*:456 (Abstr.), 1971.
195. Rapaport, F. T., and Dansset, J. (Eds.): "Human Transplantation." Grune and Stratton, New York, 1968.
196. Rapaport, F. T., Shimada, T., and Watanabe, K.: Fed. Proc. *30*:456 (Abstr.), 1971.
197. Rau, R.: Dtsch. Med. Wochenschr. *96*:992, 1971.
198. Reiner, J., and Sontham, C. M.: Nature *210*:429, 1966.
199. Richter, P., Calamera, J. C., Morgenfeld, M. C., Kierszenbaum, A. L., Lavieri, J. C., and Mancini, R. E.: Cancer *25*:1026, 1970.
200. Rosenthale, M. E., and Gluckman, M. I.: Experientia *24*:1229, 1968.
201. Rosenthale, M. E., Datko, L. J., Kassarich, J., and Schneider, F.: Arch. Int. Pharmacodyn. Ther. *179*:251, 1969.
202. Rosenthale, M. E., Datko, L. J., Kassarich, J., and Rosanaff, E.: J. Pharmacol. Exp. Ther. *180*:501, 1972.
203. Rosenthale, M. E., and Nagra, C. L.: Proc. Soc. Exp. Biol. Med. *125*:149, 1967.
204. Salvin, S. B., and Liauw, H. L.: J. Immunol. *101*: 33, 1968.
205. Sanderson, R. P., McKenna, J. M., and Blakemore, W. S.: Nature *205*: 479, 1965.
206. Santos, G. W.: Fed. Proc. *26*:907, 1967.
207. Schein, P. S., Davis, R. D., Carter, S., Newman, J., Schein, D. R., and

Rall, D. P.: Clin. Pharmacol. Ther. *11*:3, 1970.

208. Scheinman, J. L., and Stamler, F. W.: J. Pediatr. *74*:117, 1969.
209. Schneck, S. A., and Penn, I.: Lancet *1*:983, 1971.
210. Shotton, D., and Movie, I. W.: J. Am. Med. Assoc. *186*:74, 1963.
211. Schwartz, R. S.: Prog. Allergy *9*:246, 1965.
212. Schwartz, R. S. (Ed.) : Fed. Proc. *26*:879, 1967.
213. Schwartz, R. S.: Fed. Proc. *26*:914, 1967.
214. Schwartz, R. S.: In "Human Transplantation," F. T. Rapaport and J. Dausset, eds. Grune and Stratton, New York, 1968, p. 440.
215. Schwartz, R. S.: Nature *224*:275, 1969.
216. Schwartz, R. S., and Borel, Y.: In "Textbook of Immunopathology," P. A. Miescher and H. J. Müller-Eberhard, eds. Grune and Stratton, New York, 1970, p. 227.
217. Schwartz, R. S., and Dameshek, W.: J. Clin. Invest. *39*:952, 1960.
218. Schwartz, R. S., Eisner, A., and Dameshek, W.: J. Clin. Invest. *38*:1394, 1959.
219. Skoglund, R. R., Schanberger, J. E., and Kaplan, J. M.: Am. J. Dis. Child. *121*:531, 1971.
220. Sokal, J. E., and Lessmann, E. M.: J. Am. Med. Assoc. *172*:1765, 1960.
221. Spiegelberg, H. L., and Miescher, P. A.: J. Exp. Med. *118*:869, 1963.
222. Stevens, J. E., and Willoughby, D. A.: J. Pathol. *97*:367, 1969.
223. Stewart, P. B., and Bell, R.: J. Immunol. *105*:1271, 1970.
224. Stewart, P. B., and Cohen, V.: Science *164*:1082, 1969.
225. Strong, J. S., Bartholemew, B. A., and Smyth, C. J.: Ann. Rheum. Dis. *32*:233, 1973.
226. Surjan, M., and Surjan, L., Jr.: Z. Immunitaetsforsch. *140*:366, 1970.
227. Sutton, W. T., Van Hagen, F., Griffith, H. B., and Preston, F. W.: Arch. Surg. *87*:840, 1963.
228. Swanson, M., and Schwartz, R. S.: N. Engl. J. Med. *227*:163, 1967.
229. Syeklocha, D., Simonovitch, L., Till, J. E., and McCulloch, E. A.: J. Immunol. *97*:472, 1966.
230. Thomson, J. D., and Austin, R. W.: Proc. Soc. Exp. Biol. Med. *111*:121, 1962.
231. Tripathy, S. P., and Mackaness, G. B.: J. Exp. Med. *130*:1, 1969.
232. Trnavsky, K., and Lapárová, V.: Med. Pharmacol. Exp. *16*:171, 1967.
233. Turk, J. L.: Int. Arch. Allergy Appl. Immunol. *24*:191, 1964.
234. Turk, J. L.: "Delayed Hypersensitivity." North Holland, Amsterdam, 1967.
235. Turk, J. L., and Parker, D.: Immunology *24*:751, 1973.
236. Turk, J. L., and Poulter, L. W.: Clin. Exp. Immunol. *10*:285, 1972.
237. Turk, J. L., and Willoughby, D. A.: Lancet *1*:249, 1967.
238. Urowitz, M. B., Gordon, D. A., Smythe, H. A., Pruzanski, W., and Ogryzlo, M. A.: Arthritis Rheum. *3*:419, 1971.
239. Urowitz, M. B., Hunter, T., Bookmann, A. A. M., Gordon, A. D., Smythe, H. A., and Ogryzlo, M. A.: J. Rheumatol. *1*:274, 1974.
240. Urso, P., and Makinodan, T.: J. Immunol. *90*:897, 1963.
241. Uteshev, B. S., Pinegin, B. V., Babichev, V. A., and Kalinkovich, A. G.: Zh. Mikrobiol. Epidemiol. Immunobiol. *46*:136, 1969.
242. Uy, Q. L., Srinivasin, T., Santos, G. W., and Owens, A. H., Jr.: Exp. Hematol. *10*:5, 1966.
243. Uyeki, E. M.: Biochem. Pharmacol. *16*:53, 1967.

244. Uyeki, E. M., and Long, J.: J. Pharmacol. Exp. Ther. *158*:365, 1967.
245. Vanselow, N. A., Kelly, J. R., Meyers, M. C., and Johnson, A. G.: J. Allergy *37*:145, 1966.
246. Varkarakis, M. J., Sampson, D., Brede, H. D., and Murphy, G. P.: Transplantation *13*:42, 1972.
247. Vogel, G. L., and Calabresi, P.: Proc. Soc. Exp. Biol. Med. *131*:251, 1968.
248. Vogel, C. L., De Vita, V. T., Lisak, R. P., and Kies, M. W.: Cancer Res. *29*:2249, 1969.
249. Walker, D., Gill, J. J., and Carson, J. M.: J. Am. Med. Assoc. *215*:2084, 1971.
250. Walz, D. T., and Berkoff, C. E.: Proc. Exp. Biol. Med. *135*:760, 1970.
251. Walz, D. T., Di Martino, M. J., and Misher, A.: J. Pharmacol. Exp. Ther. *178*:223 1971.
252. Ward, P. A.: Am. J. Pathol. *64*:521, 1971.
253. Ward, J. R., Cloud, S., Kravitt, E. L., and Jones, R. S.: Arthritis Rheum. *7*:654, 1964.
254. Weir, D. M.: "Handbook of Experimental Immunology," 2nd edition. Blackwell, Oxford, 1973.
255. Weisberger, A. S., and Wolfe, S.: Fed. Proc. *23*:976, 1964.
256. Weitzel, G., Schneider, F., Fretzdorf, A. M., Seynsche, K., and Finger, H.: Hoppe-Seyler's Z. Physiol. Chem. *336*:271, 1964.
257. Weksler, M. E., and Weksler, B. B.: Immunology *21*:137, 1971.
258. Wheeler, G. P.: Fed. Proc. *26*:885, 1967.
259. Whittington, H.: Br. J. Pharmacol. *40*:167P, 1970.
260. Willoughby, D. A., Coote, E., and Turk, J. L.: J. Pathol. Bacteriol. *97*:295, 1969.
261. Wilson, D. B.: J. Exp. Med. *122*:167, 1965.
262. Wilson, J. D.: Immunology *21*:233, 1971.
263. Wong, K. T., Baron, S., Levy, H. B., and Ward, T. G.: Proc. Soc. Exp. Biol. Med. *125*:65, 1967.
264. Worth, P. H. L.: Br. Med. J. *3*:182, 1971.
265. Yu, D. T. Y., and Peter, J. B.: Semin. Arthritis Rheum. *4*:25, 1974.
266. Zweiman, B., and Phillips, S. M.: Science *169*:284, 1970.
267. Zweiman, B., and Silberg, D. H.: Int. Arch. Allergy. *41*:428, 1971.

Immunoregulant Agents

The term "immunoregulant" is used here to define compounds of various chemical structures, differing in their modes of action from traditional non-specific immunosuppressants and characterized by their discrete enhancement or inhibition of the cellular or humoral immune response.

Many laboratories are turning their attention to these compounds and a new generation of immunoregulants is likely to emerge soon. Some of them are undergoing intensive experimental and clinical evaluation as potential new antirheumatic agents. To further explore this area, new experimental assays must be developed to characterize the action on immune responses and the antiarthritic potential of these compounds.

A more valuable clinical feedback is also needed in order to understand "inter alia" the clinical significance of the parameters measured in the screening assays and the correlation of the animal models with human diseases.

The clinical evaluation of new agents of this type is likely to present new problems concerning, for instance, the parameters of disease activity to be measured, the selection of patients, the optimization of dosing regimens.

The nature of these new agents also requires extreme caution in the evaluation of toxicological aspects to avoid irreversible side effects and delayed carcinogenesis. Despite the many difficulties involved, efforts in this area will probably prove to be rewarding both in terms of expanded knowledge and clinical benefits.

A common feature of several of these compounds is their ability to enhance the cell-mediated immune response. If rheumatoid arthritis is regarded as a chronic inflammatory reaction maintained by the presence of an antigen and by the inability of the committed cells to remove or conceal the antigen, then stimulation of the immune system might be more beneficial than its suppression. There is some experimental evidence to support this hypothesis. For instance, D-penicillamine, an effective agent in the treatment of rheumatoid arthritis, has been shown to enhance cell-mediated immune responses (see Chapter 19) and an immunostimulant, levamisole has proved beneficial in rheumatoid patients.

This chapter presents a brief summary of the biological properties of those immunoregulants on which attention has been recently focused. Their chemical structures are reported in Fig. 40. In view of the large volume of data available on D-penicillamine, this compound, likely to be an immunoregulant, is discussed in a separate chapter.

1. LEVAMISOLE

Levamisole is a broad-spectrum antihelmintic agent now under extensive and intensive evaluation for its immunoregulant activities. It was originally found to increase or reduce the number of plaque-forming cells reacting to sheep red blood cells, depending on the dose and on the time of administration in relation to antigen stimulus (45). Levamisole enhances the pertussis vaccine reaction (5,17), the secondary lesions of adjuvant arthritis (4), the allogeneic stimulation in mixed lymphocyte cultures (58) and—under appropriate experimental conditions—the basal and lectin-stimulated incorporation of thymidine into rat lymphocytes (3). It shows, however, variable effects on human lymphocyte cultures stimulated by mitogens (51,56) and in the immune response to different ex-

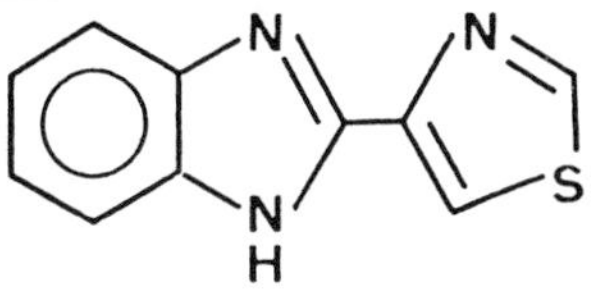

Thiabendazole

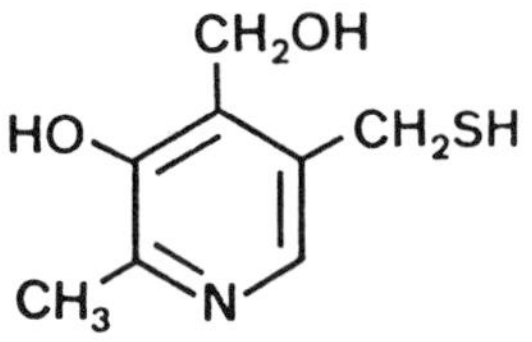

5-mercaptopyridoxine

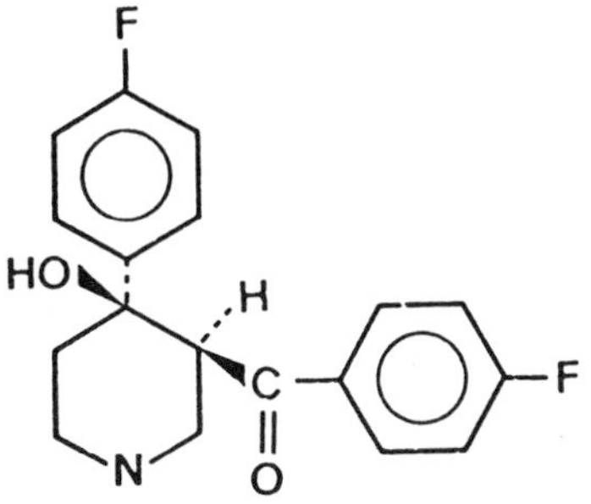

Flazalone

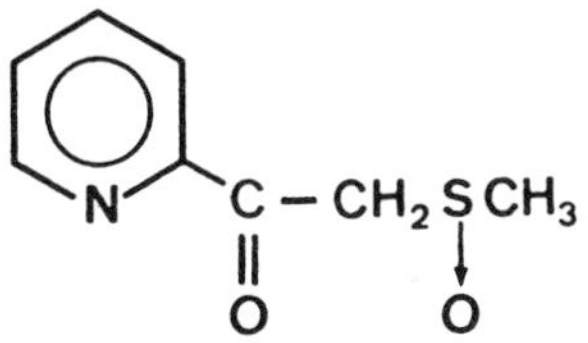

Oxisuran

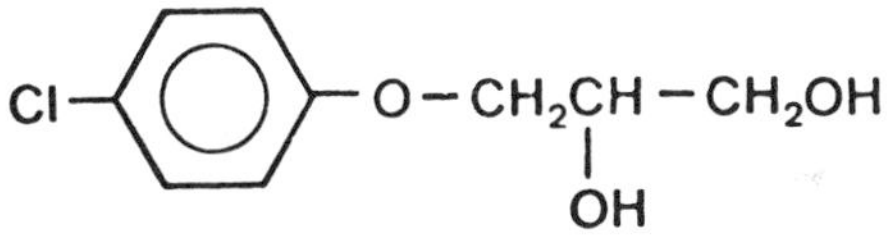

Chlorphenesin

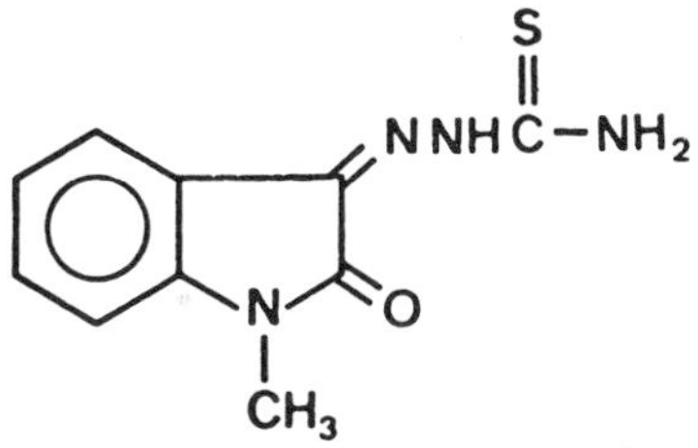

Methisazone

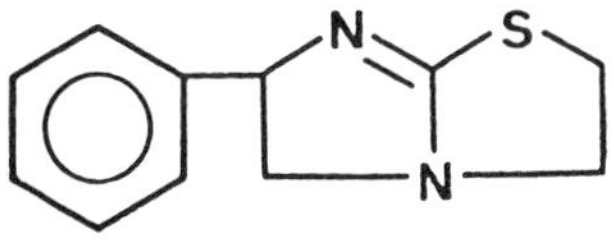

Levamisole

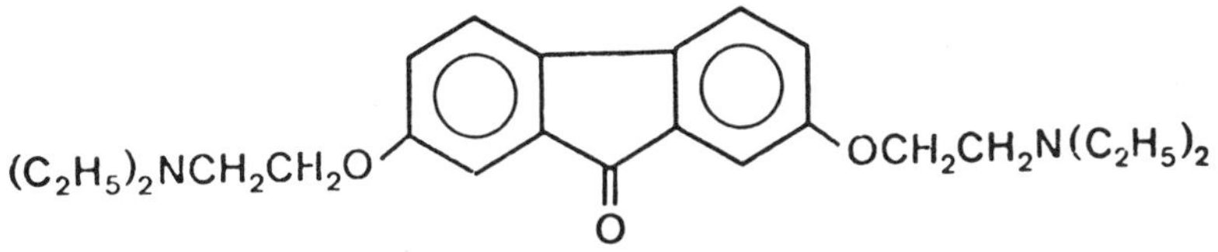

Tilorone

FIG. 40. Chemical structure of immunoregulants

perimental tumors (44). Other investigations indicate that levamisole inhibits metastases of cells transformed by herpes simplex virus (47) and prolongs the survival of leukemic mice (42). In man, it increases the delayed hypersensitivity skin recation to tuberculin and DNCB (8,52,54). Beneficial effects have been reported in patients with rheumatoid arthritis (27,48).

2. THIABENDAZOLE

This is an agent with broad-spectrum antihelmintic properties, currently under evaluation in immunological systems. It has been reported to exert moderate antiinflammatory and analgesic activity in man (10). In a model of delayed hypersensitivity reaction, the pertussis vaccine edema, it has been found to have an enhancing effect (3). Numerous thiabendazole analogs have been evaluated for their antiinflammatory effects: there appears to be no correlation of this activity with their antiparasitic or antifungal activities.

3. FLAZALONE

At a dose of 50-100 mg/kg, this drug inhibits a variety of experimental acute inflammations (carrageenin, yeast, dextran, serotonin edemas) but it is scarcely active in adjuvant arthritis. It inhibits the blueing reaction in passive cutaneous anaphylaxis in rat (3). It has no activity in experimental allergic encephalomyelitis, the Arthus reaction in rat, or the graft versus host reaction in mouse, but it inhibits DNA and RNA synthesis of lymphocytes in vitro at 0.5 mM (57).

4. OXISURAN

This compound has been described as a non-cytotoxic selective suppressant of cell-mediated hypersensitivity (22). In mice (22, 19) rats (19,26) and dogs (19), oxisuran significantly prolonged allograft survival, and in guinea pigs, mice, rats and rabbits it suppressed delayed skin reactions (20). Phytohemoagglutinin and one-way mixed lymphocyte reactions of cells from animals treated with oxisuran were found to be markedly depressed. Humoral antibody formation was not decreased (19,21,22,26). More detailed studies of the humoral response suggested that oxisuran acts on thymus-derived lymphocytes associated with cell-mediated immunity and immunological memory, to favor the latter activity rather than the former (18,19,21,22). Extensive pharmacokinetic and pharmacometabolic investigations performed in rat, dog, monkey and man (11,12,14,15) led to the identification of oxisuran metabolites: some of them, diasteroisomeric-reduced alcohols, have a simular activity as is oxisuran and one, a sulfone, has the opposite effect in enhancing both humoral antibody formation and allograft rejection. The plasma half-life of oxisuran is longer in man than in rat and dog. Preliminary investigations in man described a marked inhibition of cell-mediated immunity (prolongation of skin allograft survival) without evidence of cytotoxicity (43).

5. METHISAZONE

This antiviral drug is reported to be an inhibitor of the 7S and 19S antibody-forming cell responses to sheep red blood cells in mice, at daily doses of 25 μg. It also inhibits the reaction of hemopoietic-colony-forming cells to adjuvant stimulation in vivo, but has no effect on subsequent colony development (37). These findings suggest that methisazone interferes with specific stages of cellular differentiation.

6. CHLORPHENESIN

Chlorphenesin has been reported to suppress humoral antibody response, without affecting the antigenic priming of the immunocompetent cells (6,7). It also inhibits passive cutaneous anaphylaxis and elevates the level of cAMP in treated cells (35). Chlorphenesin has been shown to exert a therapeutic activity in several experimental tumors (49). It is non-cytotoxic but may enhance cell-mediated immune response of the host, possibly through an interference with the synthesis or binding of enhancing antibody to tumor cells.

7. TILORONE

Tilorone was first described as an orally and parenterally active broad-spectrum antiviral agent, its activity being associated with interferon induction (16,29,36,50). As interferon is one of the lymphokine components produced by sensitized lymphocytes, it is not surprising that tilorone and its analogs also influence lymphocytes in immunological systems. It has been reported that tilorone enhances the primary immune response to sheep red blood cells in mice, and the antibody response to several types of antigens (13, 25). In addition, evidence of antitumor activity has been presented (1,2). Cell-mediated immune responses associated with T-lymphocyte function, as in experimental allergic encephalomyelitis, tuberculin skin reaction, adjuvant arthritis, and transplant reaction are inhibited by tilorone administration (38,40). This compound has also been reported to prevent the inflammation elicited by non-immune agents (39). Tilorone induces a marked but transient lymphopenia, with depletion of lymphocytes in the T-cell areas of spleen, lymph node and Peyer's patches (33,59). Nude athymic mice failed to develop this effect (24). The antiviral activity detected in athymic mice was significant, although somewhat less than that found in treated normal mice (24). These findings suggest that the suppression of cell-mediated immunity is likely to depend on the specific effect on T lymphocytes. This effect may also be responsible for the stimulatory activity of tilorone on antibody response since it is known that certain T cells may inhibit the B-lymphocyte response to antigens.

8. OTHER POSSIBLE APPROACHES

Several other agents of a more or less complex nature have been described as being able to interfere by different and largely unknown mechanisms with the cellular and/or humoral components of the immune response.

In order to indicate some possible future research directions, a few of these agents are mentioned below.

5-Mercaptopyridoxine has a marginal B_6 antagonistic activity and an antiinflammatory effect. Like D-penicillamine, it enhances the delayed hypersensitivity response to pertussis vaccine and, under appropriate experimental conditions, the basal and lectin-stimulated thymidine incorporation into rat lymphocytes (3). A recent U.S. patent claims that 5-mercaptopyridoxine has a D-penicillamine-like antirheumatic action in man (28).

Ribonucleic acids and *polyanions RNA* exert broad effects on the immune response (23).Synthetic analogs amplify the antibody response, probably through an interference with cyclic nucletoides.

Poly I:Poly C is an interferon inducer in animals and is more active in man than Poly A:Poly U. This latter is, however, more effective in stimulating antibody production. Both these compounds and other polyanions seem to be B-cell mitogens (46,55).

Transfer factor. There are a number of reviews on this subject (9,31,32; see also Chapter 10). Briefly, transfer factor is a soluble product of activated lymphocytes. It acts as a de-repressor of a select small population of normal circulating lymphocytes which, after exposure to transfer factor become responsive to antigen, transform and undergo clonal proliferation. The factor thus transmits to a previously insensitized individual the immunological information necessary for the mobilization of a specific part of the immune system. Thus this individual, upon receipt of the transfer factor, is able to mount a strong secondary response upon his first exposure to the antigen.

In view of the above, attempts have been made to experiment with transfer factor in conditions related to defective cell-mediated immune responses (34,41,53) and it has been shown to be beneficial. More recently, improvement in the general conditions of patients with juvenile rheumatoid arthritis receiving transfer factor has been reported (30).

REFERENCES

1. Adamson, R. H.: Lancet *1*:398, 1971.
2. Adamson, R. H.: J. Natl. Cancer Inst. *46*:431, 1971.
3. Arrigoni-Martelli, E.: Unpublished.
4. Arrigoni-Martelli, E., Bramm, E.: Rheum. Rehabil. *15*:207, 1976.
5. Arrigoni-Martelli, E., Bramm, E., Huskisson, E. C., Willoughby, D. A., and Dieppe, P. A.: Agents Actions, *6*:613, 1976.
6. Berger, F. M., Fukin, G. M., De Angelo, H., and Chandlee, G. C.: J. Immunol. *102*:1024, 1969.
7. Berger, F. M., Kletzkin, M., and Spencer, H. J.: Fed. Proc. *31*:578, 1972.
8. Brugmans, J., Schuermans, Y., Re Cock, W., Thienpont, D., Janssen, P., Verhaegen, H., Van Nimmen, L., Lougwagie, A. C., and Stevens, E.: Life Sci. *13*:1499, 1973.
9. Burnet, F. M.: J. Allergy Clin. Immunol. *54*:1, 1974.
10. Campbell, W. C.: J. Am. Med. Assoc. *216*:2143, 1971.
11. Crew, M. C., Melgar, M. D., Haynes, L. J., Gala, R. L., and Di Carlo, F. J.: Xenobiotica *2*:431, 1972.
12. Crew, M. C., Vesel, E. S., Passananti, G. T., Gala, R. L., and Di Carlo, F. J.: Clin. Pharmacol. Ther. *14*:1013, 1973.
13. Diamantstein, T.: Immunology *24*:771, 1973.
14. Di Carlo, F. J., Crew, M. C., Haynes, L. J., and Gala, R. L.: Xenobiotica *2*: 159, 1972.

15. Di Carlo, F. J., Melgar, M. D., Haynes, L. J., and Crew, M. C.: J. Reticulo-endothel. Soc. *14*:387, 1973.
16. De Clercq, F., and Merigan, T. C.: J. Infect. Dis. *123*:190, 1971.
17. Dieppe, P. A., Willoughby, D. A., Huskisson, E. C., and Arrigoni-Martelli, E.: Agents Actions, *6*:618, 1976.
18. Fox, A. E., and Freedman, H. H.: J. Immunol. *112*:1394, 1974.
19. Fox, A. E., Gawlak, D. L., Ballantyne, D. L., and Freedman, H. H.: Transplantation *15*:389, 1973.
20. Fox, A. E., Gingold, J. L., and Freedman, H. H.: Infect. Immun. *8*:549, 1973.
21. Freedman, H. H., and Fox, A. E.: J. Reticuloendothel. Soc. *13*:33, 1973.
22. Freedman, H. H., Fox, A. E., Shavel, F., Jr., and Morrison, G. C.: Proc. Soc. Exp. Biol. Med. *139*:909, 1972.
23. Friedman H. (Ed.) : Ann. N. Y. Acad. Sci. *207*:1, 1973.
24. Gibson, J. P., Megel, H., Camyre, K. P., and Michael, J. G.: Proc. Soc. Exp. Biol. Med. *151*:264, 1976.
25. Hoffman, P. F., Ritter, H. W., and Krueger, R. F.: In "Advances in Antimicrobial and Antineoplastic Chemotherapy," M. Hejzlar, M. Semonsky, and S. Masak, eds. Urban and Schwarzenberg, Munich, 1972, p. 217.
26. Husberg, B., and Penn, L.: Proc. Soc. Exp. Biol. Med. *145*:669, 1974.
27. Huskisson, E. C., Scott, J., Balme, H. W., Dieppe, P. A., Trapanell, J., and Willoughby, D. A.: Lancet *1*:393, 1976.
28. Jaffe, I. A.: U. S. Pat. *3*:852, 454—1974.
29. Krueger, R. F., and Mayer, G. D.: Science *169*:1213, 1970.
30. Kass, E., Frøland, S. S., Natvig, J. B., Blichfeldt, P., Høyeraal, H. M., and Munthe, E.: Scand. J. Rheumatol. *3*:113, 1974.
31. Lawrence, H. S.: Adv. Immunol. *11*:195, 1969.
32. Lawrence, H. S.: N. Engl. J. Med. *283*:411, 1970.
33. Levin, S., Gibson, J. P., and Megel, H.: Proc. Soc. Exp. Biol. Med. *146*: 245, 1974.
34. Levin, A. S., Spitler, L. E., and Fundenberg, H. H.: Ann. Rev. Med. *24*: 175, 1973.
35. Malley, A., and Baecher, L.: J. Immunol. *107*:586, 1971.
36. Mayer, G. D., and Krueger, R. F.: Science *169*:1214, 1970.
37. McNeil, T. A., Fleming, W. A., McClure, S. F., and Kihen, M.: Antimicrob. Agents Chemother. *1*:1, 1972.
38. Megel, H., Raychaudhuri, A., Goldstein, S., Kinsolving, C. R., Shemano, I., and Michael, J. G.: Proc. Soc. Exp. Biol. Med. *145*:513, 1974.
39. Megei, H., Raychauduri, A., Shemano, I., Beaver, T. H., and Thomas, L. I.: Proc. Soc. Exp. Biol. Med. *149*:89, 1975.
40. Mobraaten, L. E., De Maeyer, E., and De Maeyer-Guignard, J.: Transplantation *16*:415, 1973.
41. Pabst, H. F., and Swanson, R.: Br. Med. J. *2*:442, 1972.
42. Perk, K., Chirigos, M. A., Fuhrman, F., and Pettigrew, H.: J. Natl. Cancer Inst. *54*:253, 1975.
43. Pirofsky, B., Nolte, M. T., and Baidana, E. J.: Transplant. Proc. *8(1)*:411, 1975.
44. Potter, C. W., Carr, I., Jennings, R., Rees, R. C., McGinty, F., and Richardson, V. M.: Nature *249*:567, 1974.
45. Renoux, G., and Renoux, M.: J. Immunol. *113*:779, 1974.

46. Rühl, H., Vogt, W., Bochart, G., and Diamantstein, T.: Immunology *26*: 937, 1974.
47. Sadowski, J. M., and Rapp, F.: Proc. Soc. Exp. Biol. Med. *149*:219, 1975
48. Schuermans, Y.: Lancet *1*:111, 1975.
49. Spencer, H. J., Runser, R. H., Berger, F. M., Tarnowski, G. S., and Mathé, G.: Proc. Soc. Exp. Biol. Med. *140*:1156, 1972.
50. Stringfellow, D. A., and Glasgow, C. A.: Antimicrob. Agents Chemother. *2*:73, 1972.
51. Thulin, H., Thestrup-Pedersen, K., and Ellegard, J.: Acta Allergol. (Kbh) *30*:9, 1975.
52. Tripodi, D., Parks, L. C., and Brugmans, J.: N. Engl. J. Med. *289*:354, 1973.
53. Vandvik, B., Frøland, S. S., Høyeraal, H. M., Stien, R., and Degré, M.: Scand. J. Immunol. *2*:367, 1973.
54. Verhaegen, H., Verbruggen, F., Verhaegen-Declercq, M. L., and De Cree, J.: Nouv. Presse Med. *9*:2483, 1974.
55. Vogt, W., Rühl, H., Wagner, B., and Diamantstein, T.: Eur. J. Immunol. *3*:493, 1973.
56. Wachi, K. K., Kimura, L. H., Perreiva, S., Yokama, Y., Perri, S., and Palumbo, N.: Res. Commun. Chem. Pathol. Pharmacol. *8*:681, 1974.
57. Whitehouse, M. W.: Proc. West. Pharmacol. Soc. *14*:55, 1971.
58. Woods, W., Fliegelman, M. J., and Chirigos, M. A.: Proc. Soc. Exp. Biol. Med. *148*:1048, 1975.
59. Zbinden, G., and Emch, E.: Acta Haematol. (Basel) *47*:49, 1972.

Chapter 19

D-Penicillamine

Penicillamine is so named because it is a degradation product of penicillin, prepared by hydrolysis. Chemically it is β, β-dimethylcysteine. It has been used for several years in heavy metal poisoning or cystinuria. Recently the D-isomer has developed into a widely investigated agent for the treatment of rheumatoid arthritis. D-Penicillamine is neither analgesic nor antiinflammatory. Its action is specific for rheumatoid arthritis and it does more than simply suppress the symptoms and signs of the disease (25). As mentioned in the previous chapter, experimental evidence suggests that D-penicillamine may be an immunoregulant and that this property may be relevant to its beneficial effects in rheumatoid arthritis (Fig. 41).

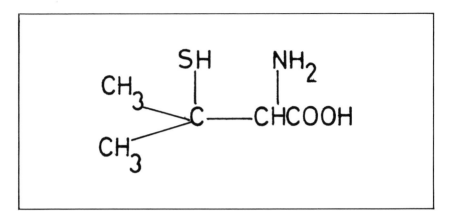

FIG. 41. Chemical structure of penicillamine

1. D-PENICILLAMINE IN RHEUMATOID ARTHRITIS AND OTHER RHEUMATIC DISEASES

The efficacy of D-penicillamine in rheumatoid arthritis was first reported in 1970 (38). In this study, its effects were evaluated in 49 patients with sustained disease activity. The treatment lasted at least 12 months and, in some cases, was reinstituted at variable intervals. The great majority of these treatment periods resulted in at least 50% improvement in the manifestations of active disease, accompanied by a fall in erythrocyte sedimentation rate and in the titer of rheumatoid factor (35). Changes in laboratory parameters occurred much later in some patients than did clinical improvement (38) which usually began after 3-4 months of treatment.

Several other clinical investigations reported encouraging results (13,19,30,49,68). In a double-blind parallel group trial of D-penicillamine and placebo, statistically significant or highly significant differences in favor of the drug were observed in terms of pain, duration of morning stiffness, grip strength, articular index and functional capacity (52). As a result of these experiences, D-penicillamine is not only being used more widely, but is currently being tried in patients with earlier, less debilitating forms of the disease (39).

D-penicillamine has also been compared with gold and the results obtained after 6-18 months of treatment were very similar (29). No significant differences were found between the clinical effects of D-penicillamine and azathioprine although there was a trend in favor of D-penicillamine (9). The latter was clearly superior to salicylates and prednisolone after 6 months of treatment (54). Other trials showed a reduction in the need for analgesic drugs and also corticosteroids in patients receiving D-penicillamine (19,38).

Moreover D-penicillamine is beneficial in some cases of palindromic rheumatism and ankylosing spondylitis (18). It has been claimed that it is effective in patients with active scleroderma (22) and in Still's disease but with a lower incidence of responses than in adult rheumatoid arthritis (61).

Non-articular manifestations of rheumatoid arthritis show improvement in patients receiving D-penicillamine; the size of rheumatoid nodules is reduced (30,38) and the Multicenter Trial Group noted improvement in tenosynovitis and lymphoadenopathy (52). Cardiac manifestations of rheumatic disease are not affected (3). Several authors have commented on the beneficial effects of D-penicillamine in patients with vasculitis (19,30,38) but controlled studies are lacking and are unlikely to be performed.

A proportion of patients (approximately 25%) fails to respond to D-penicillamine therapy. It is impossible to predict which subjects will fail to respond; no relation has been found between age, sex and duration of the disease (13,29). Seropositive patients respond as well as those who are seronegative (29). The dominant factor determining the results obtained is probably the severity of anatomical changes in the joints (13,19).

2. SIDE EFFECTS

Side effects are frequent in D-penicillamine-treated patients and are an important cause of therapy withdrawal. They are in general more likely to occur in the first few months of treatment and less so after 18 months. The Multicenter Trial Group noted an incidence of 63% in the first 3 months, compared to 34% in controls, while after 12 months, the incidence was equal in the two groups (52). Side effects are much more common in patients receiving D-penicillamine than in those on gold therapy during the first 3 months of treatment (29), subsequently, the incidence is similar in both groups. Withdrawal of patients from D-penicillamine therapy because of adverse reactions ranged from 26 to 47% after 12-18 months in three different clinical trials (15,26,52).

It has been observed that adverse reactions occur at predictable times during the course of treatment (25).

The more common side effect in the first few months of treatment is the so called "early rash" which resembles the allergic rash seen with other drugs, such as ampicillin (26). It is of interest in this connection that ampicillin yields appreciable amounts of penicillamine during its metabolic degradation (41,66). This early rash is generalized, morbilliform and itchy. It disappears within days after treatment discontinuation and does not occur when therapy is resumed at a low dose. Other types of rashes occurring later during treatment have been reported (7,23,55,65).

Gastrointestinal side effects are also common in the first few months of therapy but do not occur thereafter (29). They are quite unlike those produced by antiinflammatory drugs; very seldom does D-penicillamine initiate or exacerbate peptic ulceration (47). According to the Multicenter Trial Group, gastrointestinal disturbances are equally frequent in D-penicillamine- and placebo-treated patients (52).

Loss of taste is found in about 25% of cases in the first 2 months of treatment. Taste returns later whether D-penicillamine therapy is continued or not (36). Mouth ulcers are rare but may be severe when they occur and may lead to drug withdrawal (24,26).

Nephropathy and thrombocytopenia are fairly common problems in D-penicillamine therapy. About 15% of patients with rheumatoid arthritis develop proteinuria which begins after at least 4 months of treatment with this drug but seldom after more than 18 months. Of the patients who develop proteinuria, 30% will become nephrotic. Even if treatment is stopped as soon as proteinuria appears, it may take as long as a year for a complete recovery (30). It is unwise to continue D-penicillamine therapy in patients who become nephrotic and in those with proteinuria of 5 g daily or more (44). Proteinuria is usually caused by immune complex nephritis. Electronmicroscopy shows the presence of dense deposits on the surface of the basement membrane. Deposits of IgG and complement were also revealed by immunofluorescent staining (19,30,36).

A mean fall of 27% in the platelet count has been reported in patients receiving D-penicilamine. In many cases, platelet counts fall but never to a dangerous level and often recover even though the drug is continued (52).

Myasthenia gravis (6,12) and systemic lupus erythematosus (13) are rare complications and both rapidly respond to withdrawal of the drug.

3. DOSAGE

The rule that the starting dose of D-penicillamine should be 250 mg daily or less is absolute, because a few patients react even to this dose by high fever, acute dermatitis, persistent vomiting, thrombocytopenia or neutropenia. Violent reactions like these preclude further use of the drug by such hypersensitive patients. If tolerated, the dosage can be gradually increased at a two-weekly interval up to a maintenance dose, 1 g being sufficient for most patients (38,68). Slower introduction of D-penicillamine has been advocated since it was suggested that this reduced the incidence of side effects (15,24).

4. MODES OF ACTION

D-Penicillamine exerts a variety of biological actions and it is, therefore, extremely difficult but at same time rewarding, to determine which of these effects is responsible for its efficacy in rheumatoid arthritis.

D-Penicillamine chelates a number of metals, including copper, lead, mercury, gold, manganese, iron, zinc, and cadmium (60). It is, therefore, used in Wilson's disease (5,48), in patients with cystinuria (4) and in various types of heavy metal poisoning. Patients with rheumatoid arthritis and other inflammatory diseases have higher than normal levels of copper and ceruloplasmin (50). The more favorable results with D-penicillamine therapy were obtained in subjects with higher initial serum copper levels (50). However, copper supplement given with the drug did not affect the response (52) and changes in ceruloplasmin levels were not related to clinical improvement (68).

D-Penicillamine antagonizes pyridoxine (14,37,40). Both the chelation of copper and the antagonistic effect on pyridoxine could lead to a decreased production of rheumatoid factor. However, isoniazid, another antagonist of pyridoxine, did not cause any decrease in rheumatoid factor while the latter was reduced by a simultaneous administration of D-penicillamine and pyridoxine.

It is also known that D-penicillamine influences the maturation of collagen in the body, i.e., the transformation of neutral salt-soluble collagen into its non-soluble mature form (11,21,53). The cleavage of labile cross-links of newly formed collagen has obvious potential in scleroderma and it is possible that, in rheumatoid arthritis, benefit would accrue from preventing the collagen formation in inflamed joints. It would be difficult, however, to explain effects on extra-articular manifestations of the disease (25). Collagen-like protein is present in plasma of rheumatic patients, its level seems to correlate with the activity of the rheumatic process and it has the property of an antigen (45,51). It has been shown that the administration of D-penicillamine is followed by a decrease in the plasma level of the collagen-like protein (51).

In vitro or in the knee joint of a patient with rheumatoid arthritis, D-penicillamine promptly dissociated rheumatoid factor (32). Continued oral administration of the drug produced no effect at first, but later caused a slow reduction in the titer of rheumatoid factor, which persisted after therapy was discontinued (33). This pattern of titer change was then repeatedly observed and was often associated with clinical improvement and a return to normal values of parameters of disease activity (35). Many other investigations confirmed these findings and further suggested that prolonged administration of D-penicillamine to rheumatoid patients not only reduces rheumatoid factor, as determined serologically, but other classes of immunoglobulins as well (20,34,36,56,68). The pattern of reduction of rheumatoid factor suggests an effect on its production rather than on circulating macroglobulins (25,41). On the other hand, no correlation between changes in titer and clinical measurements of disease activity has been found (27,29,68). Rheumatoid factor may well be the result of the rheumatoid process rather than its cause and this explains why changes in rheumatoid factor follow improvement in the disease, produced by D-penicillamine.

There are certain similarities between the effects of D-penicillamine and immunosuppressive agents. All of these drugs suppress rheumatoid arthritis, diminish the requirement for other medication, reduce titers of rheumatoid factor and affect extra-articular manifestations of the disease.

An immunosuppressive effect of the racemate DL-penicillamine has been reported (31,63). Because of the different properties of L-penicillamine in intermediate metabolism (64), these observations cannot be compared to more recent findings showing no effect of D-penicillamine on the synthesis of hemoagglutinating antibodies and plaque-forming cells (58). However, a striking inhibition of immune rosette formation has been demonstrated (58). Reactions of D-penicillamine with cell surface structures or with components of the metabolism of cells involved in immunological processes are a likely possibility. Cultivated bone-marrow cells (62) and fibroblasts (43,46) are inhibited by D-penicillamine. HeLa cells also were dose-dependently inhibited by the drug (59). Moreover, it has been reported that D-penicillamine prevents the stimulation of human (42, 57) and murine (59) lymphocytes by phytohemoagglutinin and by mixed lymphocyte cultures. More recent findings suggest, however, a more complex interaction of this agent with the process of basal and lectin-stimulated incorporation of ^{3}H-thymidine into rat lymphocytes (10). The uptake of ^{3}H-thymidine by non-stimulated lymphocytes incubated for 48 hours with relatively high concentrations of D-penicillamine is enhanced. This affect is much more evident when the lymphocytes are preincubated for 24 hours with D-penicillamine, the drug is then removed and the cells cultured for an additional 48 hours. Concanavallin A stimulation is inhibited in the presence of D-penicillamine but is enhanced in preincubated lymphocytes. This inhibition does not seem to be concentration dependent, thus suggesting that it is probably due to a non-specific interference with binding of concanavallin A to the cell membrane (58). Since simple thiols, such as 2-mercaptoethanol, do not enhance concanavallin A stimulated ^{3}H-thymidine uptake in preincubation experiments but increase the basal uptake, a "thiol effect" cannot explain these findings. They suggest that D-penicillamine interferes with the functions of cells involved in immune responses (Fig. 42).

The results of in vivo experiments provide evidence that, under appropriate conditions, this drug is able to stimulate delayed hypersensitivity reactions. In fact, D-penicillamine, like levamisole, enhances the severity of the secondary lesions of adjuvant arthritis and increases their incidence (1) (Figs. 43 and 44).

A typical delayed hypersensitivity reaction, the skin response to tuberculin, is increased in rheumatoid patients treated with D-penicillamine (8).

Since there is much evidence to implicate delayed hypersensitivity as being partly responsible for the chronic inflammatory changes in rheumatoid arthritis (67), simple models of immunologically induced inflammation are being developed (2,3,16) as a testing ground for penicillamine-like drugs and to aid our understanding of their mode of action. These models—the pertussis vaccine-induced edema or pleurisy—have been described above (see Chapter 12). When administered around the sensitization or challenge times, D-penicillamine enhances the delayed hypersensitivity reaction but reduces the response when it is administered for relatively long periods prior to sensitization and continued throughout the reaction (2,3,16) (Figs. 45 and 46).

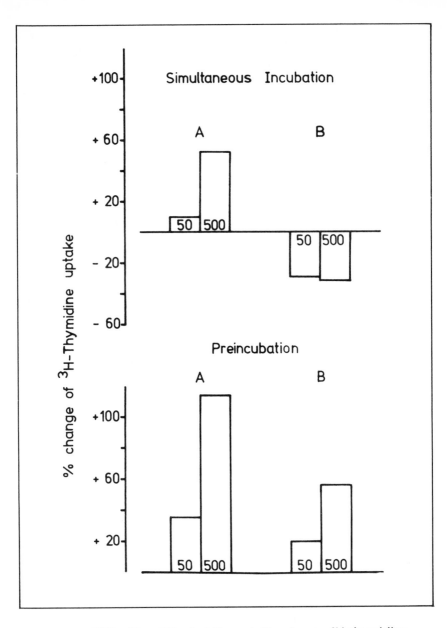

FIG. 42. Effect of D-penicillamine on ³H-thymidine uptake by rat lymphocytes
    A = Basal   B = Concanavallin A stimulated
The figures in the column indicate D-penicillamine concentrations (γ/ml)

FIG. 44. Effect of D-penicillamine and levamisole on the incidence of secondary lesions in adjuvant arthritis

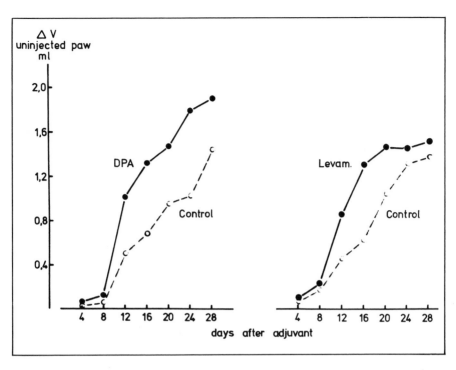

FIG. 43. Effect of D-penicillamine and levamisole on the severity of secondary lesions in adjuvant arthritis

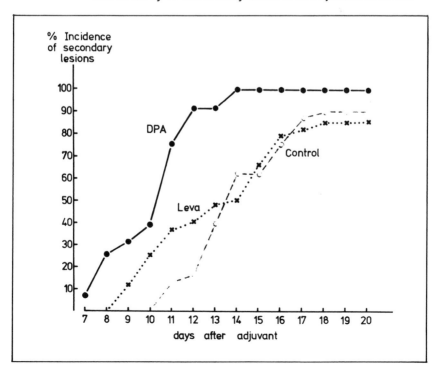

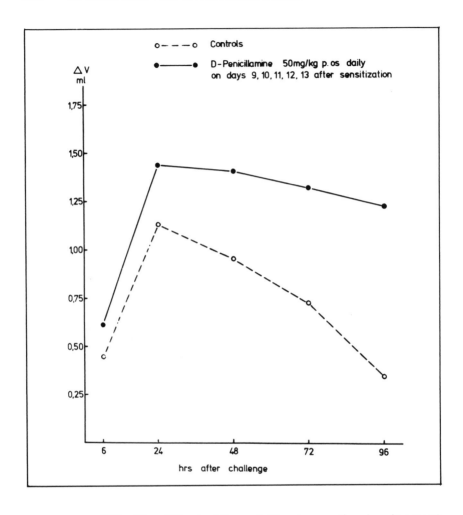

FIG. 45. Effect of D-penicillamine on the development of pertussis vaccine reaction

Levamisole, a known immunostimulant drug (17), efficacious in rheumatoid arthritis (28), exerts similar actions.

It seems, therefore, that D-penicillamine and levamisole may have a positive effect on some aspect of the immunological response. It may be speculated that such an effect is relevant to the therapeutic activity of these agents in rheumatoid arthritis.

It must be stressed, however, that the mode of action of D-pen-

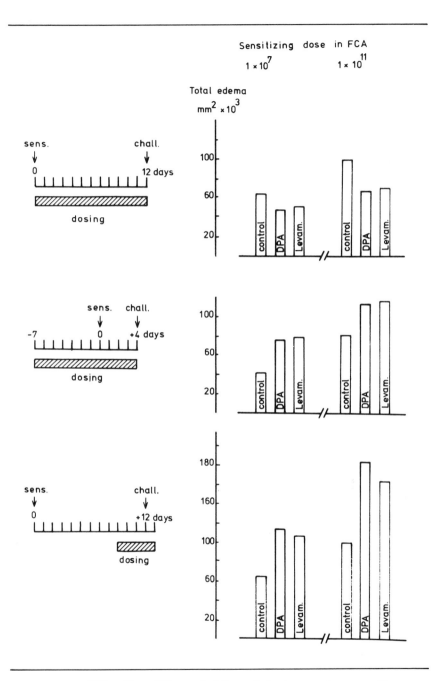

FIG. 46. Effect of different dosing regimens with D-penicillamine and levamisole on development of pertussis vaccine reaction in rats sensitized with high and low doses of antigen

icillamine is not yet clearly understood and remains open to many interpretations.

It is hoped that further research on D-penicillamine shall open the way for the development of other drugs with a specific effect in rheumatoid arthritis.

REFERENCES

1. Arrigoni-Martelli, E., and Bramm, E.: Agents Action *5*:264, 1975.
2. Arrigoni-Martelli, E., and Bramm, E.: Rheum. Rehabilit. *15*:207, 1976.
3. Arrigoni-Martelli, E., Bramm, E., Huskisson, E. C., Willoughby, D. A., and Dieppe, P. A.: Agents Actions, *6*:613, 1976.
4. Bach, F. H., and Amos, D. B.: Science *156*:1506, 1967.
5. Bach, F. H., and Hirschhorn, K.: Science *143*:813, 1964.
6. Balint, G., Szobor, A., Temesvári, P., Zahumensky, Z., and Bozsóky, S.: Scand. J. Rheumatol. *4* (Suppl. 8) : 21-12, 1975.
7. Beer, W. E., and Cooke, K. B.: Br. J. Dermatol. *79*:123, 1967.
8. Berry, H., and Huskisson, E. C.: In press, 1976.
9. Berry, H., Liyanage, S. P., and Durance, R. A.: Scand. J. Rheumatol. *4* (Suppl. 8) : 21-06, 1975.
10. Binderup L., and Arrigoni-Martelli, E.: Agents Actions. In press, 1977.
11. Bloch, H. S., Prasad, A., Anastasi, A., and Briggs, D. R. J.: J. Lab. Clin. Med. *56*:212, 1960.
12. Buchnall, R. C., Dixon, A. St. J., Glick, E. N., Woodland, J., and Zutchi, D. W.: Br. Med. J. *1*:600, 1975.
13. Camus, J. P., Cronzet, J., Guillieu, P., Benichou, C., and Lievre, J. A.: Ann. Med. Interne (Paris) *125*:9, 1974.
14. Crawhall, J. C., and Thompson, C. J.: Science *147*:1459, 1965.
15. Day, A. T., Golding, J. R., Lee, P. N., and Butterworth, A. D.: Br. Med. J. *1*:180, 1974.
16. Dieppe, P. A., Willoughby, D. A., Huskisson, E. C., and Arrigoni-Martelli, E.: Agents Actions, *6*:618, 1976.
17. Editorial: Lancet *1*:151, 1975.
18. Golding, D. N.: Scand. J. Rheumatol. *4* (Suppl. 8) : 21-18, 1975.
19. Golding, D. N., Wilson, J. W., and Day, A. T.: Postgrad. Med. J. *46*:599, 1970.
20. Goldberg, I. S., and Barnett, E. V.: Arch. Intern. Med. *125*:145, 1970.
21. Harris, E. D., and Sjoerdsma, A.: Lancet *2*:996, 1966.
22. Herbert, C. M., Lindberg, K. A., and Jackson, M. I. V., Bailey, A. J.: Lancet *1*:187, 1974.
23. Hewitt, J., Lesoana-Leibowitch, M., Benveniste, M., and Saporta, L.: Ann. Med. Interne (Paris) *122*:1003, 1971.
24. Hill, H. E. H.: Curr. Med. Res. Opin. *2*:573, 1974.
25. Huskisson, E. C.: Pharmatherapeutica *1*:24, 1976.
26. Huskisson, E. C., Balme, H. W., Berry, H., Scott, J., Burry, H. C., Gibson, T. J., Grahame, R., Henderson, D. R. F., Hart, F. D., and Woitulewski, J. A.: In "International Symposium on Penicillamine," 1975. In press.
27. Huskisson, E. C., and Berry, H.: Postgrad. Med. J. *50* (Suppl. 2) : 59, 1974.

28. Huskisson, E. C., Scott, J., Balme, H. W., Dieppe, P. A., Trapanell, J., Willoughby, D. A.: Lancet *1*:393, 1976.
29. Huskisson, E. C., Gibson, T. J., Balme, H. W., Berry, H., Burry, H. C., Grahame, R., Hart, F. D., and Woitulewski, J. A.: Ann. Rheum. Dis. *33*: 532, 1974.
30. Huskisson, E. C., and Hart, F. D.: Ann. Rheum. Dis. *31*:402, 1972.
31. Hübner, K. F., and Gengozian, N.: Proc. Soc. Exp. Biol. Med. *118*:561, 1965.
32. Jaffe, I. A.: J. Lab. Clin. Med. *60*:409, 1962.
33. Jaffe, I. A.: Ann. Rheum. Dis. *22*:71, 1963.
34. Jaffe, I. A.: Ann. Intern. Med. *61*:556, 1964.
35. Jaffe, I. A.: Arthritis Rheum. *8*:1064, 1965.
36. Jaffe, I. A.: Postgrad. Med. J. *44* (Suppl. Oct.) : 15, 1968.
37. Jaffe, I. A.: Ann. N. Y. Acad. Sci. *166*:57, 1969.
38. Jaffe, I. A.: Arthritis Rheum. *13*:436, 1970.
39. Jaffe, I. A.: N. Engl. J. Med. *288*:630, 1973.
40. Jaffe, I. A., Altman, K., and Merryman, P.: J. Clin. Invest. *43*:1869, 1964.
41. Jaffe, I. A., and Kerrebijn, K. F.: Lancet *1*:245, 1970.
42. Junge, U., Hauswal, St. Ch., and Perings, E.: Verh. Dtsch. Ges. Inn. Med. *79*:616, 1973.
43. Junge, U., Perings, E., and Lubrich, E.: Klin. Wochenschr. *52*:794, 1974.
44. Karp, M., Lurie, M., and Yonis, Z.: Arch. Dis. Child. *41*:684, 1966.
45. Kriegel, W., Langness, V., Jahn, P., and Müller, W.: Z. Rheumaforsch. *19*: 173, 1970.
46. Kühn, K.: Arzneim. Forsch. *24*:225, 1974.
47. Lyle, W. H.: Lancet *2*:285, 1974.
48. McCall, J. T., Goldstein, N. P., and Randall, R. W.: Am. J. Med. Sci. *254*: 35, 1967.
49. Miehlke, K.: Arzneim. Forsch. *21*:1815, 1971.
50. Miehlke, K., Kohlhardt, J., and Wirth, B.: Z. Rheumaforsch. *27*:445, 1968.
51. Morsches, B., Holzmann, H., and Schlaudecker, A.: Arzneim. Forsch. *21*: 421, 1967.
52. Multicenter Trial Group: Lancet *1*:280, 1973.
53. Nimni, M. E., and Bavetta, L. A.: Science *150*:905, 1965.
54. Ott, V. R., and Schmidt, K. L.: In "International Symposium on Penicillamine," 1975. In press.
55. Pass, F., Goldfischer, S. G., Sternlieb, I., and Scheinberg, I. M.: Ann. Intern. Med. *82*:673, 1975.
56. Payne, R. W., and Cahill, C. L.: J. Okla. Med. Assoc. *62*:487, 1969.
57. Roath, S., and Wills, R.: Postgrad. Med. J. *50* (Suppl.) : 2, 56.
58. Schumacher, K., Maerker, Alzer, G., and Schaaf, W.: Arzneim Forsch. *25*: 600, 1975.
59. Schumacher, K., Maerker, Alzer, G., and Preuss, R.: Arzneim. Forsch. *25*: 603, 1975.
60. Siegmund, P., Körber, F., and Hasenback, G.: Z. Klin. Chem. *4*:307, 1960.
61. Stocker, E., and Schairer, H.: In "International Symposium on Penicillamine," 1975. In press.
62. Tisman, G., Herbert V., Teng, G. O. L., and Bremer, L.: Proc. Soc. Exp. Biol. Med. *139*:355, 1972.
63. Tobin, M. S., and Altman, K.: Proc. Soc. Exp. Biol. Med. *115*:225, 1964.

64. Wacker, A., Chandra, P., and Heyl, E.: Arzneim. Forsch. *16*:825, 1966.
65. Walshe, J. M.: Postgrad. Med. J. *44* (Suppl. 6) : 1968.
66. Webster, A. W., and Thompson, R. A.: Clin. Exp. Immunol. *18*:553, 1974.
67. Yu, D. T. J., and Peter, J. B.: Semin. Arthritis Rheum. *4*:25, 1974.
68. Zuckner, J., Ramsey, R. H., Doner, R. W., and Gantner, G. E.: Arthritis Rheum. *13*:131, 1970.

Chapter 20

Gold Compounds

Through the years, conflicting reports on the efficacy of gold compounds in the treatment of rheumatoid arthritis have accumulated. A well-controlled double-blind study with gold sodium thiomalate was performed by the Empire Rheumatism Council in a large patient population (19,20). According to the results of this multicenter clinical trial, clinical improvement occured in about 25% of the patients after 1-3 months of treatment, with weekly injection of 50 mg of gold sodium thiomalate, and only very few patients were improved after more prolonged therapy (19,20). Positive radiological evidence of improvement was subsequently reported (68) and other studies (24,25) confirmed the efficacy of chrysotherapy. More recent investigations of the American Rheumatism Association (4) were in agreement with previous results. A comparative trial of sodium aurothiomalate with azathioprine and cyclophosphamide under double-blind conditions showed that a gold compound produced over 18 months clinical improvement, comparable to that achieved with the two immunosuppressants (13).

1. MECHANISM OF ACTION

The introduction of gold therapy for rheumatoid arthritis was based on the belief that this disease was due to tubercle bacilli and on the observation that gold compounds have a bactericidal effect on these micro-organisms. Tubercle bacilli have been ruled out as possible causative agents but they have been replaced in this role by other micro-organisms, such as PPLO, which have been repeatedly isolated from rheumatic joints (6,37,50,76). The decrease in rheumatoid factor titers in rheumatoid patients but not in animals with experimental arthritis, under the influence of gold compounds, strenghtened the hypothesis of an "anti-infectious" mechanism of their action (46,57). The reduction of rheumatoid factor could be due to the elimination of an infectious agent serving as antigenic stimulus for its synthesis (46,57).

A number of investigators have shown that gold sodium thiomalate suppresses the growth of mycoplasma in vitro (14,53,60,72), but the results are frequently variable (53,60,72).

Arthritis caused in rodents by PPLO (59,77,84) or other infectious agents (38,61) is suppressed by gold compounds. However, these compounds are also active on primary and secondary lesions of adjuvant arthritis (5,52,82,83) and on several types of acute experimental inflammations (5,33,62,79).

The antimicrobial activity of gold compounds seems, therefore, of scanty relevance to their antiarthritic effect.

It is possible that they exert their therapeutic effects by altering the immune response or inhibiting the discharge of lysosomal hydrolases, which is the consequence of the interaction of immune complexes with different cell types.

Aurothiopolypeptide prolongs the survival time of skin homografts in mice (65), gold thioglucose inhibits the Schwartzmann phenomenon (74), gold sodium thiomalate and gold thioglucose delay the onset of experimental allergic encephalomyelits (30). The lymphocytes of patients treated with gold compounds do not respond to the blastogenic effect of streptolysin S (22). However, it was also reported that gold sodium thiomalate fails to affect the delayed hypersensitivity in guinea pig (57) or the production of antibody (56), though a reduction of histamine release from mast cells of gold-treated rats sensitized to horse serum was observed

(56). Recently, gold therapy has been shown to exert no action on abnormal IgG and IgM metabolism in rheumatoid arthritis (51). Taking into account the effect of gold compounds on both the non-immune and immune lesions of adjuvant arthritis (5,52,82,83) and on different models of non-immunologically mediated inflammations (5,33,62,79), it seems that the positive results obtained in certain immunological responses are caused by the inhibition of enzyme release or activity.

As a matter of fact, it has been proved that acid phosphatase, β-glucuronidase and cathepsin are inhibited by gold sodium thio-malate at concentrations comparable to those found in plasma during chrysotherapy (21,58). These findings also indicate that gold compounds are actively concentrated in lysosomes (58). The access of gold to cells involved in phagocytosis might be facilitated by its binding to various serum proteins, including immunoglobulins (47) thought to be instrumental in the pathogenesis of rheumatoid arthritis. The reduced enzymatic activity is not caused by a release inhibition (21). It has been suggested that the mechanism of gold inhibition is via the binding of sulfhydryl groups since the gold drugs are heavy metal mercaptides (21). This hypothesis has been experimentally confirmed: in fact, gold sodium thiomalate produces a potent dose-dependent inhibition of the sulfhydryl-disulphide interchange reaction both in vitro and in vivo (81).

Enzymes involved in connective tissue metabolism have also been reported to be inhibited by gold compound both in vivo (10) and in vitro (26). The synthesis of glycosamine-6-phosphate, a limiting step in the biosynthesis of mucopolysaccaride, is blocked by gold concentrations attainable during chrysotherapy (10). An effect on trace-metal metabolism has been claimed to be responsible for such an activity (54).

Gold has also been reported to react with collagen, causing a cross-linkage of the fibrils (1,2,3). The ensuing increased stability of collagen reduces its susceptibility to denaturation and to subsequent enzymatic degradation, with the formation of products that may act as antigens.

2. TOXICITY

In man, the most frequently encountered toxic effects are dermatological (23,24,25). They usually appear when a cumulative dose of approximately 400 mg of gold has been reached and include non-specific dermatitis (7,63,70,75), exfoliative dermatitis (46) and local rash (46). Most serious side effects are blood dyscrasias which may be fatal (49) but are less frequent (41). Other adverse reactions include eosinophilia (27,63,67), leukopenia (7,63), granulocytopenia (63) and trombocytopenia (23,63, 64). There have also been reports of nephrotic syndrome, nephritis, and nephrosis associated with chrysotherapy (45,75,78,85) as well as of ocular toxicity (8).

A number of theories have been proposed to explain the pathogenetic properties of gold compounds: the most likely of these is that the side effects are allergic phenomena (9,24,25). The prevalence of skin reactions, sometimes occurring after a single dose of gold, and the frequence of eosinophilia tend to support this concept. It should be noted that the exact allergen, supposed to be a protein-gold complex (24), has not been identified (16,25,45,71). Kidney damage is one of the few consistently reproducible toxic effects in laboratory animals; it has been observed after administration of gold sodium thiomalate, gold sodium sulfate, gold thioglucose and gold chloride but not with colloidal gold preparations (17,38,80, 83). Eosinophilia and allergic manifestations have been described in rabbits receiving gold sodium thiomalate over a long period of time (55).

Teratogenic effects were produced in rats by gold sodium thiomalate administered during mid-pregnancy, with doses resulting in gold levels comparable to those seen in rheumatoid patients treated with this compound (43). Many reports deal with toxic effects of gold thioglucose, which include gastric mucosal lesions (17,80), hyperglycemia and glycosuria (18,35,42), and thyroid hypofunction (35,66). Some toxicity is, however, associated with hypothalamic lesions produced by this drug, which are postulated as being caused by a specific affinity of the ventromedial nucleus for the glucose moiety of gold compound (11,12,15).

3. METABOLISM

The currently used gold preparations are poorly absorbed from the gastrointestinal tract; thus, in order to obtain significant therapeutic activity they must be administered parenterally.

After intramuscular injection of an aqueous solution of gold salts, there is a rapid rise in serum gold levels followed by a decline. Published data on the rate of decline show apparent contradictions, some suggesting a uniform and relatively slow pattern (29,48), and others indicating several phases, with a short half-life (69). Using a whole-body radiation counter, it has been shown that the serum clearance of the tracer conforms to first-order kinetics. Half-times were 4.4-7.4 days, initial volumes of distribution 4.9-9.3 liters (28). Investigators also differ in reporting either no change in the weekly excretion of gold during chrysotherapy (25) or an increase (48). Recent results obtained, utilizing atomic absorption spectroscopy (34,48), suggest that there are two different phases of disappearance of gold from blood. The first rapid phase may be due to tissue absorption, the second slow phase —to excretion. A rapid rate of tissue absorption of gold has been demonstrated both in patients and animals (31,39,40,44). Gold is excreted chiefly in urine. With cumulative doses, renal clearance of gold increases (34,48). Since the daily dose eliminated is constant within each patient, it appears that the increasing amount of excreted gold comes from tissue deposits (32). It has been found, however, that a considerable portion is eliminated in feces (48) although the amount varied considerably among patients. Only 50% of fecal gold comes from bile (41). After chrysotherapy is terminated, gold is found in the blood and excreta for a long period, whose duration depends on the size of the weekly dose. The gradual build up and subsequent prolonged excretion of gold are believed to be responsible for the delayed and long-term benefits, and toxicity observed in chrysotherapy.

4. GOLD COMPOUNDS IN USE

Gold compounds in use today (Fig. 47) are complexes of aurous gold with different sulfur-containing ligands, such as thiomalic acid (Myochrysine), thioglucose (Solganal) and sodium thiosulphate (Sanocrysine, Crisalbine). Because they are not absorbed orally, these agents are administered by the intramuscular route.

Recently, a series of compounds (Fig. 47) has been prepared in which aurous gold is combined with trialkylphosphine (51). One of these new gold compounds—SK&F-36914—is claimed to produce antiarthritic activity and serum gold levels are seen after oral administration to adjuvant arthritic rats (83). It has also been found equipotent with parenterally administered gold sodium thiomalate in delaying the onset and decreasing the severity of experimental allergic encephalomyelitis in rats (30).

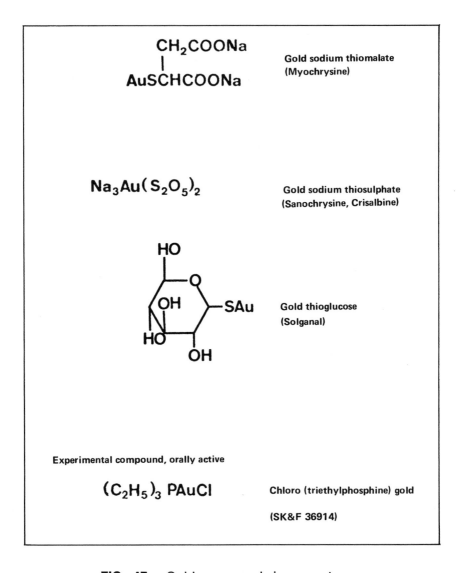

FIG. 47. Gold compounds in current use

REFERENCES

1. Adam, M., Bartl, P., Deyl, Z., and Rosmus, J.: Experientia 20:203, 1964..
2. Adam, M., Bartl, P., Deyl, Z., and Rosmus, J.: Ann. Rheum. Dis. 24:378, 1965.
3. Adam, M., and Kühn, K.: Eur. J. Biochem. 3:407, 1968.
4. American Rheumatism Association: Arthritis Rheum. 16:353, 1973.
5. Arrigoni-Martelli, E., and Bramm, E.: Agents Actions 5:264, 1975.
6. Bartholomew, L. E.: Arthritis Rheum. 8:376, 1965.
7. Bayles, T. B., and Fremont-Smith, P.: Ann. Rheum. Dis. 15:394, 1954.
8. Behrend, T., and Rodenhauser, J. H.: Z. Rheumaforsch. 28:441, 1969.
9. Block, W. D., and Van Goor, K.: In "Metabolism, Pharmacology and Therapeutic Use of Gold Compounds," A. C. Curtis, ed. Charles C. Thomas, Springfield, Ill., 1959, p. 39.
10. Bollett, A. J., and Shuster, A.: J. Clin. Invest. 39:1114, 1960.
11. Brecher, G., Laqueur, G. L., Cronkite, E. P., Edelman, P. M., and Schwartz, I. L.: J. Exp. Med. 121:395, 1965.
12. Chang, R. J., and Persellin, R. H.: Proc. Soc. Exp. Biol. Med. 129:598, 1968.
13. Currey, H. L. F., Harris, J., Mason, R M., Woodland, J., Beveridge, T., Roberts, C. J., Vere, D. W., Dixon, A. S. J., Daries, J., and Owen-Smith, B.: Br. Med. J. 3:763, 1974.
14. Davidson, M., and Thomas, L.: Antimicrob. Agents Chemother. 6:312, 1966.
15. Debous, A. F., Silver, L., Cronkite, E. P., Johnson, H. A., Brecher, G., Tenzer, D., and Schwartz, I. L.: Am. J. Physiol. 202:743, 1962.
16. Denman, A. M., Huber, H., Wood, P. H. N., and Scott, J. T.: Ann. Rheum. Dis. 24:278, 1965.
17. Deter, R. L., and Liebelt, R. A.: Gastroenterology 43:575, 1962.
18. Edelman, P. M., Schwartz, I. L.: Cronkite, E. P., Brecher, G., and Livingston, L.: J. Exp. Med. 121:403, 1965.
19. Empire Rheumatism Council: Ann. Rheum. Dis. 19:95, 1960.
20. Empire Rheumatism Council: Ann. Rheum. Dis. 27:756, 1968.
21. Ennis, R. S., Granda, J. L., and Posner, A. S.: Arthritis Rheum. 11:756, 1968.
22. Fikrig, S. M., and Smitwick, E. M.: Arthritis Rheum. 11:478, 1968.
23. Forestier, J.: Arch. Interam. Rheumatol. 6:15, 1963.
24. Freyberg, R. H.: In "Arthritis and Allied Conditions," J. L. Hollander, ed. Lea and Febiger, Philadelphia, 1966, p. 302.
25. Freyberg, R. H.: In "Arthritis and Allied Conditions," J. L. Hollander, ed. Lea and Febiger, Philadelphia, 1972, p. 455.
26. Fujihira, E., Tsubota, N., and Nakazawa, M.: Chem. Pharm. Bull. (Tokyo) 19:190, 1971.
27. Garrel, M.: Arch. Intern. Med. 106:874, 1960.
28. Gerber, R. C.: J. Lab. Clin. Med. 83:778, 1974.
29. Gerber, R. C., Paulus, H. E., and Bluestone, R.: Arthritis Rheum. 15:652, 1972.
30. Gerber, R. C., Whitehouse, M. W., and Orr, K. J.: Proc. Soc. Exp. Biol. Med. 140:1379, 1972.
31. Gottlieb, N. L., Smith, P. M., and Smith, E. M.: Arthritis Rheum. 15:16, 1972.

32. Gottlieb, N. L., Smith, P. M., and Smith, E. M.: Arthritis Rheum. *15*:582, 1972.
33. Guiral, M. J., and Saxena, P. N.: Indian J. Med. Res. *44*:657, 1956.
34. Hart, M.: Clin. Pharmacol. Ther. *15*:354, 1974.
35. Hazama, F.: Folia Endocrinol. Jpn. *40*:385, 1965.
36. Hill, D. F.: Med. Clin. N. Am. *52*:733, 1968.
37. Jansson, E., Mäkisara, P., Vainio, K., Vainio, U., Snellman, O., and Tuuri, S.: Ann. Rheum. Dis. *30*:506, 1971.
38. Jasmin, G.: J. Pharmacol. Exp. Ther. *120*:349, 1957.
39. Jeffery, R. M., Freundlich, H. F., and Bailey, D. M.: Ann. Rheum. Dis. *17*: 52, 1958.
40. Kantor, T. C., Harley, N., and Bishko, F.: Arthritis Rheum. *14*:392, 1971 (Abstr.).
41. Kapelowitz, R. F., Nelp, W. M., and Healay, L. A.: Arthritis Rheum. *7*: 319, 1964 (Abstr.).
42. Katsuki, S., Hirata, Y., Horino, M., Ito, M., Ishimoto, M., Makino, N., and Hososako, A.: Diabetes *11*:209, 1962.
43. Kidston, M. E., Beck, F., and Lloyd, J. B.: Proc. Anat. Soc. G. Br. Ireland *108*:590, 1070.
44. Lawrence, J. S.: Ann. Rheum. Dis. *20*:341, 1961.
45. Lee, J. C., Dushkin, M., Eyring, E. J., Engelman, E. P., and Hopper, J., Jr.: Arthritis Rheum. *8*:1, 1965.
46. Lewis, D. C., and Ziff, M.: Arthritis Rheum. *9*:682, 1966.
47. Lorber, A., Bovy, R. A., and Chang, C. C.: Nature (New Biol.) *236*:250, 1972.
48. Mascarenhas, B. R., Granda, J. L., and Freyberg, R. H.: Arthritis Rheum. *15*:391, 1972.
49. McCarty, D. J., Brill, J. M., and Harrop, D.: J. Am. Med. Assoc. *179*:655, 1962.
50. Moore, R. W., and Redmond, H. E.: Arthritis Rheum. *8*:458, 1965.
51. Mouridsen, H. T., Baerentsen, O., Rossing, N., and Jensens, K. B.: Arthritis Rheum. *17*:391, 1974.
52. Newbould, B. B.: Br. J. Pharmacol. *21*:127, 1963.
53. Newsham, A. G., and Chu, H. P.: J. Hyg. (Camb.) *63*:1, 1965.
54. Niedermeier, W., Brillmann, W. W., and Griggs, J. H.: Arthritis Rheum. *14*:533, 1971.
55. Nineham, A. W.: Arch. Interam. Rheumatol. *6*:113, 1963.
56. Norn, S.: Acta Pharmacol. Toxicol. *26*:470, 1968.
57. Persellin, R. H., Hess, E. V., and Ziff, M.: Arthritis Rheum. *10*:99, 1967.
58. Persellin, R. H., and Ziff, M.: Arthritis Rheum. *9*:57, 1966.
59. Preston, W. S., Block, W. D., and Freyberg, R. H.: Proc. Soc. Exp. Biol. Med. *50*:253, 1942.
60. Robinson, L. B., Wichelhausen, R. H., and Brown, T. McP.: J. Lab. Clin. Med. *39*:290, 1952.
61. Rothbord, S., Angevine, D. M., and Cecil, R. L.: J. Pharmacol. Exp. Ther. *72*:164, 1941.
62. Sancilio, L. F.: J. Pharmacol. Exp. Ther. *168*:199, 1969.
63. Saiyanen, E., and Laaksonen, A. L.: Ann. Paediat, Fenn. *8*:105, 1962.
64. Saphir, J. R., and Ney, R. G.: J. Am. Med. Assoc. *195*:782, 1966.
65. Scheiffart, F., Baenkler, H. W., and Islinger, M.: Z. Gesamte. Exp. Med.

Exp. Chir. *152*:125, 1970.
66. Schindler, W. J., and Liebelt, R. A.: Endocrinology *80*:387, 1967.
67. Sievers, K., Hurvi, L., and Sievers, U. M.: Acta Rheumatol. Scand. *9*:56, 1963.
68. Sigler, J. W., Bluhm, G. B., Duncan, H., Sharp, J. T., Ensign, D. C., and McCrum, W. R.: Arthritis Rheum. *15*:125, 1972.
69. Silvberg, D. A., Kidd, E. C., and Shuitka, T. K.: Arthritis Rheum. *13*:812, 1970.
70. Smith, R. T., Peak, W. P., Kron, K. M., Hermann, I. F., and Deltoro, R. A.: J. Am. Med. Assoc. *167*:1197, 1958.
71. Stavem, P., Stromme, J., and Bull. O.: Scand. J. Haematol. *5*:271, 1968.
72. Stewart, S. M., Bernet, M. W., and Young, J. E.: J. Med. Microbiol. *2*:287, 1969.
73. Sutton, B. M., McGusty, E., Walz, D. T., and DiMartino, M. J.: J. Med. Chem. *15*:1095, 1972.
74. Szilágyi, T., Tóth, S., Muszbek, L., Lévai, G., and Laczko, J.: Acta Microbiol. *15*:331, 1968.
75. Sørensen, A. W.: Acta Rheumatol. Scand. *9*:122, 1963.
76. Thomas, P.: Rheumatology *1*:29, 1967.
77. Tripi, H. B., and Kuzell, W.: Stanford Med. Bull. *5*:98, 1947.
78. Vanden Broek, H., and Han, M. G.: N. Engl. J. Med. *274*:210, 1966.
79. Vykydal, M., Klabusay, L., and Tonavsky, K.: Arzneim. Forsch. *6*:568, 1956.
80. Wagner, J. W., and DeGroot, J.: Proc. Soc. Exp. Biol. Med. *112*:33, 1963.
81. Walz, D. T., and DiMartino, M. J.: Proc. Soc. Exp. Biol. Med. *140*:263, 1972.
82. Walz, D. T., DiMartino, M. J., and Misher, A.: Ann. Rheum. Dis. *30*:303, 1971.
83. Walz, D. T., DiMartino, M. J., Sutton, B., and Misher, A.: J. Pharmacol. Exp. Ther. *181*:292, 1972.
84. Wiesinger, D.: In "International Symposium on Non-Steroidal Anti-Inflammatory Drugs," S. Garattini and M. N. G. Dukes, eds. Excerpta Medica, Amsterdam, 1965, p. 221.
85. Wilkinson, R., and Eccleston, D. W.: Br. Med. J. *2*:772, 1970.

Chapter 21

Antiinflammatory
Proteins

1. ENZYMES

The use of proteases and nucleases as therapeutic agents in inflammation presents some drawbacks in view of the general uncertainty about their possible mode of action, the small number of well-controlled clinical trails, and the recognized capacity of several proteolytic enzymes to cause inflammation.

Different types of intra- and extracellular enzymes participate, indeed, in different phases of inflammation (4,16,24). The appearance of different proteases at the site of inflammation is related to tissue type, severity of the inflammatory stimulus and time (5). Although local enzymes of tissue and cell origin apparently contribute to the inflammatory process, injected proteolytic enzymes of exogenous origin inhibit different types of experimental inflammation. Since the injected enzymes are irritants, the observed effect on inflammation may be mediated via systemic processes and, therefore, regarded as a non-specific counterirritant action. It has been suggested, however, that other mechanisms are implicated in the antiinflammatory effect of proteolytic enzymes (2,5,21). In addition, various types of proteases, orally administered, have been found to inhibit different types of edema (48). The response to these proteases is of the all-or-none type, rather than dose related (34).

Natural protease inhibitors have also been identified as being able to regulate the activity of intracellular proteases and those involved in blood-clotting processes. The two major inhibitors are a_1-antitrypsin and a_2-macroglobulin. The former combines with trypsin, resulting in its enzymatic inactivation (44), modulating excessive proteolysis, and interfering with fibrinolytic processes (11). It has also been suggested that a_1-antitrypsin may play a systemic role in affecting the antiinflammatory activity of exogenously administered enzymes (30,47). Unlike the trypsin complex with a_1-antitrypsin, the enzyme complex with a_2-macroglobulin, although retaining little proteolytic activity, still maintains about 90% of the original esterolytic effects (38).

Although there is some evidence that exogenous enzymes may alter the titer of these natural protease inhibitors (30,38) and that the complexes formed may somehow reduce some phases of the inflammatory process (1,18,38), it is still uncertain whether this simply involves some form of complement depletion.

Using diverse clinical criteria, a number of investigators have reported evidence for the effectiveness of enzymes as antiinflammatory agents (13,29,37,40,42,45). Proof of oral absorption has been claimed for trypsin and chymotrypsin (1,3,26,32,33), and for bromelain (6,31,41), both in man and animals. However, the evidence of clinical efficacy has been challenged for a variety of reasons, the principal of these being the lack of specific, objective quantitative parameters to back up the subjective criteria of effectiveness (10,12,27) (Table 47).

2. CHALONES

When tissue is injured, cellular mitotic activity is enhanced resulting in an increase in the specific cells needed to replace those damaged, in order to restore and maintain the structural integrity of the tissue.

When a sufficient number of new cells has been produced,

TABLE 47. Animals models used to evaluate the antiinflammatory activity of enzymes

Assay	Procedure	References
Rat paw edema:	Serotonin egg white carrageenin dextran brewers yeast	34
Granuloma pouch (rat)	Croton oil	19 23
Scals size (rabbit)	UV light	41

mitotic activity subsides. At least, two different mechanisms controlling the enhanced mitotic activiy could exist. Thus, the existence of a mitotic stimulator released from damaged cells has been proposed (36). A second hypothesis suggests the presence of a depressor substance whose depletion enhances mitotic activity: when restoration of tissue integrity is achieved, mitotic activity subsides because of an increase in this inhibitory substance (7,8,9).

This depressor substance has been designated as a "chalone," i.e., an internal secretion produced by a tissue to control—by inhibition—the rate of cell production in that tissue (8,9). The chalone is tissue specific, but studies on chalones obtained from different species revealed that they are not species specific (8,9,20), thus raising the possibility that they could be utilized in therapy.

A variety of chalones have been isolated from different tissues (14,15,28,46), namely, epidermis (7,8,9), blood erythrocytes (25), granulocytes (35), lymphocytes (17,22), spleen, thymus, and liver (43.)

The epidermal chalone has been characterized as a protein, degradable by trypsin but not by pepsin (7,8,9). The lymphoid chalone has probably a similar molecular weight—approximately 40.000 Daltons—and it is also trypsin degradable (22) while the granulocyte chalone is a dialyzable polipeptide of a lower molecular weight (25).

It has been suggested that a functional similarity exists between histones and chalones, both of them inhibiting DNA which serves as a template for RNA synthesis (43). Because of tryptic degradation of chalones, the presence of a trypsin-like activity in inflammatory exudates may be of importance—by removing these inhibitory substances, it would trigger the reparative processes (39).

REFERENCES

1. Ambrus, C. M., Black, N., and Ambrus, J. L.: Circ. Res. *10*:161, 1962.
2. Atkinson, D. C.: Arch. Int. Pharmacodyn. Ther. *193*:391, 1971.
3. Avakian, S.: Clin. Pharmacol. Ther. *5*:712, 1964.
4. Bazin, S., and Delannay, A.: J. Dent. Res. *51(1)*:244, 1972.
5. Bertelli, A.: J. Dent. Res. *51(2)*:235, 1972.
6. Bodi, T.: Exp. Med. Surg. (Suppl.) :51, 1965.
7. Bullough, W. S.: Biol. Basis Med. *1*:311, 1968.
8. Bullough, W. S., and Laurence, E. B.: Exp. Cell Res. *33*:176, 1964.
9. Bullough, W. S., Laurence, E. B., Iversen, O. H., and Elgic, K.: Nature *214*:578, 1964.
10. Calnan, J., Kulatilake, A. E., and Saad, M. N.: Br. J. Surg. *3*:743, 1963.
11. Chakrabarti, H., Hocking, E. D., and Feonly, G. R.: J. Med. Pathol. *22*: 659, 1969.
12. Council on Drugs: J. Am. Med. Assoc. *188*:857, 1964.
13. De Fiebre, C. W., Ramsay, A. G., Goldberg, R. I., and Schuman, F. I.: In "Drugs of Animal Origin," A. Leonardi and J. Walsh eds. Ferro, Milano, 1967, p. 103.
14. Elgic, K., Laerum, O. D., and Edgehill, W.: Virchows Arch. (Cell Pathol.) *B8*:277, 1971.
15. Elgic, K., Laerum, O. D., and Edgehill, W.: Virchows Arch. (Cell Pathol.) *B10*:299, 1972.
16. Foster, J.: J. Dent. Res. *51(1)*:257, 1972.
17. Garcia-Giralt, E., Lasalvia, E., Florentin, I., and Mathé, G.: Eur. J. Clin. Biol. Res. *15*:1012, 1970.
18. Gaurot, K.: Biochim. Biophys. Acta *295*:245, 1973.
19. Hakim, A. A., Dailey, V. P., and Lesh, J. B.: In "Non-Steroidal Antiinflammatory Drugs," S. Garattini and M. N. G. Dukes, eds. Excerpta Medica Foundation, Amsterdam, 1965, p. 265.
20. Halprin, K. M., and Taylor, J. K.: Adv. Clin. Chem. *14*:319, 1971.
21. Horáková, Z., Muratová, J.: In "Non-Steroidal Antiinflammatory Drugs," S. Garattini and M. N. G. Duges eds. Excerpta Medica Foundation, Amsterdam, 1965, p. 237.
22. Houck, J. C., Inranusquin, H., and Leikin, S.: Science *173*:1139, 1971.
23. Innerfield, I., Cohen, H., and Zweil, T.: Proc. Exp. Biol. Med *123*:871, 1966.
24. Janoff, A.: Annu. Rev. Med. *23*:172, 1972.
25. Kivilaakso, E., and Rytomaa, T.: Cell Tissue Kinet. *4*:1, 1971.
26. Kobacoff, B. L., Wholman, A., Umhey, M., and Avakian, S.: Nature *199*: 815, 1963.
27. Korlof, B., Ponten, B., and Ugland, O.: Scand. J. Plast. Reconstr. Surg. *3*:27, 1960.
28. Laurence, E. G., Randers-Hansen, E., Christophers, E., and Rytomaa, T.: Rev. Eur. Etud. Clin. Biol. *17*:133, 1972.

29. Lie, K. K., Larsen, R. D., and Posch, J. L.: Surg. Gynecol. Obstet. *125*: 595, 1967.
30. Margetts, G., Barber, K., Christie, R. B., Jones, W. E., and Bowdder, W. T.: Br. J. Clin. Pract. *26*:293, 1972.
31. Martin, G. J.: In "Symp. Non-Steroidal Antiinflammatory Drugs," S. Garattini and M. N. G. Dukes, eds. Excerpta Medica Foundation, Amsterdam, 1965, p. 90.
32. Miller, J. M.: Clin. Med. *75*:35, 1968.
33. Moriya, H., Moriwaki, C., Akamoto, S., Yamaguchi, K., and Iwadare, M.: Chem. Pharm. Bull. *15*:1662, 1967.
34. Netti, C., Bandi, G. L., and Pecile, A.: Farmaco (Prat.) *27*:453, 1972.
35. Pankovits, W. R.: Cell Tissue Kinet. *4*:539, 1972.
36. Pashkis, K. E.: Cancer Res. *18*:981, 1958.
37. Rathgeber, W. F.: S. Afr. Med. J. *45*:181, 1971.
38. Rinderknecht, H., and Glokas, M. C.: Biochim. Biophys. Acta *295*:233, 1973.
39. Schilling, J. A.: Physiol. Rev. *48*:374, 1968.
40. Schwinger, U.: Wien. Med. Wochenschr. *36*:1, 1970.
41. Seneca, H.: Exp. Med. Surg. (Suppl.) :63, 1965.
42. Shaw, P. C.: Br. J. Clin. Pract. *23*:25, 1969.
43. Sluyser, M.: In "Regulation of Nucleic Acid and Protein Biosynthesis," V. V. Koningsberger and L. Bosch, eds. Elsevier, New York, 1967, p. 225.
44. Trans, J. and Coan, M. H.: In "Pulmonary Emphysema and Proteolysis," C. Mittman ed. Academic Press, New York, 1972, p. 341.
45. Tsomides, J. and Goldberg, R. I.: Clin. Med. *76*:40, 1969.
46. Voorhess, J. J., and Duell, E. A.: Arch. Dermatol. *104*:352, 1971.
47. Whitehouse, M. W.: Pure Appl. Chem. *19*:35, 1969.
48. Winter, C. A., Risley, E. A., and Nuss, G. W.: Fed. Proc. *23*:284, 1964.

Chapter 22

Antigout Agents

The term "gout" denotes a group of defects in purine metabolism, each of which results in an overproduction of urate. It also includes deficiencies in urate elimination that have the same effect as urate overproduction, i.e., hyperuricemia (31). "Secondary gout" refers to those forms of hyperuricemia which are caused by a mechanism other than a metabolic defect or impaired urate elimination. The long list of sources (45) of secondary gout includes lead poisoning, tuberculostatic drugs (pyrazinamide), diuretic agents which produce hyperuricemia by interfering with renal handling of urate, and myeloproliferative disease that results in hyperuricemia because of a high rate of nucleic acid turnover.

Numerous investigations on gout have elucidated the etiological role of sodium urate, so that this disease is now the one more thoroughly understood among the inflammatory conditions (25).

A parallel development occurred in the area of antigout agents, with great advances being made in clarifying the mechanism of action of colchicine and introducing allopurinol, probenecid and sulfinpyrazone into gout therapy.

The actual symptomatology of an acute attack of gout is a result of the intrasynovial presence of microcrystalline monosodium urate (44). The examination of gouty joints consistently reveals the presence of this salt in microcrystalline form and the injection of synthetic crystalline urate—but not of the amorphous form—into the synovial cavity produces an inflammatory response (12,62). It has been observed that calcium pyrophosphate can also trigger an attack of gout and it has been suggested that the decisive factor is not the chemical nature of the material but its physical state. Therefore, it has been proposed that classical gout should be considered as one member of a family of "crystal deposition disease" (51).

The presence of polymorphonuclear leukocytes (PMN) within the synovial cavity is essential for an acute attack of gout to occur. In fact, in dogs depleted of PMN, the intra-articular injection of urate crystals does not elicit a response (50). The crystals are phagocytozed into PMN; the vacuole containing the ingested material fuses with lysosomes and then the crystals interact by hydrogen bonding with the lysosome membrane, causing its rupture. Subsequently, lysosomal materials are released, eliciting the inflammatory reaction (70).

Significant participation of kinins in gouty arthritis seems unlikely (50). Chemotactic substances are released by PMN following phagocytosis of urate (48). It has also been suggested that urate by itself could stimulate random motility of PMN (64,65) (Fig. 48).

1. COLCHICINE

The most significant biological properties of colchicine are its ability to inhibit mitosis in metaphase and its effectiveness in alleviating acute attacks of gout. In recent years, it has became increasingly evident that both these actions derive from a more fundamental property of the drug, i.e., its interaction with microtubule protein.

The antimitotic activity of colchicine, recognized for a long time, is a function of its ability to bind to a protein submit of microtubules (41), a major element of the spindle fibers of the mitotic apparatus (8). As a consequence of this binding, mitosis is blocked.

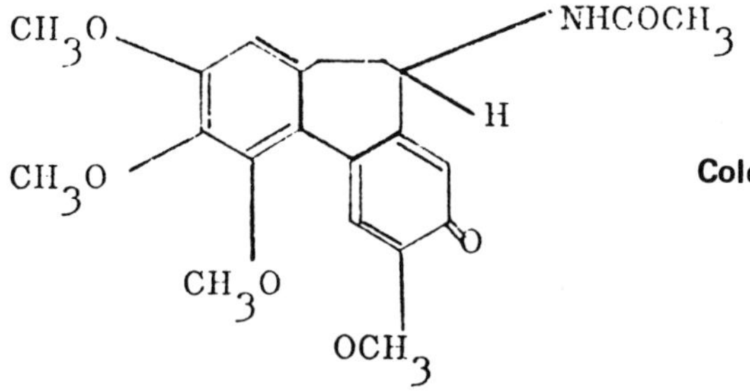

Colchicine

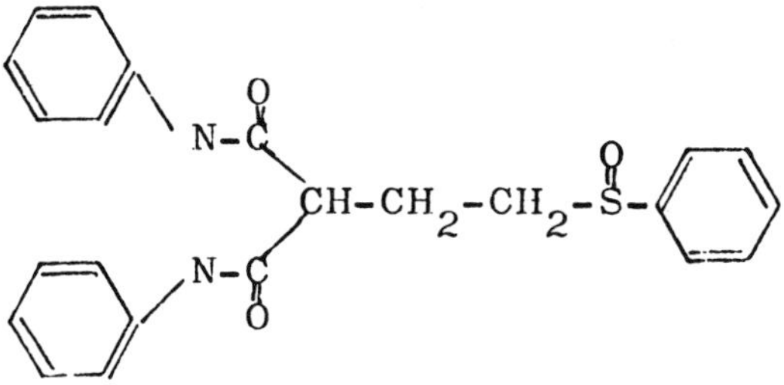

Sulfinpyrazone

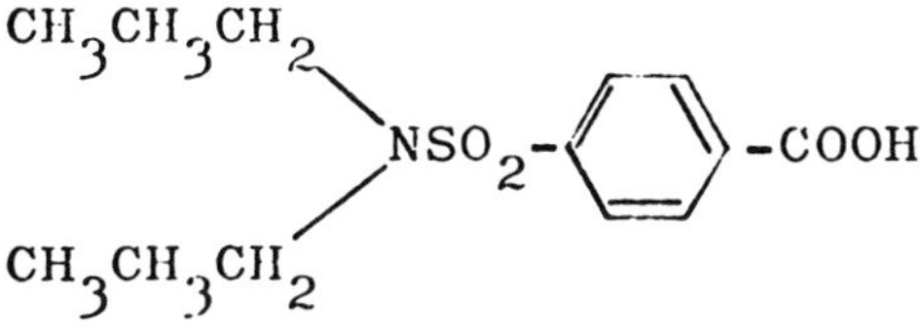

Probenecid

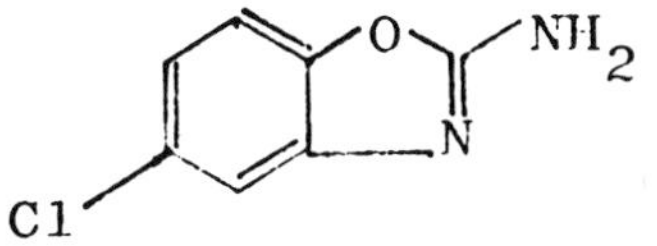

Zoxazolamine

FIG. 48. Chemical structure of antigout agents

The disappearance of microtubules from the isolated mitotic apparatus parallels, in fact, the appearance of a colchicine-binding protein in the extracts of these specimens (1,2,32).

Microtubules are not only involved in the mitotic process but in other cellular functions as well. These include degranulation and secretion (20,38,40,52,71), their relevance in inflammatory-mediator release having been previously discussed (Chapter 1). The functional state of microtubules, possibly regulated by the intracellular level of cAMP, has been shown to be also responsible for granule movement in many cell types, including human PMN (19, 22,70) and, therefore, for the translocation of lysosomes to the phagocytic vacuoles. Investigations on colchicine-treated PMN showed that microtubules were no longer present in these cells (39). Moreover, it has been demonstrated that colchicine inhibits the increased metabolism associated with phagocytosis and the subsequent fusion of lysosomes with the vacuoles and their degranulation (41). Because colchicine does not stabilize the lysosomes (68), this effect may be mediated through microtubule disruption. Low concentrations of colchicine (10^{-6}M) reduce the uptake of zymosan particles by murine macrophages (69) and decrease the phagocytosis of urate crystals by human PMN (49). At lower concentrations, colchicine inhibits the random motility of PMN, induced by dissolved urate (47), and the production of chemotactic factor (48). It seems likely, therefore, that colchicine's interference with PMN functions reflects its ability to bind to microtubule protein, thereby, reducing the contribution of this cell to the inflammatory process. It should be mentioned in this connection that several investigations (7,15,63,67,75) demonstrated a good correlation between the antimitotic activity of many colchicine derivatives and their efficacy in human gout and in different animal models of the disease. These findings further support the hypothesis that the antimitotic and antiinflammatory activities of colchicine share a common mechanism of action.

2. ALLOPURINOL

Allopurinol was originally prepared as a potential antitumoral agent because it represented an isomeric purine molecule (57). This compound and several other related substances are inhibitors of xantine oxidase, the enzyme responsible for the conversion of hypoxantine to uric acid (13). Xantine oxidase is an enzyme widely distributed in nature; although it is present in several tissues, in man the highest concentration is found in liver. It is an enzyme of rather low specificity with regard to substrates and electron acceptors. It has been ascertained that the oxidative mechanism involves enzyme-bound molybdenum, flavine nucleotide and non-heme iron associated with labile sulfide (35,42). Both flavin and non-heme iron sulfur chromofores of the enzyme are reduced by allopurinol (43). The oxidation product of allopurinol, alloxantine, is unable to reduce xantine oxidase under conditions favorable to reduction by allopurinol or xantine. However, it is able to inactivate xantine oxidase in the presence of xantine (43) and it has been suggested that alloxantine rather than allopurinol is primarily responsible for xantine oxidase inhibition in vivo (10). In addition to its ability to lower urate formation, allopurinol is claimed to have inhibitory effects on some experimental models of inflammation, such as exudate formation caused by turpentine and kaolin-induced paw swelling in rats (56). No activity against the paw swelling of adjuvant arthritis was observed in contrast to colchicine (9). Antinociceptive activity in mice has also been reported (28).

Allopurinol was first introduced clinically as adjunct therapy in patients receiving 6-thiopurine for leukemia (159). Since these patients showed reduction in both serum and urinary uric acid values (59,72), a trial of this agent in gout was suggested and it is now established as one of the standard forms of therapy for hyperuricemia and uric acid stones.

Administration of allopurinol to gouty patients (orally, 200-800 mg/day), for 3-5 days, effectively lowers serum urate to normal levels (58,60). A corresponding drop in urinary excretion of urate occurs, but the urinary output of oxypurines is not as great as expected, probably because of reutilization of hypoxantine and xantine in the biosynthesis of nucleic acids and because of feedback inhibition in purine biosynthesis, resulting from the accumulation of intermediate products.

Serious complications from allopurinol therapy are not frequent. Approximately 5% of patients find it necessary to discontinue the drug (37). Allopurinol may lead to the development of gastrointestinal intolerance (74), skin rashes, sometimes with fever (33), leukopenia, thrombocytopenia, hepatitis, and vasculitis (29). It is not clear whether these are related to hypersensitivity or to a toxic effect of the drug. So far no development of xantine crystalluria or lithiasis has been observed in any patient treated with allopurinol.

Allopurinol has also some other metabolic effects. Among these, the inhibition of orotidine-5'-phosphate decarboxilase should be mentioned, which catalizes a step in the conversion of orotic acid to uridine-5'-monophosphate (16,30). Such an inhibition leads to a striking increase in the excretion of orotidine and orotic acid (16, 30). There are several potentially important drug interactions involving allopurinol. Purine analogs, 6-mercaptopurine and azathioprine, are potentiated by the xantine oxidase inhibition. Furthermore, allopurinol has an inhibitory effect on the microsomal drug-metabolizing enzymes (66) which prolong the half-life of antipyrine, bishydroxycoumarin and probenecid (66). It has been also observed that the concomitant administration of allopurinol is associated with a threefold higher incidence of an ampicillin-related rash (3).

3. URICOSURIC DRUGS

A large number of drugs with different chemical and pharmacological properties decrease the serum urate concentration in man by enhancing renal excretion of uric acid. At present, probenecid and sulfinpyrazone are most widely used for this purpose. The renal handling of uric acid consist of its glomerular filtration and then of its reabsorption and secretion within the nephron. The uricosuric effect of a drug could, therefore, be due to an increase in filtered urate, an inhibition of reabsorption, or augmented secretion. The possibility that some uricosuric drugs, including probenecid and sulfinpyrazone, increase the quantity of urate filtered, through a displacement of binding to albumin, has received some support from in vitro studies (27,34,61) but, with the exception of salicylates, has not been confirmed in vivo (53).

Several drugs with significant uricosuric effects in man, such as probenecid and sulfinpyrazone, are weak organic acids and it has been assumed that they inhibit tubular reabsorption of filtered urate in a competitive manner (23). Other uricosuric drugs are not organic acids; their mechanism of action is unknown, as in the case of zoxazolamine, or it is believed to be a non-specific inhibition of urate reabsorption into the proximal tubule, as in the case of chlorprotixene and tetracycline (no longer used in gout) (17), or to depend on other pharmacological effects, as in the case of glycopyrrolate (54).

TABLE 48. Drugs with uricosuric effect in man

Acetoheximide	p-Nitrophenylbutazone
Azauridine	Orotic acid
Benzbromarone	Outdated tetracyclines
Chlorprotixene	Phenylbutazone
Cinchophen	Phenylindandione
Dicumarol	Probenecid
Diflumidone	Salicylate
Clycopyrrolate	Sulfinpyrazone
Halophenate	Zoxazolamine

Probenecid consistently lowers serum urate concentrations in gout. The maintenance dose ranges from 500 mg to 3 g daily: the initial dose should be low (250 mg, b.i.d.) in order to avoid sudden mobilization of a large quantity of urate (26). It is readily absorbed by the gastrointestinal tract and bound to plasma proteins; its half-life is dose-dependent and ranges from 6 to 12 hours (6). Serious side effects are rare, but an incidence up to 18% of gastrointestinal complaints has been reported (11,14,36,55,73). A complication of therapy with probenecid (as with sulfinpyrazone) is the formation of uric acid stones (26), which can be minimized by initiating therapy with low doses, maintaining an adequate urine flow and alkalinizing the latter. Probenecid affects renal excretion, volume of distribution and/or liver uptake of a number of drugs. Thus, indomethacin should be used at lower doses in patients receiving probenecid, and aspirin and related compounds should not be given together with this drug. In fact, the latter not only delays the renal excretion of aspirin-like agents but acetylsalicylate blocks the uricosuric effect of probenecid (24). The blood level of ampicillin and penicillin are enhanced and the volumes of distribution of ampicillin and cephaloridine are reduced (18).

Sulfinpyrazone is one of the most potent uricosuric agents: 400 mg per day have an effect similar to that observed with 2 g of probenecid per day (4,73). It has an additional uricosuric action in patients receiving the maximal effective dose of probenecid and a shorter half-life than the latter (1 to 3 hours). Sulfinpyrazone is almost completely bound to plasma proteins (4,5): approximately 40% is excreted unchanged, the rest as a parahydroxyl metabolite which is also uricosuric in man (4). The incidence of gastrointestinal side effects (11,36,73) and of uric acid stone formation (26) is roughly the same as with probenecid. However, sulfinpyrazone appears to produce a higher incidence of bone-marrow changes, as compared to probenecid (21,46,73). It seems possible that sulfinpyrazone may inhibit the excretion or metabolism of many of the same compounds altered by probenecid but relatively scanty data on this subject are available at this time (Table 48).

REFERENCES

1. Bibring, T., and Baxandall, J.: J. Cell Biol. *48*:324, 1971.
2. Borisy, G. G., and Taylor, E. W.: J. Cell Biol. *34*:535, 1967.
3. Boston Collaborative Drug Surveillance Program: N. Engl. Med. *286*: 505, 1972.
4. Burns, J. F.: J. Pharmacol. Exp. Ther. *119*:418, 1957.
5. Dayton, P. G., Sicam, L. E., Landrau, M., and Burns, J. J.: J. Pharmacol. Exp. Ther. *132*:287, 1961.
6. Dayton, P. G., Yu, T. F., Chen, W., Berger, L., West, L. A., and Gutman, A. B.: J. Pharmacol. Exp. Ther. *140*:278, 1963.
7. Denko, C. W., and Whitehouse, M. W.: Pharmacology *3*:229, 1970.
8. De Harven, E., and Bernhard, W.: Z. Zellforsch. Mikrosk. Anat. *45*:378, 1956.
9. Duane Sofia, R., Knobloch, L. C., and Vassar, H. B.: J. Pharmacol. Exp. Ther. *193*:918, 1975.
10. Elion, G. B.: Ann. Rheum. Dis. *25*:608, 1966.
11. Emmerson, B. T.: Med. J. Aust. *1*:839, 1963.
12. Faires, J. S., and Mc Carty, D. J., Jr.: Lancet *2*:282, 1962.
13. Feigelson, P., Davidson, J., and Robins, R.: J. Biol. Chem. *226*:993, 1957.
14. Ferris, T. F., Morgan, W. S., and Levitin, H.: N. Engl. J. Med. *265*:381, 1961.
15. Fitzergald, T. J., Williams, B., and Uyeki, E. M.: Proc. Soc. Exp. Biol. Med. *136*:115, 1971.
16. Fox, R. M., Royse-Smith, D., and O'Sullivan, W. J.: Science *168*:861, 1970.
17. Funlop, M., and Drapkin, A.: N. Engl. J. Med. *272*:986, 1965.
18. Gibaldi, M., and Schwartz, M. A.: Clin. Pharmacol. *9*:346, 1968.
19. Gillespie, E.: J. Cell Biol. *50*:544, 1971.
20. Gillespie, E., Levine, R. J., and Malawista, S. E.: J. Pharmacol. Exp. Ther. *164*:158, 1968.
21. Glick, E. N.: Proc. R. Soc. Med. *54*:432, 1961.
22. Goodman, D. B., Rasmussen, H., Di Bella, F., and Guthrow, C. E., Jr.: Proc. Natl. Acad. Sci. USA. *67*:652, 1970.
23. Gutman, A. B.: Adv. Pharmacol. *4*:91, 1966.
24. Gutman, A. B.: Adv. Pharmacol. *4*:621, 1966.
25. Gutman, A. B.: Arthritis Rheum. *16*:431, 1973.
26. Gutman, A. B., and Yu, T. F.: Lancet *2*:1258, 1957.
27. Holmes, E. W., Kelley, W. N., and Wyngaarden, J. B.: Kidney Int. *2*:115, 1972.
28. Jacques, R., and Helfer, H.: Pharmacology *5*:49, 1971.
29. Jarzobski, J. R., Ferry, J., Womholt, D., Fitch, D. M., and Eagan, J. D.: Am. Heart J. *79*:116, 1970.

30. Kelley, W. N., and Beardmore, T. D.: Science *169*:388, 1970.
31. Kelley, W., Green, M., Rosenbloom, F., Henderson, J., and Seegmiller, J.: Ann. Intern. Med. *70*:155, 1969.
32. Kiefer, B., Sakai, H., Solari, A., and Mazia, D.: J. Mol. Biol. *20*:75, 1966.
33. Klinenberg, J. R., Goldfinger, S. E., and Seegmiller, J. E.: Ann. Intern. Med. *62*:639, 1965.
34. Klinenberg, J. R., and Kippen, I.: J. Lab. Clin. Med. *75*:503, 1970.
35. Komai, H., Massey, V., and Palmer, G.: J. Biol. Chem. *244*:1692, 1969.
36. Kuzell, W., Glower, R., Gibbs, J., and Blau, R.: Acta Rheum. Scand. (Suppl. *8*):31, 1964.
37. Kuzell, W., Seebach, C. M., Glover, R. P., and Jackman, A. E.: Ann. Rheum. Dis. *25*:634, 1966.
38. Levy, D. A., and Carlton, J. A.: Proc. Soc. Exp. Biol. Med. *130*:1333, 1969.
39. Malawista, S. E., and Bensch, W. G.: Science *156*:521, 1967.
40. Malawista, S. E., Bodel, B.: J. Clin. Invest. *46*:786, 1967.
41. Margulius, L.: Int. Rev. Cytol. *34*:333, 1973.
42. Massey, V., Brumby, P., and Komai, H.: J. Biol. Chem. *244*:1682, 1969.
43. Massey, V., Komai, H., Palmer, G., and Elion, G.: J. Biol. Chem. *245*:2837, 1970.
44. Mc Carty, D. J., Jr., and Hollander, J. L.: Ann. Intern. Med. *54*:452, 1961.
45. Mc Laughlin, G. E., Mc Carty, D. J., Jr., and Prescott, D. J.: Top. Med. Chem. *3*:263, 1970.
46. Persellin, R. H., and Schmid, F. R.: J. Am. Med. Assoc. *175*:971, 1961.
47. Phelps, P.: Arthritis Rheum. *12*:189, 1969.
48. Phelps, P.: Arthritis Rheum. *12*:197, 1969.
49. Phelps, P.: Arthritis Rheum. *13*:1, 1970.
50. Phelps, P., and Mc Carty, D. J., Jr.: J. Exp. Med. *124*:115, 1966.
51. Phelps, P., and Mc Carty, D. J., Jr.: Postgrad. Med. *45*:87, 1969.
52. Poisner, A. M., and Bernstein, J.: J. Pharmacol. Exp. Ther. *177*:102, 1971.
53. Postlethawaite, A. E., Gutman, R. A., and Kelley, W. N.: Metabolism *23*:771, 1974.
54. Postlethwaite, A. E., Ramsdell, C. M., and Kelley, W. N.: Arch. Intern. Med. *134*:270, 1974.
55. Reynolds, E. S., Schlant, R. C., Gonick, H. C., and Dammin, G. J.: N. Engl. J. Med. *256*:592, 1957.
56. Riesterer, L., and Jacques, R.: Pharmacology *2*:288, 1969.
57. Robins, R. K.: J. Am. Chem. Soc. *78*:784, 1956.
58. Rundles, R. W., Wyngaarden, J., Hitchings, G., and Elion, G.: Annu. Rev. Pharmacol. *9*:345, 1969.
59. Rundles, R. W., Wyngaarden, J. B., Hitchings, G. H., and Elion, G. B.: Ann. Intern. Med. *60*:717, 1963.
60. Rundles, R. W., Wyngaarden, J. B., Hitchings, G. H., Elion, G. B., and Silberman, H.: Trans. Assoc. Am. Physicians. *76*:126, 1963.
61. Schlosstein, L. H., Kippen, I., Whitehouse, M. W., Bluestone, R., Paulus, H. E., and Klinenberg, J. R.: J. Lab. Clin. Med. *82*:412, 1973.
62. Seegmiller, J. E., Howell, R. R., and Malawista, S. E.: J. Am. Med. Assoc. *180*:469, 1962.
63. Trnavsky, K., and Kopecky, S.: Med. Exp. *15*:322, 1966.
64. Tse, R. L., and Phelps, P.: J. Lab. Clin. Med. *76*:403, 1970.
65. Tse, R. L., and Phelps, P.: Arthritis Rheum. *14*:418, 1971.

66. Vesell, E. S., Passananti, G. T., and Greene, F. E.: N. Engl. J. Med. *283*: 1484, 1970.
67. Wallace, S. L.: Arthritis Rheum. *2*:389, 1959.
68. Weissmann, G.: Arthritis Rheum. *9*:834, 1966.
69. Weissmann, G., Dukor, P., and Zurier, R. B.: Nature (New Biol.) *231*:131, 1971.
70. Weissmann, G., Zurier, R. B., Spjeler, P. J., and Goldstein, I. M.: J. Exp. Med. *134*:1495, 1971.
71. Williams, J. A., and Wolff, J.: Proc. Nat. Acad. Sci. USA *67*:1901, 1970.
72. Wyngaarden, J. B., Rundles, R. W., Silberman, H. R., and Hunter, S.: Arthritis Rheum. *6*:306, 1963.
73. Yu, T. F., Burns, J. J., and Gutman, A. B.: Arthritis Rheum. *1*:532, 1958.
74. Yu, T. F., and Gutman, A. B.: Am. J. Med. *37*:885, 1964.
75. Zweig, M. H., Maling, H. M., and Webster, M. E.: J. Pharmacol. Exp. Ther. *182*:344, 1972.

Index